Recent Results in Cancer Research 125

F. Raue (Ed.)

Medullary Thyroid Carcinoma

With 57 Figures and 25 Tables

Springer-Verlag
Berlin Heidelberg New York
London Paris Tokyo
Hong Kong Barcelona
Budapest

Prof. Dr. Friedhelm Raue

Abteilung Innere Medizin I – Endokrinologie
und Stoffwechsel, Klinikum
Ruprecht Karls-Universität Heidelberg
Luisenstraße 5, W-6900 Heidelberg, FRG

ISBN 3-540-55372-X Springer-Verlag Berlin Heidelberg New York
ISBN 0-387-55372-X Springer-Verlag New York Berlin Heidelberg

Library of Congress Cataloging-in-Publication Data.
Medullary thyroid carcinoma/F. Raue (ed.). p. cm. – (Recent results in cancer research; 125) Includes bibliographical references and index.
ISBN 3-540-55372-X (alk. paper). – ISBN 0-387-55372-X (alk. paper)
1. Thyroid gland-Cancer. I. Raue, F. (Friedhelm) II. Series
[DNLM: 1. Carcinoma. 2. Thyroid Neoplasms. WK 270 M493] RC261.R35 vol. 125 [RC280.T6] 616.99'4 s-dc20 [616.99'444] DNLM/DLC 92-2297

Typesetting: Best-set Typesetter Ltd., Hong Kong
25/3130-5 4 3 2 1 0 – Printed on acid-free paper.

Preface

Thirty-two years after medullary thyroid carcinoma was first described by Hazard and colleagues, pathological and biochemical techniques make it possible to reliably distinguish it from other thyroid cancers. Medullary thyroid carcinoma is a malignancy of the C cells, which originate from the neural crest and are located adjacent to but outside the thyroid follicle. The clinical spectrum includes several special features: for example, the secretion of various peptides, such as production of the calcitonin gene family; the association with other endocrine tumors, such as the multiple endocrine neoplasia type 2; and the familial appearance.

In 1987 the *Studiengruppe medulläres Schilddrüsencarcinom* (Study group for medullary thyroid carcinoma) was established by the authors to stimulate cooperative research and provide a forum to discuss progress in research (F. Raue, R.F. Gagel, Multiple endocrine neoplasia type 2. *Hormone and Metabolic Research Supplement* 21, 1989). After 5 years of national and international cooperation information from the biological, medical, and surgical investigators has accumulated rapidly, making it an appropriate time to review recent research progress in this rare malignancy. This volume focuses on two aspects:

1. The cellular, molecular and genetic features of this tumor, which provide exciting perspectives to further the understanding of tumor biology and pathology.
2. The clinical management of patients with familial and sporadic medullary thyroid carcinoma. The authors provide a comprehensive overview of established and experimental concepts.

Heidelberg, May 1992 C. Herfarth

Contents

*List of Contributors**

---

* The address of the principal author is given on the first page of each contribution.

[1] Page on which contribution begins.

Regulation of Calcitonin Secretion and Calcitonin Gene Expression*

F. Raue, A. Zink, and H. Scherübl**

Abteilung für Innere Medizin I – Endokrinologie und Stoffwechsel, Universität Heidelberg, Luisenstraße 5, W-6900 Heidelberg 1, FRG

Introduction

Medullary thyroid carcinoma (MTC) is a tumor of the calcitonin (CT)-secreting cells (C-cells or parafollicular cells). During embryogenesis C-cells migrate from the neural crest to the last branchial pouch and ultimately into the thyroid. In contrast to the follicular cells of the thyroid gland that produce the thyroid hormones under the control of thyroid-stimulating hormone (TSH), the C-cells secrete CT and related peptides under different control systems (Deftos and Roos 1989). CT helps to maintain the calcium homeostasis and as a feedback, physiological changes in blood-calcium concentration directly regulate CT secretion. In addition, 1,25 $(OH)_2D_3$ is involved in CT secretion and synthesis. CT release is also closely tied to feeding and gastrointestinal activity; gastrointestinal hormonal factors including gastrin, cholecystokinin (CCK), and glucagon participate in promoting CT release. Moreover neuroendocrine factors may be involved in the control of CT secretion. β-Adrenergic agonists stimulate CT secretion, while α-adrenergic agonists and dopamine inhibit it, which suggests a participation of the autonomic nervous system in the regulation of CT secretion. Somatostatin appears to have a paracrine or autocrine regulatory function as it is secreted by C-cells and it is able to inhibit CT secretion. While these phenomena can be studied in vivo, emphasizing their physiological relevance, the cellular and molecular mechanisms underlying regulation of CT secretion, synthesis, and transcription can only be studied in in vitro systems. The available in vitro systems include rat thyroid explants (Cooper et al. 1977), primary cell cultures of MTC (Raue et al. 1989), and

* This work was supported by a research grant from the Deutsche Forschungsgemeinschaft (Ra 327/1-4) and a DFG fellowship to Hans Scherübl.
** Present address: Abteilung für Innere Medizin/Gastnoenterologie, Freie Universität Berlin, Hindenburgdamm 30, 1000 Berlin 45, FRG.

Recent Results in Cancer Research, Vol. 125

permanent C-cell carcinoma cell lines (human TT: Leong et al. 1981; rMTC 6–23: Gagel et al. 1980). Cellular signaling processes thought to be involved in initiation of C-cell neoplasia and subsequent cellular changes during tumor progression are activation of adenylate cyclase, protein kinase C, and oncogenes.

Control of CT Secretion and Synthesis in Vivo

Calcium

CT secretion from C-cells is clearly regulated by plasma calcium (Ca) levels. When plasma Ca rises acutely, there is a proportional increase in plasma CT. This is the basis for using calcium infusion as a provocative test for CT release in patients with suspected MTC. In contrast, the effect of chronic hypercalcemia and hypocalcemia are controversial, and contradictory results have been reported. Normal, elevated, and decreased basal levels of CT have been observed in hyperparathyroidism, whereas CT reserve can be normal or decreased (Tiegs et al. 1986; Tørring et al. 1985). During chronic hypercalcemia a reversible exhaustion of CT content was observed in rats, while basal serum CT levels remained unchanged (Raue et al. 1984). In contrast chronic hypocalcemia enhanced CT storage and secretion in the rat. The serum Ca levels showed an inverse relationship to CT storage and CT response to acute stimuli (Raue et al. 1988).

Gastrointestinal Factors

The most important CT secretagogues apart from Ca probably are the gastrointestinal hormones, gastrin, CCK, glucagon, and secretin. Gastrin is the most effective of these, and the gastrin analog pentagastrin is also used for provocative tests in patients with MTC. However, the physiological significance of the regulation of CT secretion by these hormones is unclear since large doses have been used in most studies. An increase in plasma CT after meals or an oral Ca load could be demonstrated in only a few clinical and experimental studies (Deftos and Roos 1989).

Gender and Age

Both sex and age appear to influence CT secretion in humans. Higher than normal plasma levels for adults have been reported in pregnant women, children, and newborn infants. CT levels appear to decrease with age in humans, in contrast to rats. Women have been shown to have lower basal plasma CT levels and reduced responses to i.v. Ca or pentagastrin compared to men. These findings have led many to postulate that lower CT levels in women might contribute to the higher female prevalence of symptomatic osteoporosis (McDermott and Kidd 1987). When evaluating the relationship of CT secretion to osteoporosis, variable findings have been reported: lower (Reginster et al. 1989), unchanged, or even elevated basal CT levels with normal (Body et al. 1989) or impaired CT response. Replacement of estrogen resulted in increased or unchanged basal CT levels and in augmented CT response to Ca stimulation. The discrepancies presumably reflect the use of different estrogens, different treatment periods, and different CT assays. The role of CT in the pathogenesis of osteoporosis is still questionable.

Regulation of CT Gene Expression in Vivo

Other steroid hormones like glucocorticoids or 1,25 $(OH)_2D_3$ are also involved in CT secretion and synthesis. Dexamethasone increases CT messenger ribonucleic acid (mRNA) in adrenalectomized rats within 5 days (Besnard et al. 1989) while 1,25 $(OH)_2D_3$ decreases CT mRNA in rats (Naveh-Many and Silver 1988) within 6h; 1–2h after injection of 1,25 $(OH)_2D_3$, CT serum levels increase (Raue et al. 1983) and a transient rise in translatable CT mRNA activity is observed (Segond et al. 1985). A similar rapid increase in translatable CT mRNA is observed immediately after injection of Ca into rats, which probably acts at the post-transcriptional level (Segond et al. 1989), whereas after 6h of Ca infusion into rats no effect on total CT mRNA is seen (Naveh-Many and Silver 1989). Elevating the plasma potassium concentration has an acute effect on CT secretion and CT mRNA within 30min in female rats. This effect is most likely mediated through a rise in $[Ca^{2+}]_i$ of the C-cell (Jousset et al. 1988). A similar positive effect on CT mRNA 1h after Ca injection was seen in adrenalectomized rats treated with dexamethasone (Besnard et al. 1989).

Control of CT Secretion and Synthesis in Vitro

As seen in vivo, the extracellular calcium concentration ($[Ca^{2+}]_e$) tightly regulates CT secretion in vitro. Various gastrointestinal and hypothalamic peptide hormones trigger CT release by acting via different intracellular second messenger systems, like cyclic adenosine monophosphate (cAMP), diacylglycerol, protein kinase C, or Ca. Steroid hormones exert their effects on CT secretion and storage by binding to specific nuclear receptors, thereby directly regulating CT gene transcription.

Calcium-Dependent CT Secretion

Extracellular Calcium and Calcium Channels

An acute elevation of $[Ca^{2+}]_e$ evokes a prompt release of preformed CT from C-cells of the carcinoma cell lines rMTC 6–23 or rMTC 44–2. There is a strong positive relationship between $[Ca^{2+}]_e$ and CT secretion. Even a small acute decrease of $[Ca^{2+}]_e$ causes a decreases in CT release in rat thyroid explants. It is an essential function of C-cells to monitor $[Ca^{2+}]_e$ and to respond to changes in $[Ca^{2+}]_e$ by regulating CT secretion which in turn regulates serum Ca. This tight linkage between $[Ca^{2+}]_e$ and CT secretion is mediated by changes in intracellular cytosolic free calcium ($[Ca^{2+}]_i$) (Fried and Tashjian 1986). A small increase in $[Ca^{2+}]_e$ causes a distinct rapid elevation in $[Ca^{2+}]_i$ via Ca influx through dihydropyridine-sensitive Ca channels. The essential role of these voltage-dependent Ca channels could be confirmed by applying Ca channel activators (BAY K 8644), Ca channel blockers (nifedipine, verapamil), or by depolarization of the plasma membrane by high external potassium. BAY K 8644-stimulated CT secretion can be completely inhibited by equimolar concentration of nifedipine or by chelating $[Ca^{2+}]_e$ (Hishikawa et al. 1985; Raue et al. 1989). In the human MTC cell line (TT), a rise of $[Ca^{2+}]_e$ does, however, neither affect $[Ca^{2+}]_i$ nor the secretion of CT, which indicates a defect in the Ca^{2+} signal transduction in TT cells (Haller-Brem et al. 1987). These findings have strongly suggested a prominent role for dihydropyridine-sensitive Ca channels in the Ca sensitivity of C-cells.

Electrophysiological Studies

Electrophysiological studies on rMTC cells now provide direct evidence for voltage-dependent, dihydropyridine-sensitive Ca^{2+} currents with a steady state conductivity for Ca^{2+} even at the normal resting membrane potential (Scherübl et al. 1990). While rMTC cells showed this slowly decaying Ca^{2+} inward current, C-cells of the "defective" TT cell line exhibited only a transient Ca^{2+} current. Thus, the steady state conductivity for Ca^{2+} is a prerequistie for C-cells to be able to monitor $[Ca^{2+}]_e$.

Calmodulin

The anticonvulsant agent phenytoin which can inhibit the Ca channel activity and also inhibits calmodulin, also inhibits CT release (Cooper et al. 1988). Similar actions are described for other more or less specific calmodulin inhibitors such as W7, trifluoperazine, chlorpromazine, and haloperidol (Cooper and Borosky 1986). Other agents which increase $[Ca^{2+}]_i$ by enhancing Ca influx or by mobilization of intracellular Ca enhance CT release. This has been reported for the Ca ionophores ionomycin, and A23187 (Haller-Brem et al. 1988; Seitz and Cooper 1989). These findings again indicate that changes in $[Ca^{2+}]_i$ play a functional role in CT secretion in C-cells.

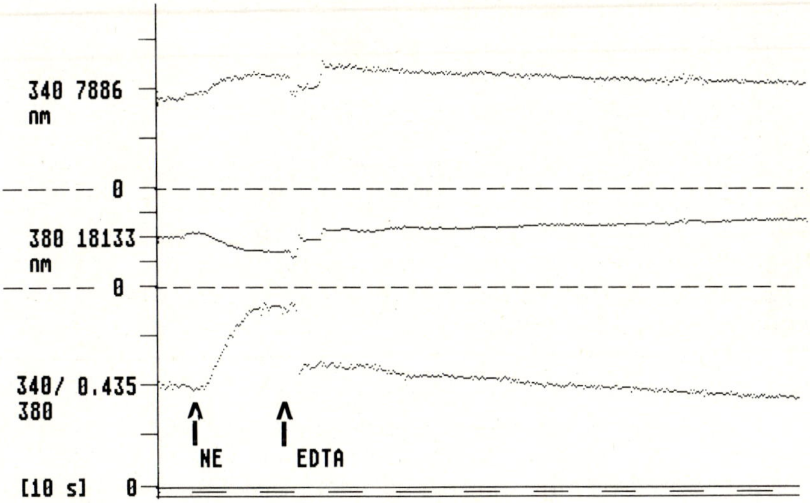

Fig. 1. Blocking effect of extracellular addition of EGTA (*right arrow*) on norepinephrine (*NE*)-induced increase in intracellular calcium (*left arrow*) in a single rMTC 6–23 cell

Neuroendocrine Factors

Not only $[Ca^{2+}]_e$ but also biogenic amines and neuropeptides are able to stimulate CT secretion. Norepinephrine (NE) and the neuropeptide rat growth hormone-releasing hormone (rGRF) increase CT secretion in rMTC cells not only via the cAMP-dependent pathway but also via an increase of $[Ca^{2+}]_i$. They caused a biphasic response in $[Ca^{2+}]_i$ consisting of a rapid spike within 5 s and a second phase with a decline in $[Ca^{2+}]_i$ to a plateau that was always higher than baseline. rGRF and NE do not acutely increase IP3 levels, so increase of $[Ca^{2+}]_i$ seems not likely to be mediated by redistribution of intracellular Ca^{2+} stores (Fried and Tashjian 1987). The increase of $[Ca^{2+}]_i$ could be blocked by Ca channel blockers and addition of extracellular ethylene glycol-bis (β-aminoethyl ether)-N,N,N′,N′-tetraacetic acid (EGTA) indicating an influx of calcium through voltage-dependent Ca channels (Fig. 1). Similar effects of rGRF on $[Ca^{2+}]_i$ have been observed in rat somatotrophs (Lussier et al. 1991a).

Somatostatin

Somatostatin (SMS) which is produced and secreted by the C-cell itself (Aron et al. 1981) regulates the secretion of CT in an autocrine and paracrine fashion. SMS inhibits Ca-stimulated CT release in a dose-dependent manner

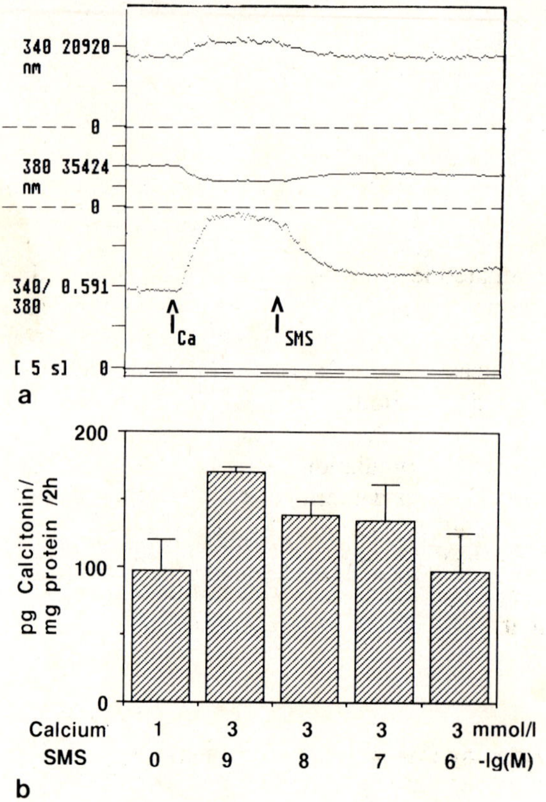

Fig. 2a,b. Inhibitory effect of somatostatin (SMS) (*right arrow*) on intracellular calcium increased by elevation of extracellular calcium from 1 to 3 mmol/l (*left arrow*) in a single rMTC 6–23 cell (**a**) and on calcium-stimulated CT secretion (**b**)

by reducing the increase of $[Ca^{2+}]_i$ (Fig. 2). This is mediated by closing Ca channels in the cell membrane (Reuter and Scholz 1977) or by influencing activation kinetics of Ca^{2+} channels. SMS is known to reduce the rate of activation of inward Ca^{2+} currents in neuronal cells (Bean 1989). Both mechanisms, decreasing the number of open Ca channels at high SMS concentrations and affecting the Ca^{2+} influx activation kinetics at low SMS concentrations are responsible for preventing an rGRF-induced $[Ca^{2+}]_i$ increase in rat somatrotrophs (Lussier et al. 1991b). Similar to that seen in GH_3 cells, SMS decreases $[Ca^{2+}]_i$ in rMTC cells involving a pertussis toxin (PT)-sensitive G protein as shown by measuring Ca current and $[Ca^{2+}]_i$ (Scherübl et al. 1991). Two possible mechanisms by which rGRF and SMS modulate the Ca channels have been described: a direct inhibition of Ca channels by G proteins as recently described in cardiac muscle cells (Yatani et al. 1987) and GH_3 cells (Lewis et al. 1986) or a G protein-dependent increase in potassium conductance (Koch et al. 1988; Koch and Schonbrunn 1988), which in turn closes voltage-dependent Ca channels and thereby reduces $[Ca^{2+}]_i$.

Chronic Elevation of $[Ca^{2+}]_e$

Similar to the in vivo findings, the long-term effect of high $[Ca^{2+}]_o$ led to a decline in CT release to unstimulated levels within 4 h in vitro. This decline proved to be reversible by lowering the high $[Ca^{2+}]_o$ concentration to basal for 2 h and then increasing Ca^{2+} again (Scherübl et al. 1989a). Thus, the Ca-induced desensitization of CT release was not due to an exhaustion of the secretory reserve in the observation period. These results suggest that a reversible modification of Ca channels of the C-cells may cause the desensitization of CT release to repetitive Ca stimulation. Also long-term exposure to BAY K 8644 over 4 days results in a decrease in CT secretion and CT content in rMTC 6–23 cells, while short-term experiments with BAY K 8644 caused a stimulation effect lasting over 6 h (Mekonnen et al. 1990). The different time course of desensitization to BAY K 8644 and $[Ca^{2+}]_c$ might be explained by different modifications of the voltage-dependent Ca channels.

Regulation of CT Gene Expression by Calcium-Dependent Pathway

An increase in $[Ca^{2+}]_i$ is the important step in the activation of the Ca-dependent metabolic processes, e.g., activation of regulatory enzymes by Ca-dependent protein kinases. Activators of protein kinase C such as phorbol esters are highly effective in acutely releasing CT within minutes (de Bustros et al. 1985). In addition, a CT-specific cytoplasmic mRNA increases within hours. Phorbol esters stimulate transcriptional activation of the CT/calcitonin gene-related peptide (CGRP) gene by *cis* elements that lie within the 5′-flanking DNA. Several potential sequences were identified for these consensus elements; one of them is the binding site for the activator protein 1 or 2, which mediate their effects through protein kinase C in other systems. In addition to phorbol ester, the activator protein 2 regulatory element is also responsive to forskolin (cAMP-dependent transcriptional enhancement) (Cote et al. 1990). The tissue-specific expression of the CT/CGRP gene is not only regulated on the level of alternative RNA processing events but also on the DNA level. A cell-specific enhancer sequence in the 5′-flanking DNA of the CT/CGRP gene has been identified that functions in cells of neuronal or C-cell origin, but not in any other cell type tested (Stolarsky-Fredman et al. 1990). An acute effect on the Ca-mediated pathway by depolarizing potassium concentration on CT mRNA has been observed within 30 min, probably due to a post-transcriptional effect (Jousset

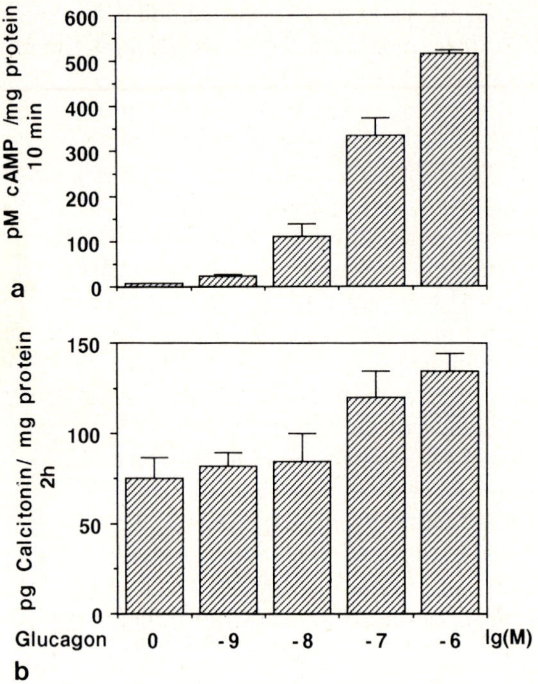

Fig. 3 a,b. Stimulatory effect of glucagon on cAMP production (**a**) and calcitonin secretion (**b**) in rMTC 6–23 cells

et al. 1988). In contrast to the acute effect, incubation with a high ionized Ca concentration (4 m*M*) for 72–96 h causes a decrease in CT secretion and also a decrease in specific CT mRNA (Zeytin et al. 1987). This demonstrates that the Ca-dependent pathway controls secretion and possibly the transcription of CT in a time-dependent fashion in the C-cell, acutely affecting exocytosis of stored proteins and chronically affecting transcription and synthesis of CT and perhaps sustained secretory response. A prolongation of ionomycin-stimulated secretion of CT by 12-O-tetradecanoylphorbol 13-acetate (TPA), a phorbol ester, could be demonstrated in the TT cell line (Haller-Brem et al. 1988). The various agents used suggest that the Ca-dependent secretory pathway involve plasma membrane Ca channels, $[Ca^{2+}]_i$, calmodulin and protein kinase C.

cAMP-Dependent CT Secretion

Glucagon

Glucagon is one of the classical peptide hormones which act upon the cell surface to stimulate the formation of cAMP by activation of adenylate cyclase (AC). The effect of cAMP on cellular metabolism is mediated by protein kinase A, which in turn stimulates hormone secretion (CT in rMTC cells) (Fig. 3). This cAMP-dependent CT secretion could be imitated by cAMP analogs (8-Br-cAMP, dibutyryl-cAMP) or substances like forskolin, a diterpene which enhances protein kinase A activity by stimulating the catalytic subunit of AC. Other protein kinase A-activating substances are cholera toxin which stimulates ADP ribose transfer to the G protein with consequent inhibition of its GTPase activity and prolonged activation of AC, or theophylline (or 3-isobutyl-1-methylxanthine, IBMX), which inhibits phosphodiesterase and thereby the endogenous degradation of cAMP.

Neuroendocrine and Gastrointestinal Factors

AC and thereby CT secretion is also stimulated by catecholamines (epinephrine, norepinephrine) and peptide hormones like GRF, vasoactive intestinal polypeptide (VIP), gastrin, and CCK in C-cells. Hormones can exert inhibitory as well as stimulatory effects on AC. This dual control of hormone-sensitive AC is mediated by specific guanyl nucleotide-binding regulatory proteins (G proteins) in the plasma membrane, stimulatory G_s and inhibitory G_i proteins. cAMP production in rMTC cells stimulated by glucagon or rGRF could be dose dependently inhibited by SMS and *N*-6-phenylisopropyladenosine (PIA) an agonist on the adenosine A_1 receptor. This inhibition of AC could be neutralized by PT (Fig. 4). Thus, the AC of the C-cells is controlled by a dual regulation and the inhibitory pathway involves a PT-sensitive G protein (Höflich et al. 1990). In parallel to inhibition or stimulation of AC, CT secretion is inhibited or stimulated. SMS appears to inhibit CT release by a second, cAMP-independent mechanism, as it reduces Ca-stimulated CT secretion (Endo et al. 1988).

Regulation of CT Gene Expression by cAMP-Dependent Pathway

Not only secretion but also synthesis of CT is regulated by cAMP. cAMP binding to the regulatory unit of protein kinase A appears to be necessary for activation of both secretion and synthesis. A cAMP regulatory element binding (CREB) protein as a transregulatoring factor has been identified (Cote et al. 1990) as well as a *cis* cAMP regulatory element (CRE) at the 5′-flanking DNA of the CT gene. Phosphorylation of CREB protein by protein kinase A and interaction with specific *cis* elements 5′ to the CT gene results in enhanced transcription.

Interaction Between Calcium- and cAMP-Dependent Pathways

There are lots of interactions and "cross talks" between the two main intracellular messenger systems, cAMP and $[Ca^{2+}]_i$, at the different cellular

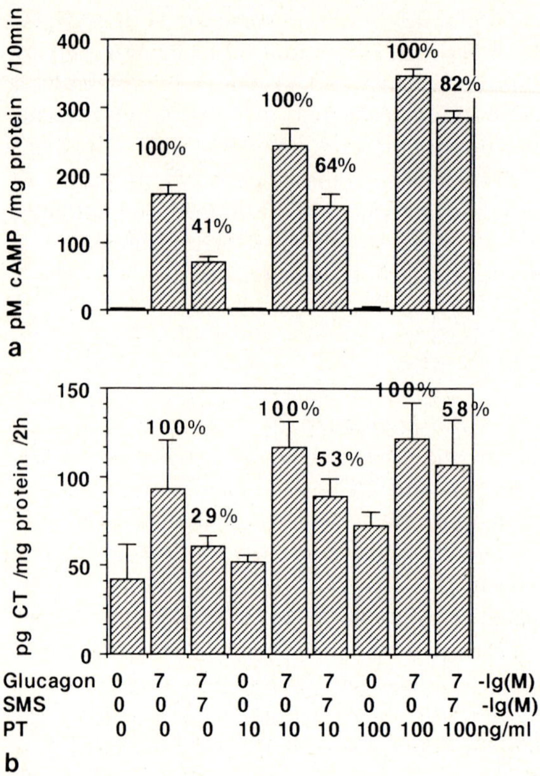

Fig. 4 a,b. Effect of pertussis toxin (*PT*) on the inhibitory action of somatostatin (*SMS*) on glucagon-stimulated cAMP production (**a**) and on glucagon-stimulated CT secretion (**b**)

levels. These interactions of effector systems are responsible for the spectrum of individual target cell responses. Many hormones interact with both intracellular pathways and exert a rapid and a slow action that exerts both acute secretion and long-term growth effect via transcription. Epinephrine, for instance, acts simultaneously on cAMP- and Ca-dependent pathways (Fried and Tashjian 1987). $[Ca^{2+}]_i$ has an important effect on AC activity (Scherübl et al. 1989b) and phosphorylation and conversely, the cAMP pathway acts by modulation of $[Ca^{2+}]_i$.

Oscillation of $[Ca^{2+}]_i$

Interaction of both pathways can result in a new signal, the oscillation: after activating the cAMP pathway by glucagon or Br-cAMP, $[Ca^{2+}]_i$ in C-cells started to oscillate when $[Ca^{2+}]_e$ was raised. These fluctuations in $[Ca^{2+}]_i$

could be stopped by chelating the $[Ca^{2+}]_e$ with EGTA or by adding Ca channel blockers (Eckert et al. 1989). This points to a major role of voltage-dependent Ca channels in maintaining the oscillations of $[Ca^{2+}]_i$ in C-cells. A cAMP- and $[Ca^{2+}]_i$-dependent mechanism at the inner mouth of Ca channels may be proposed. The activity of voltage-dependent Ca^{2+} channels and thereby the Ca influx is regulated by the membrane potential, and in some tissue by phosphorylation of the channel protein or a regulatory component by protein kinases. cAMP-dependent phosphorylation of Ca channels as a prerequisite for channel opening has recently been reported for pituitary cells (Armstrong and Eckert 1987; Croxton et al. 1988). Besides Ca channel modulation by phosphorylation another more direct mechanism has become apparent by which extracellular signals acting via G protein-coupled receptors influence the action of voltage-dependent Ca channels (Rosenthal et al. 1988). In rMTC cells, SMS and adenosine (via A_1 receptor) cause an inhibition of Ca^{2+} currents and thereby lower $[Ca^{2+}]_i$ via a PT-sensitive G protein (Scherübl et al. 1992). The inhibiting agonists SMS and PIA inhibit AC via receptors coupled to PT-sensitive G_i proteins. This inhibition of AC was, however, not causal for the observed inhibition of Ca^{2+} currents, the decrease in $[Ca^{2+}]_i$ and CT secretion, because SMS inhibited the $[Ca^{2+}]_o$-induced increase in $[Ca^{2+}]_i$ and CT secretion, which does not involve changes in the intracellular cAMP levels.

The combination of the two secretagogues Ca and glucagon has been reported to result in higher CT release than would be expected from the sum of the effects of each stimulant alone (Aron et al. 1981). A synergistic effect of both intracellular pathways on CT secretion could be confirmed in other C-cell systems, while in rMTC 6–23 only an additive stimulatory effect was observed (Scherübl et al. 1989b). It appears that regulatory pathways affecting exocytosis of stored proteins differ from the ones that have a direct effect on exocytosis and transcription. Activators of protein kinase C (phorbol ester), and cAMP have been demonstrated to increase the transcriptional rate of the CT gene by *cis* regulatory elements in the 5′-flanking DNA. There seem to be several potential regulatory sequences, which enhances the transcription efficiency, and it is likely that cAMP transcription enhancement may occur through protein kinase C regulatory element (Murray et al. 1988).

Steroid Hormone Regulation of CT Secretion and Gene Expression

In their target tissue, steroid hormones elicit specific cell responses by stimulating the expression of genes. The first step is binding to specific receptors that are present in the target cell followed by an activation of the hormone receptor complex that increases the affinity of the complex for nuclear binding sites. Estrogen and 1,25 $(OH)_2D_3$ receptors are well documented in C-cells (Yang et al. 1988; Freake et al. 1982). 1,25 $(OH)_2D_3$ has a negative effect on CT gene transcription: CT mRNA decreases and consequently CT content and CT secretion is reduced (Cote et al. 1987). This inhibition of transcription is specific, as the inactive analog 24,25 $(OH)_2D_3$ has no effect on CT content and secretion. Dexamethasone, a synthetic glucocorticoid, has a stimulatory effect on CT gene transcription, CT content and secretion in different MTC cell lines (Cote and Gagel 1986). It seems to directly regulate CT gene expression, since it does not alter the stability of CT mRNA in the TT cell line. By combining the agonistic effect of dexamethasone and the antagonistic effect of 1,25 $(OH)_2D_3$, the stimulatory activity of dexamethasone could be abolished by 1,25 $(OH)_2D_3$. The explanation of this interaction might be a modulation of 1,25 $(OH)_2D_3$ receptor levels by glucocorticoids or interference with the action of transcriptional factors on the levels of the DNA binding sites (Lazaretti-Castro et al. 1990). The combination of the two agents only led to a reduction of the CT mRNA and did not abolish the dexamethasone effect (Grauer et al. 1991).

There is no direct stimulatory effect of estrogen on CT secretion in the C-cell carcinoma cell line in vitro, neither after short-term (within 3 h) nor after long-term (up to 6 days) exposure. But there is a significant dose-dependent increase on total cellular protein content. In contrast, a dose-dependent transient inhibition of CT secretion and content with a nadir at 24 h could be demonstrated (Raue et al. 1990; Lazaretti-Castro et al. 1991). This discrepancy with the in vivo studies, which demonstrate a stimulatory effect of estrogen on CT secretion (Greenberg et al. 1986), might be best explained by the more complex environment with interfering factors due to the presence of other cell types.

Tumorigenesis and Tumor Progression in MTC

Tumorigenesis

The MTC is an important model for understanding the molecular steps in the genesis of neoplasia, the events in tumor progression and peptide hormone gene expression. Twenty-five percent of patients with MTC have an autosomal dominant inherited form of the disease. Recent findings using DNA restriction fragment length polymorphism have linked the germline genetic abnormality for multiple endocrine neoplasia (MEN) 2 to the centromeric region of chromosome 10 (Mathew et al. 1987; Simpson et al. 1987). But in contrast to other heritable cancers like retinoblastoma, no loss of heterozygosity for the DNA marker in the involved region of chromosome 10 was found. The "two hit" hypothesis of carcinogenesis that has been shown to occur in retinoblastoma, where a first hit, i.e., the germline genetic defect of one allele, makes cells susceptible to a second hit, namely, the loss of the remaining normal allele during somatic development, does not occur in MEN 2. A mechanism similar to that proposed for familial polyposis, in which the mutation in the hereditary gene results in hyperplastic cell growth and subsequent events involving genes at other loci result in further progressive neoplastic changes has been suggested (Nelkin et al. 1989b). C-cell hyperplasia and hyperplasia of the adrenal chromaffin and parathyroid cells may be the manifestation of the initial heritable mutation of chromosome 10, while a second event occurring in hyperplastic tissue at another locus on either the same or a different chromosome is responsible for converting hyperplastic cells to cancer cells.

Tumor Progression

Tumor progression to more malignant states as a consequence of heritable mutation might be induced by activation of oncogenes, which are involved in regulation of growth and differentiation. A large number and variety of oncogenes and proto-oncogenes have been defined which might be responsible for the mechanism of transformation, a process whereby a normal cell is converted to a state of uncontrolled proliferation. Introduction of the Simian virus 40 (SV40) large T oncogene gave rise to transgenic mice with a distinct predisposition to MEN. Malignant tumor growth was consistently seen in all endocrine tissue (Reynolds et al. 1988). Pheochromocytomas and C-cell hyperplasia developed in transgenic mice carring the *mos* proto-oncogene (Schulz et al. 1990).

Tumor Differentiation

Oncogenes do not only regulate proliferation but also differentiation. Introduction of the viral Harvey *ras* oncogene into DMS 53 cells, a human small cell lung cancer cell line, via retroviral infection, results in increased feature of neuroendocrine differentiation, increased CT secretion and gene expression, but markedly diminished cellular proliferation (Mabry et al. 1989). The molecular mechanism by which *ras* genes influence endocrine cell differentiation may relate to signal transduction events mediated by *ras* gene products. The *ras* genes activate the protein kinase C signal transduction pathway in a similar way to phorbol ester. A dramatic differentiation response characterized by slowing of cell growth, increased transcription of the CT gene, alteration of the CT gene mRNA splicing events with high CT mRNA and low CGRP mRNA and the appearance of abundant mature cytoplasmic neurosecretory granules is seen (Nakagawa et al. 1987). The variation of the ratio of CT/CGRP mRNA as a function of growth has been shown in the human MTC TT cell line, such that CT mRNA is lowest and CGRP mRNA is highest during rapid growth (Nelkin et al. 1989b). C-*myc* oncogene expression induced by 1,25 $(OH)_2D_3$ is accompanied by an increase in proliferation and a decrease in CT mRNA expression (Baier et al. 1991). These RNA processing changes represent an important type of regulation pathway for cell growth and may be involved in autocrine control of growth of neoplastic C-cells. Human MTC is usually a slow-growing well-differentiated endocrine tumor which produces high levels of CT. Patients with aggressive MTC and widespread, steadily growing metastases have markedly diminished CT content or immunohistochemically detectable CT in their metastases and decreased serum CT levels (Saad et al. 1984).

Conclusion

Serum Ca seems to be the most important regulator of CT secretion. The underlying mechanism appears to be a voltage-dependent calcium channel that works as a calcium sensor by allowing transmembranous Ca^{2+} influx even under steady state conditions. Acute changes in $[Ca^{2+}]_e$ are thus converted into changes of cytosolic free Ca, which mediate CT secretion and other cell processes. Beside this Ca-dependent intracellular pathway, the cAMP-mediated pathway, activated by intestinal and hypothalamic hormones and inhibited by adenosine (A_1) or SMS, is involved in the regulation of secretion and gene transcription. Interactions between the two pathways on every cellular level occur and modify the response. 1,25 $(OH)_2D_3$ acts directly on gene transcription and has a negative effect on CT secretion. Two feedback relationships between the C-cells and the whole organism could be postulated: an acute rise in serum Ca is the adequate stimulus for secretion of CT, which in turn normalizes serum Ca, and a more prolonged interrelationship, whereby 1,25 $(OH)_2D_3$ inhibits CT synthesis and secretion, while CT stimulates 1,25 $(OH)_2D_3$ synthesis in the kidney (Jaeger et al. 1986). An autosomal dominant genetic defect is responsible for development in the inherited form of MTC. Oncogenes might be responsible for tumor progression and differentiation.

References

Armstrong D, Eckert R (1987) Voltage-activated calcium channels that must be phosphorylated to respond to membrane depolarisation. Proc Natl Acad Sci USA 84:2518–2624

Aron DC, Muszynski M, Birnbaum RS, Sabo SW, Roos BA (1981) Somatostatin elaboration by monolayer cell cultures derived from transplantable rat medullary thyroid carcinoma synergistic stimulatory effects of glucagon and calcium. Endocrinology 109:1830–1834

Baier R, Lazaretti-Castro M, Grauer A, Raue F, Ziegler R (1991) 1,25 $(OH)_2D_3$ stimulates cell proliferation and C-myc oncogene transcription in a human C-cell carcinoma cell line (TT cell). Acta Endocrinol 124 [Suppl 1]:Abstr 221

Bean BP (1989) Neurotransmitter inhibition of neuronal calcium currents by changes in channel voltage dependence. Nature 340:153–155

Besnard P, Jousset V, Garel JM (1989) Additive effects of dexamethasone and calcium on the calcitonin mRNA level in adrenalectomized rats. FEBS Lett 258:293–296

Body JJ, Struelens M, Borkowski A, Mandrat G (1989) Effects of estrogens and calcium on calcitonin secretion in postmenopausal women. J Clin Endocrinol Metab 68:223–226

Cooper CW, Borosky SA (1986) Inhibition of secretion of rat calcitonin by calmodulin inhibitors. Calcif Tissue Int 38:103–108

Cooper CW, Ramp WK, Becker DI, Ontjes DA (1977) In vitro secretion of immunoreactive rat thyrocalcitonin. Endocrinology 101:304–311

Cooper CW, Yi SJ, Seitz PK (1988) Inhibition by phenytoin of in vitro secretion of calcitonin from rat thyroid glands and cultured rat C-cells. J Bone Miner Res 3:219–223

Cote GJ, Gagel RF (1986) Dexamethasone differentially affects the levels of calcitonin and clacitonin gene-related peptide mRNAs expressed in a human medullary thyroid carcinoma cell line. J Biol Chem 261:15524–15528

Cote GJ, Abruzze RV, Lips CJM, Gagel RF (1990) Transfection of calcitonin gene regulatory elements into a cell culture model of the C-Cell. J Bone Miner Res 5:165–171

Cote GJ, Rodgers DG, Huang ESC, Gagel RF (1987) The effect of 1,25-dihydroxyvitamin D_3 treatment on calcitonin and calcitonin gene-related peptide mRNA levels in cultured human thyroid C-cells. Biochem Biophys Res Commun 149:239–243

Croxton TL, Ben-Jonathan N, Armstrong WM (1988) Gonadotropin-releasing hormone induces oscillatory membrane current in rat gonadotrophes. Endocrinology 123:1783–1799

De Bustros A, Baylin SB, Berger CL, Roos A, Leony SS, Nelkin BD (1985) Phorbol ester increase calcitonin gene transcription and decrease c-myc mRNA levels in cultured human medullary thyroid carcinoma. J Biol Chem 260:98–104

Deftos LJ, Roos BA (1989) Medullary thyroid carcinoma and calcitonin gene expression. In: Peck WA (eds) Bone and mineral research 6. Elsevier, Amsterdam, pp 267–316

Eckert RW, Scherübl H, Petzelt C, Raue F, Ziegler R (1989) Rhythmic oscillations of cytosolic free calcium in rat C-cells. Mol Cell Endocrinol 64:267–270

Endo T, Saito T, Uchida T, Onaga T (1988) Effects of somatostatin and serotonin on calcitonin secretion from cultured rat and parafollicular cells. Acta Endocrinol (Copenh) 117:214–218

Freake HC, McIntyre I (1982) Specific binding of 1,25 dihydroxycholecalciferol in human medullary thyroid carcinoma. Biochem J 206:181–184

Fried RM, Tashjian AH (1986) Unusual sensitivity of cytosolic free Ca^{2+} to changes in extracellular Ca^{2+} in rat C-cells. J Biol Chem 261:7669–7674

Fried RM, Tashjian AH (1987) Action of rat growth hormone-releasing factor and norepinephrine on cytosolic free calcium and inositol trisphosphate in rat C-cells. J Bone Miner Res 2:579–585

Gagel RF, Zeytinoglu FN, Voelkel EF, Tashjian AH (1980) Establishment of a calcitonin-producing rat medullary carcinoma cell line. II. Secretory studies of the tumor and cells in culture. Endocrinology 107:516–523

Grauer A, Baier B, Lazaretti-Castro M, Raue F, Ziegler R (1991) 1,25 $(OH)_2D_3$ inhibits the dexamethasone induced stimulation of calcitonin gene expression in a human C-cell carcinoma cell line (TT-cell) (Abstr). Calcif Tissue Int 48 [Suppl]:26

Greenberg C, Kukreja SC, Bowser EN, Hargis GK, Henderson WJ, William GA (1986) Effect of estradiol and progesterone on calcitonin secretion. Endocrinology 118:2594–2598

Haller-Brem S, Muff R, Fischer JA (1988) Calcitonin gene-related peptide and calcitonin secretion from a human medullary thyroid carcinoma cell line: effects of ionomycin, phorbol ester and forskolin. J Endocrinol 119:147–152

Haller-Brem S, Muff R, Petermann JB, Born W, Roos BA, Fischer JA (1987) Role of cytosolic free calcium concentration in the secretion of calcitonin gene-related peptide and calcitonin from medullary thyroid carcinoma cells. Endocrinology 121:1272–1277

Hishikawa R, Fukase M, Takenaka M, Fujita T (1985) Effect of calcium channel agonist BAY K 8644 on calcitonin secretion from a rat C-cell line. Biochem Biophys Res Commun 130:454–459

Höflich M, Scherübl H, Raue F, Hoffmann J, Ziegler R (1990) Regulation of adenylate cyclase in rat C-cells (Abstr). Acta Endocrinol (Copenh) 122 Suppl 1:35

Jaeger P, Jones W, Clemens TL, Haystett JP (1986) Evidence that calcitonin stimulates 1,25-dihydroxyvitamin D production and intestinal absorption of calcium in vivo, J Clin Invest 78:456–461

Jousset U, Besnard P, Segond N, Julliene A, Garel JM (1988) Potassium administration and calcitonin mRNA levels in the rat. Mol Cell Endocrinol 59:65–169

Koch BD, Schonbrunn A (1988) Characterization of cyclic AMP independent actions of somastatin in GH cells. II. An increase in potassium conductance initiates somatostatin-induced inhibition of prolactin secretion. J Biol Chem 263:226–234

Koch BD, Dorflinger LJ, Schonbrunn A (1985) Pertussis toxin blocks both cyclic AMP-mediated and cAMP-independent actions of somatostatin: evidence for coupling of Ni to decrease in intracellular free calcium. J Biol Chem 260:13138–13145

Koch BD, Blalock JB, Schonbrunn A (1988) Characterization of the cyclic AMP-independent actions of somatostatin in GH cells. I. An increase in potassium conductance is responsible for both the hyperpolarisation and the decrease in intracellular free calcium produced by somatostatin. J Biol Chem 263:216–225

Lazaretti-Castro M, Grauer A, Raue F, Ziegler R (1990) 1,25-dihydroxyvitamin D_3 suppresses dexamethasone effects on calcitonin secretion. Mol Cell Endocrinol 71:R13–R18

Lazaretti-Castro M, Grauer A, Mekonnen Y, Raue F, Ziegler R (1991) 17ß-estradiol effects on calcitonin secretion and content in a human medullary thyroid carcinoma cell line. J Bone Miner Res 6:1191–1195

Leong SS, Horoszewicz JS, Shimoaka K, Friedmann M, Kawinski E, Song MJ, Zeigel R, Chu TM, Baylin S, Miraud EA (1981) A new cell line for study of human medullary thyroid carcinoma. In: Andreoli M, Monaco F, Robbind J (eds) Advances in thyroid neoplasia. Field Educational Italia, Rome, pp 95–108

Lewis DL, Weight FF, Luini A (1986) A guanine nucleotide-binding protein mediates the inhibition of voltage-dependent calcium current by somatostatin in a pituitary cell line. Proc Natl Acad Sci USA 83:9035–9045

Lussier BT, French MB, Moor BC, Kraicer J (1991a) Free intracellular Ca^{2+} concentration $[Ca^{2+}]_i$ and growth hormone release from purified rat somatotrophs. I. GH-releasing factor-induced Ca^{2+} influx raises $[Ca^{2+}]_i$. Endocrinology 128:570–582

Lussier BT, Wood DA, French MB, Moor BC, Kraicer J (1991b) Free-intracellular Ca^{2+} concentration $[Ca^{2+}]_i$ and growth hormone release from purified rat somatotrophs. II. Somatostatin lowers Ca^{2+} by inhibiting influx. Endocrinology 128:583–591

Mabry M, Nakagawa T, Baylin S, Pettengill O, Sorenson G, Nelkin B (1989) Insertion of the v-Ha-ras oncogene induces differentiation of calcitonin-producing human small cell lung cancer. J Clin Invest 84:194–199

Mathew CGP, Chiu KS, Easton DF, Thorpe K, Carter C, Liou CI, Fong SL, Bridge CD, Haak H, Kruseman HC, Schifter S, Hansen HH, Telenius H, Telenius-Berg M, Ponder BAJ (1987) A linked genetic marker for multiple endocrine neoplasia type 2a on chromosome 10. Nature 328:527–528

McDermott MT, Kidd GS (1987) The role of calcitonin in the development and treatment of osteoporosis. Endocr Rev 8:377–390

Mekonnen Y, Lazaretti-Castro M, Raue F, Ziegler R (1990) Long term exposure to the calcium channel agonist BAY K 8644 inhibits calcitonin secretion and content in a rat C-cell carcinoma cell line (Abstr). J Endocrinol Invest 13 Suppl 2:P 316

Murray SS, Burton DW, Deftos LJ (1988) The effects of forskolin and calcium ionophore A 23187 on secretion and cytoplasmic RNA levels of chromogranin-A and calcitonin. J Bone Miner Res 3:447–452

Nakagawa T, Mabry M, de Bustros A, Ihle JN, Nelkin BD, Baylin SB (1987) Introduction of v-Ha-ras oncogene induces differentiation of cultured human medullary thyroid carcinoma cells. Proc Natl Acad Sci USA 84:5923

Naveh-Many T, Silver J (1988) Regulation of calcitonin gene transcription by vitamin D metabolites in vivo in the rat. J Clin Invest 81:270–273

Naveh-Many T, Friedlaender M, Mayer H, Silver J (1988) Calcium regulates parathyroid hormone messenger ribonucleic acid (mRNA), but not calctionin mRNA in vivo in the rat; dominant role of 1,25 dihydroxyvitamin D. Endocrinology 125:275–280

Nelkin BD, Chen YK, de Bustros A, Boos BA, Baylin SB (1989a) Changes in calcitonin gene RNA processing during growth of a human medullary thyroid carcinoma cell line. Cancer Res 49:6949

Nelkin BD, de Bustros A, Mabry M, Baylin SB (1989b) The molecular biology of medullary thyroid carcinoma, a model for cancer development and progression. JAMA 261:3130–3135

Raue F, Deutschle I, Ziegler R (1983) Acute effect of 1,25-dihydroxyvitamin D_3 on calcitonin secretion in rats. Horm Metab Res 15:208–209

Raue F, Deutschle I, Küntzel C, Ziegler R (1984) Reversible diminished calcitonin secretion in the rat during chronic hypercalcemia. Endocrinology 115:2362–2367

Raue F, Wieland U, Weiler C, Ziegler R (1988) Enhanced calcitonin secretion in the rat after parathyroidectomy and during chronic calcium deprivation. Eur J Clin Invest 18:284–289

Raue F, Serve H, Grauer A, Scherübl H, Schneider HG, Ziegler R (1989) Role of voltage-dependent calcium channels in secretion of calcitonin from human medullary thyroid carcinoma cells. Klin Wochenschr 67:635–639

Raue F, Lazaretti-Castro M, Grauer A, Ziegler R (1990) Effect of estradiol on calcitonin secretion and storage in a human C-cell carcinoma cell line. 72nd Meeting of the Endocrine Society, Abstract 1432. Available from the Endocrine Society

Reginster JY, Deroisy R, Albert A, Denis D, Lecart MP, Collette J, Franchimont P (1989) Relationship between whole plasma calcitonin levels, calcitonin secretory capacity, and plasma levels in estrone in healthy women and postmenopausal osteoporotics. J Clin Invest 83:1073–1077

Reuter H, Scholz H (1977) The regulation of the calcium conductance of cardiac muscle by adrenaline. J Physiol (Lond) 264:49

Reynolds RK, Hoekzema GS, Vogel J, Hinrichs SH, Jay G (1988) Multiple endocrine neoplasia induced by the promiscuous expression of a viral oncogene. Proc Natl Acad Sci USA 85:3135–3139

Rosenthal W, Hescheler J, Trautwein W, Schultz G (1988) Control of voltage dependent Ca^{2+} channels by G protein-coupled receptors. FASEB J 2:2784–2790

Saad MF, Ordonez NG, Guido JJ, Samaan NA (1984) The prognostic value of immuno staining in medullary carcinoma of the thyroid. J Clin Endocrinol Metab 54:233–239

Scherübl H, Raue F, Zopf G, Hoffmann J, Ziegler R (1989a) Reversible desensitization of calcitonin secretion by repetitive stimulation with calcium. Mol Cell Endocrinol 63:263–266

Scherübl H, Raue F, Zopf G, Ziegler R (1989b) Calcitonin secretion and cAMP-efflux from C-cells, stimulated by glucagon and either calcium or BAY K 8644. Horm Metab Res Suppl 21:18–21

Scherübl H, Schultz G, Hescheler J (1990) A slowly inactivating calcium current works as a calcium sensor in calcitonin-secreting cells. FEBS Lett 273:51–54 [Errata 278:287 (1991)]

Scherübl H, Hescheler J, Schultz G, Kliemann D, Zink A, Ziegler R, Raue F (1992) Inhibition of Ca^{2+}-induced calcitonin secretion by somatostatin: roles of voltage-dependent Ca^{2+} channels and G proteins. Cell Signal 4:77–85

Schulz N, Propst F, Westphal H, Rosenberg M, Vande Wounde F (1990) Pheochromocytomas and C-cell thyroid neoplasms in transgenic C-mos mice, a transgenic model for the human familial neoplasia syndrome MEN II (Abstr). J Cancer Res Clin Oncol 116 Suppl:A 106103

Segond N, Legendre B, Tahri EH, Besnard P, Jullienne A, Moukhtar MS, Garel JM (1985) Increased level of calcitonin mRNA after 1,25-dihydroxyvitamin D_3 injection in the rat. FEBS Lett 184:268–272

Segond N, Delehage MC, Jullienne A, Taboulet J, Minvielle S, Milhaud G, Moukhtar MS (1989) Actinomycin D inhibits the rapid increase in translatable calcitonin mRNA provoked by acute calcium stimulation. Horm Metab Res 21:489–493

Seitz PK, Cooper CW (1989) Cosecretion of calcitonin and calcitonin gene-related peptide from cultured rat medullary thyroid C-Cells. J Bone Miner Res 4: 129–134

Simpson NE, Kidd KK, Goodfellow PJ, McDermid H, Myers S, Kidd JR, Jackson CE, Duncan AMV, Farrer LA, Brasch K, Castiglione C, Genel M, Gertner J, Greenberg CR, Gasella JF, Holden JJA, White GN (1987) Assignment of multiple endocrine neoplasia type 2A to chromosome 10 by linkage. Nature 328:528

Stolarsky-Fredman L, Left SE, Klein ES, Crenshow EB, Yeakley J, Rosenfeld MG (1990) A tissue specific enhancer in the rat-calcitonin/CGRP gene is active in both neural and endocrine cell types. Mol Endocrinol 4:497–504

Tiegs RD, Body JJ, Barta JM, Heath H III (1986) Plasma calcitonin in primary hyperparathyroidism: failure of C-cell response to sustained hypercalcemia. J Clin Endocrinol Metab 63:785–788

Tørring O, Bucht E, Sjöberg HE (1985) Decreased plasma calcitonin response to a calcium clamp in primary hyperparathyroidism. Acta Endocrinol (Copenh) 108:372–376

Yang K, Pearson CE, Samaan NA (1988) Estrongen receptor and hormone responsiveness of medullary thyroid carcinoma cells in continuous culture. Cancer Res 48:2760–2763

Yatani A, Codina J, Imoto Y, Reeves JP, Birnbaumer L, Brown AM (1987) A G protein directly regulates mammalian cardiac calcium channels. Science 238: 1288–1292

Zeytin FN, Rusk S, Leff SE (1987) Calcium, dexamethasone, and the anticorticoid RU-486 differentially regulate neuropeptide synthesis in a rat C-cell line. Endocrinology 121:361–370

Pathology of Sporadic and Hereditary Medullary Thyroid Carcinoma[*,**]

S. Schröder, K. Holl, and B.C. Padberg

Institut für Pathologie, Universität Hamburg (UKE), Martinistraße 52, W-2000 Hamburg 20, FRG

Historical Background and Aetiology

Although cases of "malignant goitre with amyloid stroma" had already been described by the turn of this century in the German literature (Burk 1901; Jaquet 1906; Stoffel 1910), it is only 30 years since medullary carcinoma of the thyroid (MTC) was first clearly separated from the other types of thyroid carcinoma (Hazard et al. 1959). During the following decade, the classical histological features of MTC were described (Williams et al. 1966), the thyroid C-cell as the cell of origin delineated (Williams 1966), and the link with calcitonin (CT) production demonstrated (Cunliffe et al. 1968; Milhaud et al. 1968). It was, in addition, realized that a proportion of cases of MTC were genetically determined, occurring in association with phaeochromocytoma, or with phaeochromocytoma and multiple mucosal neuromas (Williams 1965; Schimke et al. 1968; Williams and Pollock 1966). Afterwards, the terms multiple endocrine neoplasia (MEN) 2 and MEN 3 were introduced by Steiner et al. (1968) and Khairi et al. (1975), respectively, to distinguish these combinations of tumours from Wermer's syndrome (parathyroid, pituitary, and endocrine pancreatic tumours), which was given the name MEN 1 as it was described first. MEN 2 has been subsequently subdivided into MEN 2A (which includes MTC, phaeochromocytoma, and hyperparathyroidism) and MEN 2B (which refers to the neuromata syndrome including MTC, phaeochromocytoma, mucosal neuromata, gastrointestinal ganglioneuromatosis and marfanoid habitus) (Chong et al. 1975), and the term MEN 2B is now more commonly used than MEN 3 to designate the neuromata syndrome. The genetic defects

* Supported by the Deutsche Forschungsgemeinschaft, the Hamburger Krebsgesellschaft and the Hamburger Stiftung zur Förderung der Krebsbekämpfung.
** The skilful technical assistance of Mr. Jochen Koppelmeyer in preparing the micrographs is gratefully acknowledged.

leading to the development of familial MTC inherited in the setting of the MEN 2 syndromes are described in detail in R.F. Gagel et al., this volume. The aetiology and concrete pathogenesis of sporadic (non-hereditary) MTC has, in contrast, not yet been elucidated. It is, however, generally accepted that exogenous factors such as hypercalcaemia, hypervitaminoses D and A and irradiation known to be associated with higher incidence of MTC in various mammals are not carcinogenic to human C-cells (Saad et al. 1984a).

Incidence, Histogenesis and Gross Pathology

MTC is an unusual type of thyroid neoplasm. In most studies, its incidence among thyroid cancers ranges from approximately 3% to 12% (Deftos 1983). In the general population the lower figure is probably more accurate, while in institutions where kindreds with the familial forms of the disease are followed and treated, the percentage of thyroid carcinomas that are medullary lesions will be higher (LiVolsi 1990). The ratio of female-to-male involvement seems to be closer to unity than in other thyroid tumours when more comprehensive series are considered. Hence, in 73 cases of MTC out of 777 cases of thyroid cancer studied by Hill et al. (1973), the female-to-male ratio was 1.4 to 1, compared with 2.5 to 1 for other thyroid tumours.

The tumour is usually located in the area of highest C-cell concentration, i.e., the lateral upper two-thirds of the gland. In inherited cases, multiple small nodules may be detected macroscopically, and – as opposed to the majority of sporadic tumours – bilaterality of disease can nearly always be documented (Ljungberg 1972; Chong et al. 1975; Saad et al. 1984a). The tumours range in size from barely visible to several centimetres; the former variety is found in familial cases, in which the tumour is identified only through biochemical screening (LiVolsi 1990).

Most MTC are macroscopically well demarcated, although true encapsulation appears to be a rare event (Fig. 1). They have a white or white-grey colour, but some are yellow or tan. The tumours are firm but rarely hard. Granular calcification can occur; rarely, bone formation is found (Saad et al. 1984a, LiVolsi 1990).

Conventional Microscopy

As compared to the other types of thyroid cancer, the cytoarchitectural appearance of MTC is enormously variable (Figs. 2 and 3). The variability in histological structure (solid, trabecular or insular) and cellular pattern (spindle, polyhedral, angular or round shape) was already noted when MTC was first recognized as a distinct clinicopathological entity by Hazard et al. (1959). Upon investigation of 21 cases, however, these authors noted that all these tumours had in common the presence of stromal amyloid. The detec-

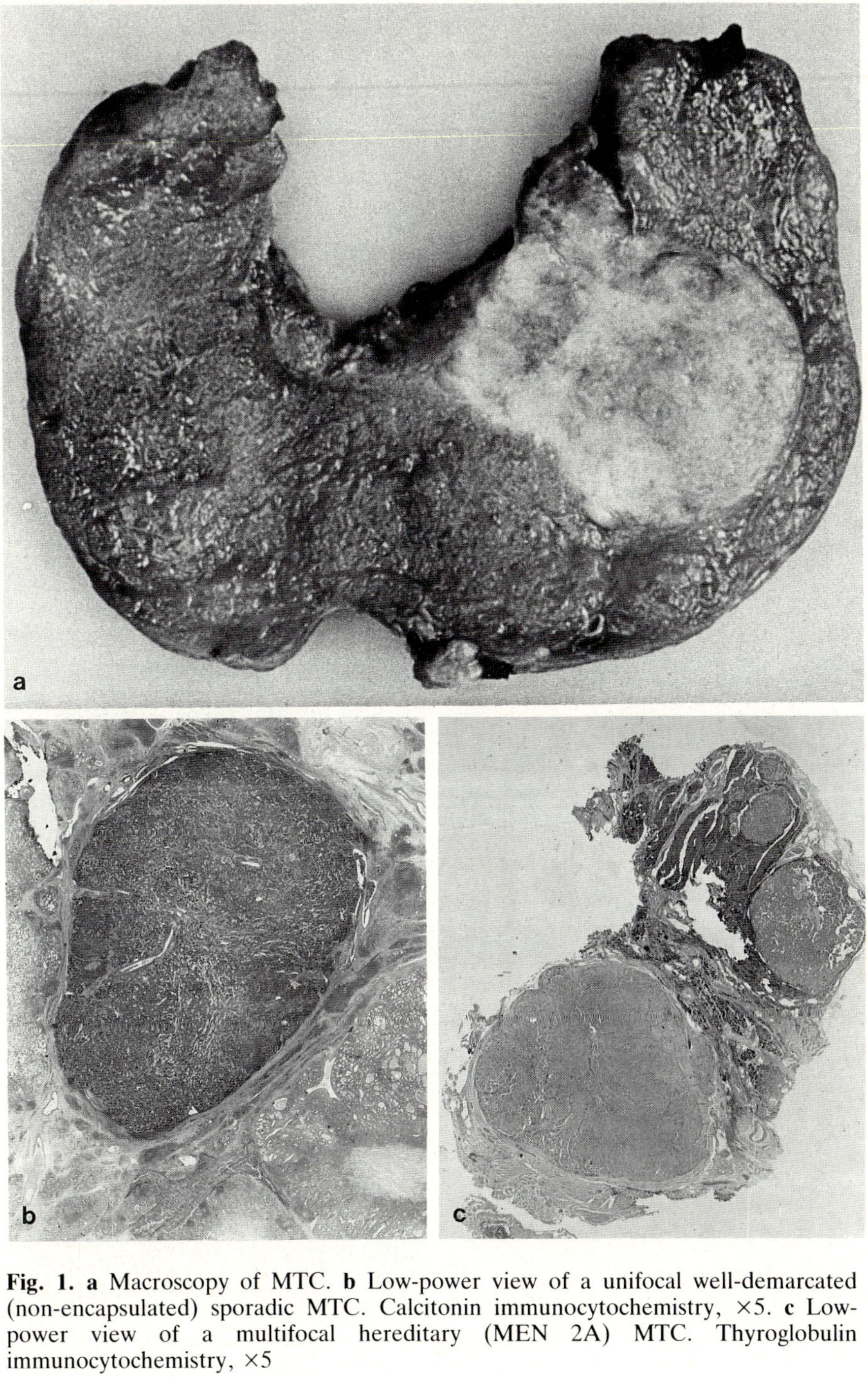

Fig. 1. **a** Macroscopy of MTC. **b** Low-power view of a unifocal well-demarcated (non-encapsulated) sporadic MTC. Calcitonin immunocytochemistry, ×5. **c** Low-power view of a multifocal hereditary (MEN 2A) MTC. Thyroglobulin immunocytochemistry, ×5

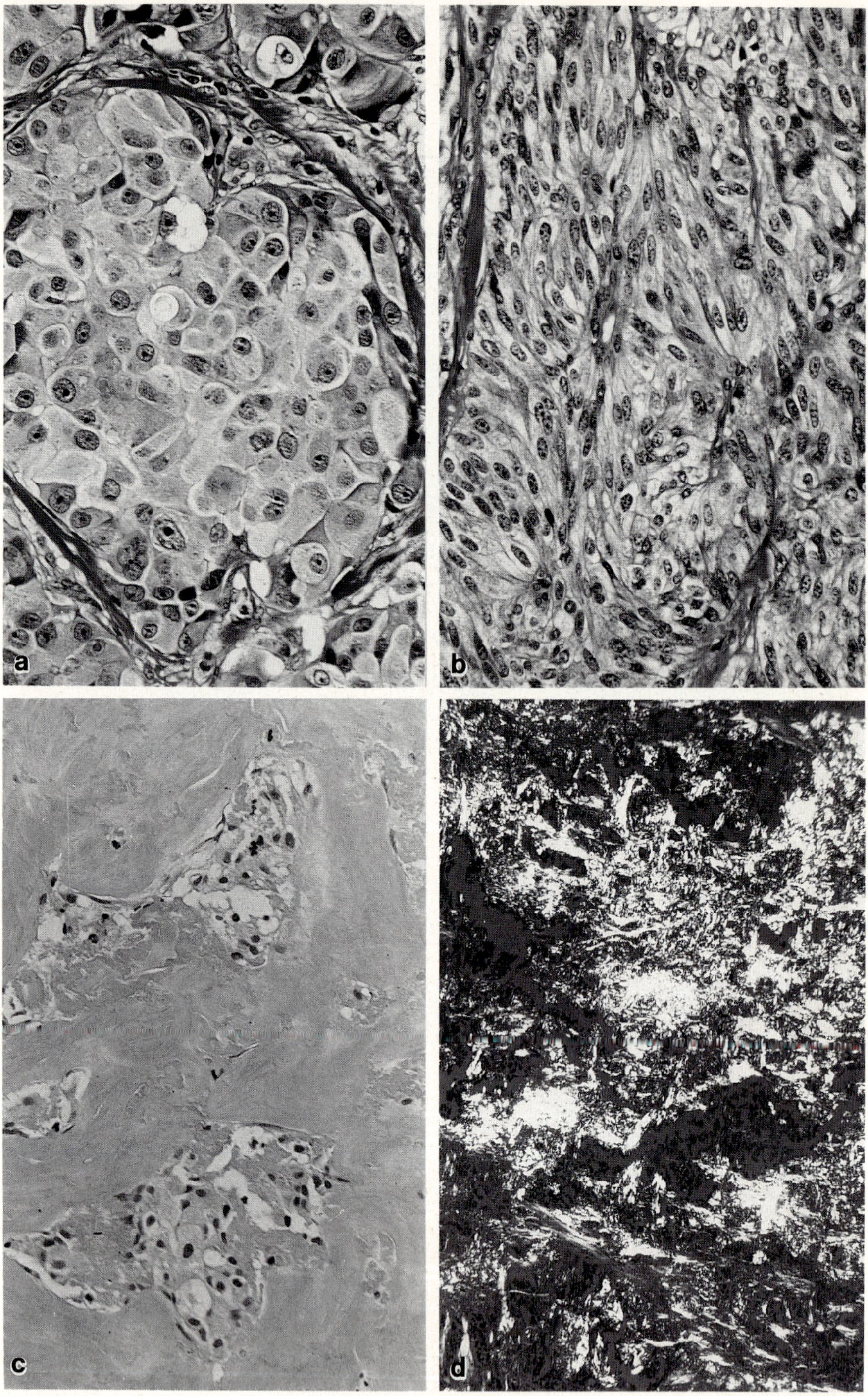

Fig. 2 a–d. Conventional histology of MTC. **a** Polygonal and **b** spindle-shaped cell type. H&E, ×270. **c** Amyloid-rich neoplasm. H&E, ×220. **d** Visualisation of Congo red-positive deposits by polariscope microscopy. Congo red stain, ×50

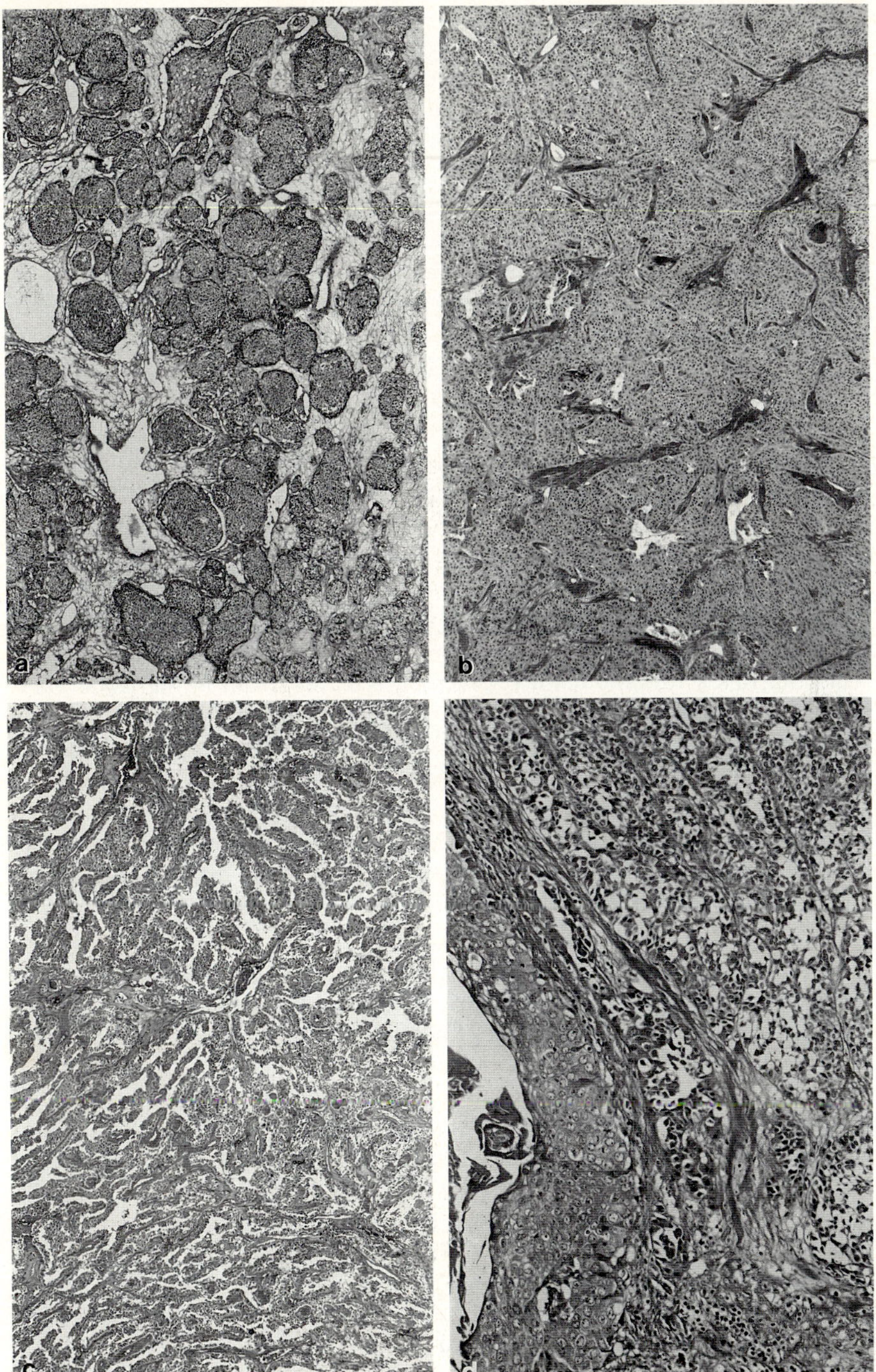

Fig. 3 a–d. Histological variants of MTC. **a** Insular (H&E, ×50), **b** trabecular (H&E, ×70) and **c** papillary architecture (H&E, ×50). **d** MTC with transition to a keratinising squamous cell carcinoma. H&E, ×100

tion of amyloid was considered to be the main auxiliary diagnostic criterion for MTC until Norman et al. (1976) upon using immunocytochemistry and electron microscopy confirmed the existence of amyloid-free MTC cases.

Ultrastructurally, MTC cells were shown to invariably possess characteristic neurosecretory granules, which are composed of a central electron-dense core, surrounded by a clear space and a single delimiting membrane. Immunoelectron microscopic studies have proved that these granules contain CT (Meyer et al. 1973). A variability in their sizes has been detected, suggesting the existence of multiple endocrine cell types in this tumour (Capella et al. 1978; Holm et al. 1989). The granules are responsible for the argyrophilia of MTC which usually can be demonstrated histochemically utilizing the Grimelius or Sevier-Munger methods (DeLellis and Balogh 1973), especially if the tissue has been fixed in Bouin's fluid.

Microscopically, the typical MTC case consists of a solid proliferation of round, polygonal or spindle-shaped cells of amphophilic or eosinophilic cytoplasm and medium-sized nucleus. The cytoplasm has ill-defined margins and may appear granular. The nuclei are uniformly round-to-oval in most of the tumours. However, there often is isolated cellcular pleomorphism, with the finding of enlarged nuclei or even multinucleated cells. Mitoses can be seen, but this a variable feature. Necrosis is a rare event in the usual MTC (Chong et al. 1975; LiVolsi 1990).

The smear of an aspirate from MTC commonly shows pleomorphic cancer cells, either isolated or in loosely cohesive groups. Their nuclei are always eccentric. A remarkable and consistent feature is the presence of intranuclear cytoplasmic inclusions. The cytoplasm generally stains pale and has a fibrillar quality. Amyloid can be seen in cytological preparations as fluffy, finely granular, or dense acellular material in the background (Kini et al. 1984).

The histological pattern of growth is of tumour cells arranged in nests separated by a highly vascular stroma, hyalinized collagen, and amyloid. As recently re-emphasized by LiVolsi (1990), the most complete and concise characterization of architectural variants can be found in a review by Saad et al. (1984a), including the following five categories: classical (nests of uniform round-to-oval cells mixed with spindle-shaped cells and separated by fibrous stroma containing small amounts of amyloid); amyloid rich (solid groups of round or spindle-shaped cells separated by large masses of amyloid); insular (carcinoid appearance in which cells are arranged in nodular solid nests); trabecular (ribbon-like structures of polygonal or spindle-shaped cells forming anastomotic cords of two or three cells in thickness); and epithelial (sheets of polygonal or cuboidal regular cells with scanty intervening stroma mimicking the appearance of carcinoma). The description of papillary (Kakudo et al. 1979), follicular (Harach and Williams 1983), oxyphilic (Harach and Bergholm 1988), clear-cell (Landon and Ordonez 1985), anaplastic (Kakudo et al. 1978; Mendelsohn et al. 1980; Martinelli et al. 1983), small cell (Albores-Saavedra et al. 1985) and squamous variants (Dominguez-Malagon et al. 1989) as well as of mucin-producing (Fernandes et al. 1982) and melanin-producing types (Marcus et al. 1982) has since widened the histopathological spectrum of MTC.

The stromal amyloid, present in about 50%–80% of MTC cases, can be stained with Congo red (resulting in apple-green birefringence when examined with polarized light), metachromatic stains such as crystal violet, and thioflavine T (DeLellis and Balogh 1973). With regard to biochemical and physiochemical properties, namely its molecular weight being twice that of CT and its immunoreactivity with anti-CT antisera, the amyloid protein in MTC is believed to be related to or represent procalcitonin, following cleavage of the preprohormone (Berger et al. 1988; Westermark and Johnson 1988).

Immunocytochemistry

Lectin histochemistry has again recently been shown to be unsuitable in discriminating between different MTC subtypes or between medullary and non-medullary carcinomas of the thyroid (Sobrinho-Simoes et al. 1990). Instead, numerous studies have proved the value of immunocytochemistry in establishing the diagnosis of MTC (Fig. 4). Regarding intermediate filament typing, virtually all cases display cytokeratin immunoreactivity, while – upon usage of paraffin-embedded material – approximately 50% or, where applicable, less than 20% of tumours stain positively for vimentin and neurofilaments, respectively (Schröder et al. 1986). Obligatory positivity of MTC has also been reported for a variety of pan-neuroendocrine markers such as neuron-specific enolase (Holm et al. 1985), chromogranin A (Sikri et al. 1985; Kimura et al. 1988; Schröder et al. 1988a) and synaptophysin (Miettinen 1987) which, like neurofilament proteins, are generally negative in non-medullary thyroid cancers (Schröder 1988). In addition, MTC differs from the follicular and papillary types of the differentiated thyroid follicle cell carcinoma by its consistent positivity for CT and its consistent negativity for thyroglobulin (TG) (Krisch et al. 1985; Schröder and Klöppel 1987a) (for exceptions see below).

It seems impossible that one could define a tumour as MTC if it were negative for CT, the specific product of C-cells. Since the introduction of immunolocalization techniques, most authors have considered CT positivity to be the prerequisite for diagnosing this condition. Thus, 265 of 266 immunocytochemically investigated cases communicated until 1988 were reported to be positively stained (DeLellis et al. 1978; Talerman et al. 1979; Wolfe et al. 1980; Lloyd et al. 1983; Saad et al. 1984b; Holm et al. 1985; Krisch et al. 1985; Sikri et al. 1985; Uribe et al. 1985; Wilson et al. 1986; Schröder et al. 1988a). LiVolsi (1990) therefore postulated that in order to accept a CT-free neoplasm of the thyroid as MTC, it should arise in a familial setting or occur in a thyroid with unequivocal C-cell hyperplasia, whereby immuno-

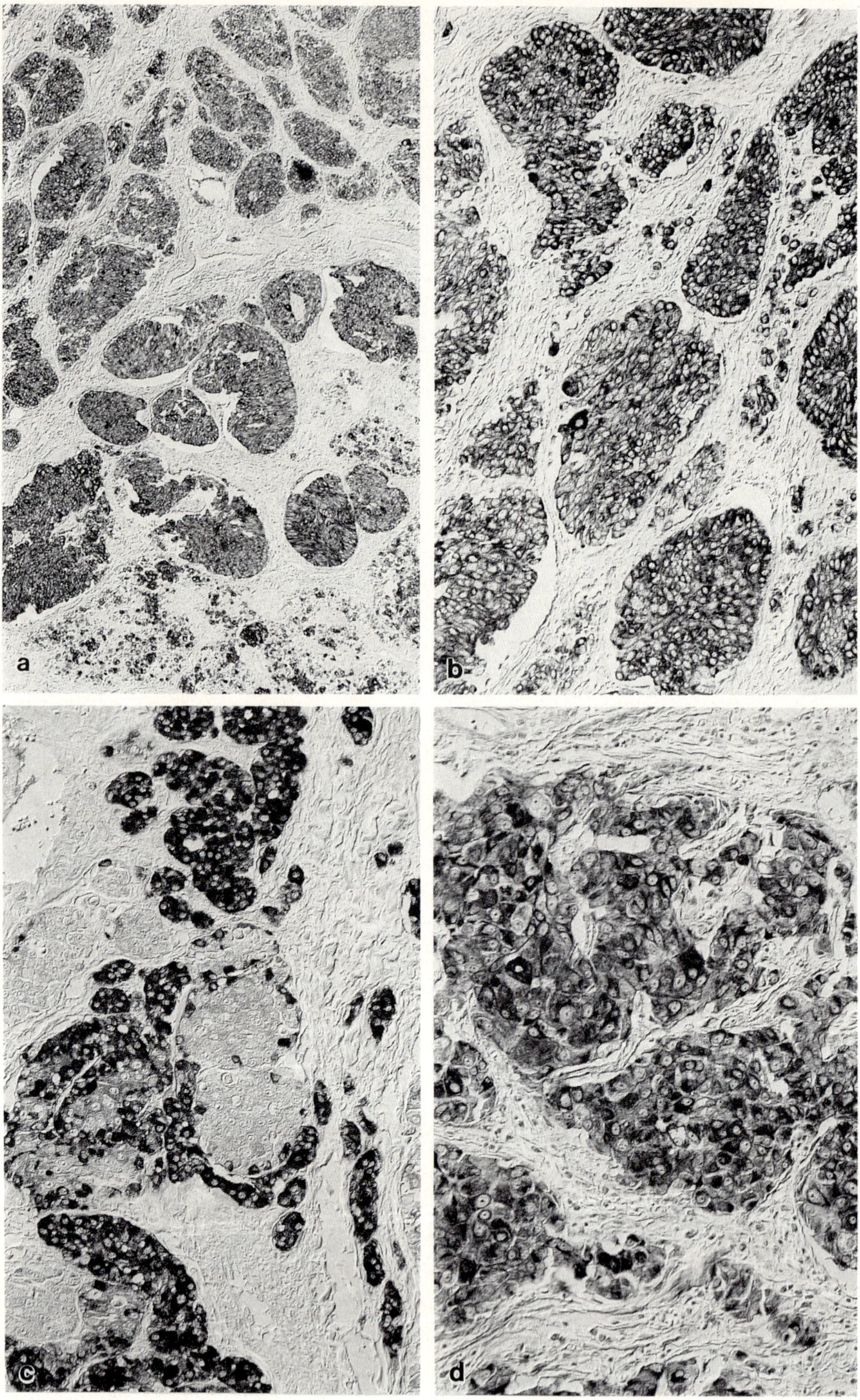

Fig. 4 a–d. Immunocytochemical features of MTC. Intense diffuse positivity for chromogranin A (**a**), ×90; calcitonin (**b**), ×220; CGRP (**c**), ×220; and CEA (**d**), ×220

reactivity for calcitonin gene-related peptide (CGRP) would provide further proof of the medullary nature of such a lesion. This author also noted that there exist occasional CT-free small cell cancers of thyroid origin which, as recently described by Eusebi et al. (1990), should be categorized as thyroid small cell carcinoma although they might represent small cell MTC without CT arising in a non-familial setting. It has yet to be stressed that rarely – 1/138 cases in our material – also non-small-cell thyroid carcinomas with a distinctly "neuroendocrine" growth pattern and immunoreactivity for pan-neuroendocrine markers occur, which regarding their negativity for both CT and TG can neither be pigeon-holed into C-cell or follicular origin. With respect to their classical appearance it appears unlikely that such neoplasms are poorly differentiated variants of MTC that have lost the capacity to produce CT. Since conceptually a histogenetic relation exists between MTC and carcinoids of other sites, such cases rather might be considered as separate "neuroendocrine carcinomas" analogous to those seen in many other organs (Rosai 1989).

Katacalcin (PDN-21), the C-terminal flanking peptide of the CT molecule, and CGRP, another major peptide, encoded by the same gene as CT, are regularly produced by MTC (Emmertsen 1985; Sikri et al. 1985; Williams 1985) and thus may be employed as additional tumour markers for C-cell carcinoma (Albores-Saavedra et al. 1985). The ability of MTC to synthesize and secrete carcinoembryonic antigen (CEA) is another point of diagnostic importance. Until 1987, the literature documented CEA immunoreactivity in 108 of 119 (91%) tumour cases (DeLellis et al. 1978; Talerman et al. 1979; Lloyd et al. 1983; Holm et al. 1985; Krisch et al. 1985; Uribe et al. 1985; Wilson et al. 1986). The considerably lower number of 77% (46/60) in our material is most likely to be due to the use of a monoclonal CEA antibody lacking reactivity with the non-specific cross-reacting antigens (NCA) 95 and 55. Since we found NCA 95 and NCA 55 to be expressed by all types of thyroid carcinoma, while CEA was present only in C-cell tumours of this organ (Schröder and Klöppel 1987a), such epitope-defined CEA-specific probes appear to provide the most consistent results in the immunocytochemical differential diagnosis of thyroid neoplasias.

Immunocytochemistry has documented MTC cases capable of synthesizing, apart from CT, PDN-21, CGRP and CEA, a wide variety of opioid and polypeptides and other hormonal and non-hormonal substances. The list of products secreted or found in MTC includes but is not limited to: adrenocorticotropic hormone (ACTH), prostaglandins, beta-endorphin, bradykinin, bombesin, somatostatin, prolactin-like activity, vasoactive intestinal polypeptide (VIP), substance P, alpha human chorionic gonadotropin (alpha-hCG), serotonin, histaminase, dopa decarboxylase, and proopiomelanocortin (for literature review see Grün and Eberle 1981; Deftos 1983; LiVolsi 1990). In some tumours many of these substances are made, and production of more than one factor by the same neoplastic cell is also well documented (Williams 1985). Since, however, only a relatively small number of MTC cases stain positively for the last-named products and considerable discrepancies come to light when comparing the results of different investigators, none of these substances by itself nor a combination of these substances has gained diagnostic significance. Yet, their occasional presence in MTC again points to the above-mentioned analogies between thyroid C-cell carcinoma and neuroendocrine tumours (carcinoids) of other sites.

Mixed Medullary-Follicular Carcinoma

As different areas within one given tumour may differ considerably concerning their architectural pattern, the new WHO classification of thyroid tumours (Hedinger et al. 1988) does not recommend formal classification of MTC into multiple different subtypes. Special mention is, however, made of the mixed medullary-follicular variant, which is described as a tumour showing "both the morphological features of medullary carcinoma together with immunoreactive calcitonin, and the morphological features of follicular carcinoma together with immunoreactive thyroglobulin". It appears that not only the partly follicularly structured thyroid carcinomas fulfill these criteria: Recently, two neoplasms were reported by Albores-Saavedra et al. (1990) which, in accordance with the WHO definition, were typed as mixed medullary-papillary carcinoma of the thyroid. Both of these conditions have to be distinguished from the simultaneous occurrence, which is just as rare, of medullary and follicular (Tanaka et al. 1989) or medullary and papillary carcinoma (Lamberg et al. 1981) in the same thyroid lobe.

Since the positive staining for TG in individual MTC cases was first noted by Hales et al. (1982), several other reports on the concurrent production of CT and TG within the same tumour (Pfaltz et al. 1983; Ljungberg et al. 1984; Holm et al. 1985; Parker et al. 1985; Uribe et al. 1985; Mills et al. 1986) and even within the same neoplastic cells (Holm et al. 1986) have been published. As a consequence, the separate origin of follicle-cell and C-cell carcinomas has been questioned (Sobrinho-Simoes et al. 1985) and the existence of a common multipotent stem cell was suggested (Holm et al. 1987). The possible precursor normal cell counterpart has, however, as yet not been identified and the origin of TG immunoreactivity in MTC is still a matter of controversial debate. Some of the cases in which the diagnosis of mixed medullary-follicular carcinoma has been entertained might well represent MTC with entrapped follicles and/or secondary incorporation of TG by the medullary carcinoma cells (Rosai 1989). It has thus been stressed by the WHO (Hedinger et al. 1988) that absolute proof of the occurrence of this lesion depends on identification of both patterns of differentiation in metastatic tumours (Fig. 5). Another fact to remember in this context is that – due to immunization procedures using peptide hormone preparations conjugated to TG – certain commercially available antisera against regulatory peptides (including CT, bombesin and neurotensin) also react with

TG (Holm et al. 1986; Williams 1986; Schröder and Klöppel 1987b). This cross-reactivity led to considerable unspecific staining (e.g., false-positive CT staining) in several of our non-medullary carcinomas, which could be completely abolished after preabsorbing the respective antisera with TG (Schröder and Klöppel 1987b). As again recently noted by Albores-Saavedra et al. (1990), a different methodology such as in situ hybridization may eventually solve the controversy surrounding these tumours by the identification of mRNA specific for CT and TG in the neoplastic cells.

Irrespective of the fact that the majority of MTC cases reported to coexpress TG and CT lacked a focal follicular architecture and thus do not comply with the above-mentioned requirements of the new WHO classification, additional questions regarding their incidence and their biological behaviour remain to be answered about these "mixed" tumours of the thyroid. The frequency of TG-positive cases among CT-positive MTC was stated to be 19% (5/27) and 37% (7/19) by Holm et al. (1985) and Uribe et al. (1985), respectively, whereas we have so far failed to identify any of 138 immunocytochemically investigated MTC as staining positively for TG. In disagreement with earlier observations of Ljungberg et al. (1984), Holm et al. (1987) stated TG-positive MTC to have a better outcome than those of the control group. On the basis of dual differentiation, the regression of individual MTC cases following administration of thyroid extract (Didolkar and Moore 1974) and the ability of some of such lesions to concentrate radioactive iodine (Hales et al. 1982) could be explained. Due to the actual rarity of mixed medullary-follicular thyroid carcinomas containing mature TG-positive follicles – the latter obviously being a prerequisite for positive radioiodine uptake (Schröder et al. 1991) – we assume only a small minority of MTC patients gain profit from these treatment procedures. Hence, the diagnosis of this tumour variant would not imply an alteration of the therapeutic strategies generally applied in patients afflicted with C-cell carcinoma of the thyroid gland.

Inherited Medullary Thyroid Carcinoma and C-Cell Hyperplasia

In approximately 20% of MTC cases the tumour occurs in syndromatic association with extrathyroidal neoplasias in the setting of MEN 2. Conversely, more than 90% of patients afflicted with the MEN 2 syndromes develop MTC, which in the majority of MEN 2A cases represents the initial symptom of the disease (Khairi et al. 1975; Heitz and Steiner 1981; Deftos 1983). Regarding histological (predominant cell type, architecture, amyloid content), immunocytochemical (expression of polypeptides) and DNA cytophotometrical parameters no systematic differences exist between hereditary and sporadic examples of MTC which in the individual case would enable a clear assignment (Saad et al. 1984a; Schröder et al. 1988a; Bergholm et al. 1989). Also the prognosis of hereditary and non-hereditary

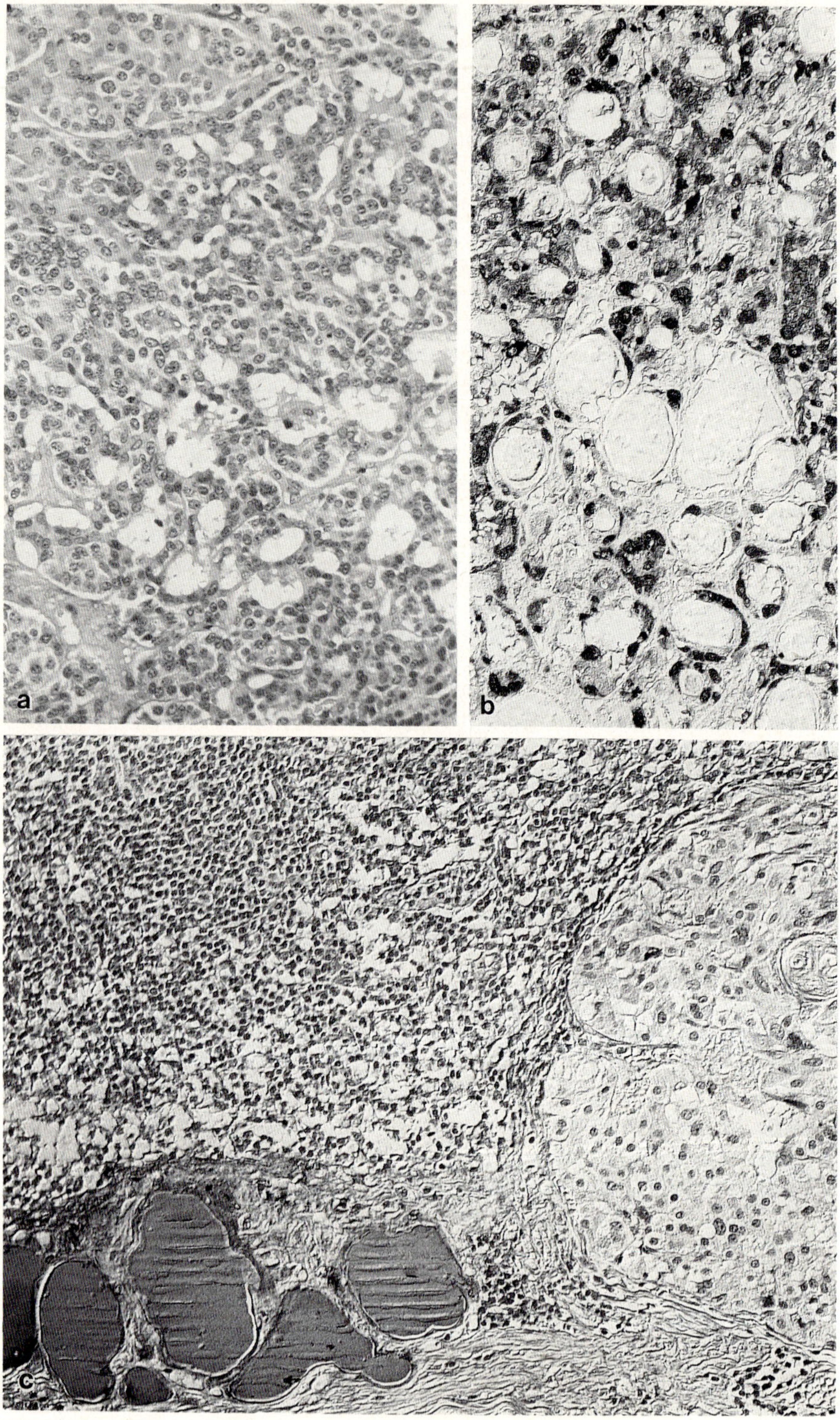
a
b
c

MTC is determined by the same parameters listed below. It has, also, to be further scrutinized whether, as suggested by the WHO (Hedinger et al. 1988), the identification of C-cell hyperplasia (CCH) in the thyroid bordering MTC renders a distinction possible.

Bilateral CCH was described by Wolfe et al. (1973) as an obligatory precursor lesions to hereditary MTC. As a continuous process, from the initial event of hypertrophy of individual C-cells CCH is supposed to proceed from focal via diffuse to nodular hyperplasia which, once the basement membrane is breached and the interstitial stroma is invaded, changes into microinvasive MTC (DeLellis et al. 1977) (Fig. 6). Focal and diffuse CCH are defined as the eccentric or circular intrafollicular proliferation of C-cells displacing the follicular epithelium centrally in the follicle. Nodular CCH represents the most advanced change in this spectrum of events, characterized by complete replacement of the thyrocytes of individual follicles by proliferating C-cells, thus resulting in solid clusters entirely consisting of parafollicular cells. Defects and gaps in the follicular basal lamina were shown to precede the development of overt stromal invasion, i.e., MTC (DeLellis et al. 1977). As has been stressed by the WHO (Hedinger et al. 1988), identification of normal and hyperplastic C-cells on H&E-stained sections is not reliable and a special technique such as CT immunolocalization should be used. Immunocytochemical procedures also appear to be a promising adjunct to discriminate between different steps in the progression of C-cell hyperplasia to C-cell neoplasia, since upon investigation of thyroid tissues from MEN 2 patients only CCH already accompanied by invasive MTC was documented to stain positively for CEA (Fig. 7) (Schröder and Klöppel 1987a), while only microinvasive MTC, but not non-invasive CCH, was reported to be histaminase positive (Baylin et al. 1979).

According to Wolfe et al. (1980) the thyroid tissue bordering MEN 2-associated MTC regularly contains residues of not yet neoplastically transformed diffuse or nodular CCH, while this finding is generally absent in sporadic MTC. Contrary to this assumption, different authors have described the occurrence of CCH in the neighbourhood of non-hereditary MTC (Ulbright et al. 1981; Uribe et al. 1985; Rosenberg-Bourgin et al. 1989), while 25% of hereditary MTC were reported to lack accompanying CCH (Rosenberg-Bourgin et al. 1989). In addition, nodular CCH can occasionally

◀ **Fig. 5 a–c.** Morphological features simulating mixed medullary-follicular carcinoma. **a** MTC with follicular structure (but lacking immunoreactivity for TG). H&E, ×220. **b** MTC with entrapped (non-neoplastic) follicles lacking immunoreactivity for CT. CT immunocytochemistry, ×220. **c** Regional metastasis of a classical (TG-negative) MTC (*right-hand side*) adjacent to non-neoplastic heterotopic (TG-positive) follicles to be seen in the marginal sinus of the lymph node (*bottom left*). TG immunocytochemistry, ×160

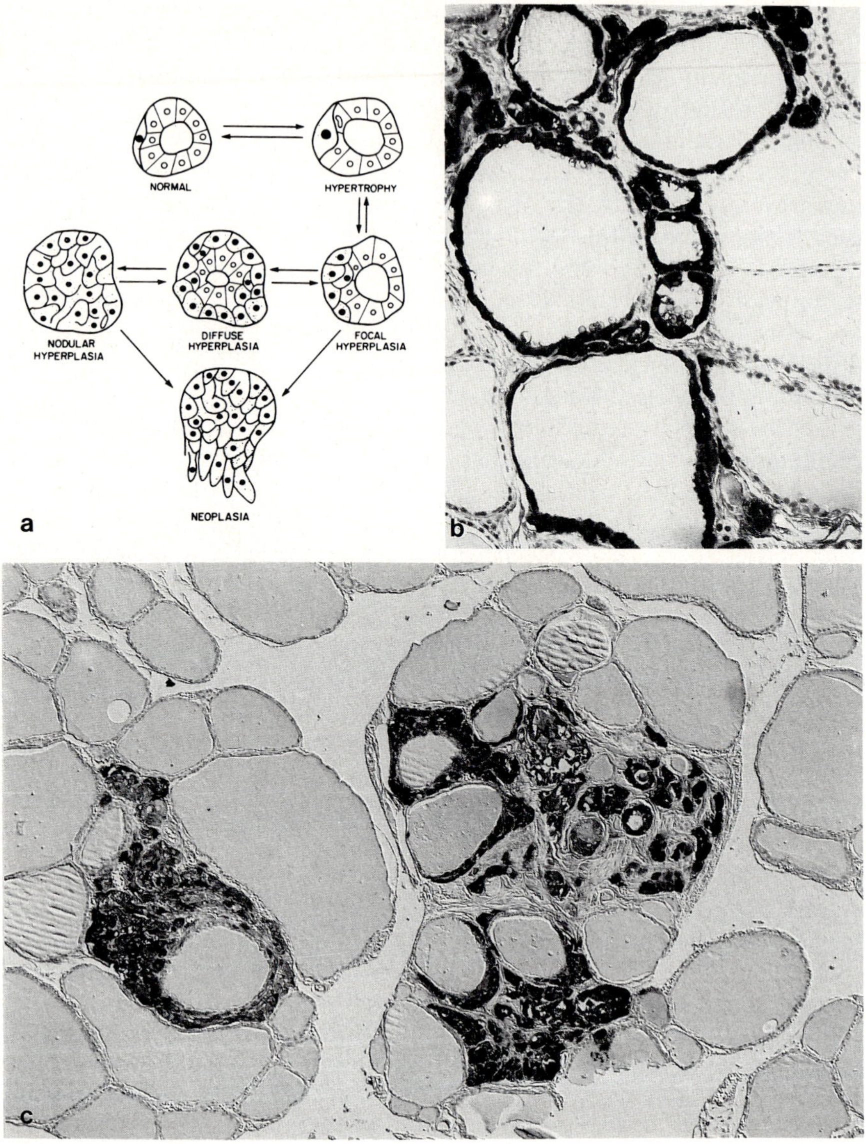

Fig. 6. a Histogenesis of C-cell hyperplasia (CCH) and hereditary MTC (from DeLellis et al. 1977). **b** Diffuse CCH (patient afflicted by MEN 2A). CT immunocytochemistry, ×150. **c** Transition from (diffuse and nodular) CCH to MTC as evidenced by overt stromal invasion (patient afflicted by MEN 2B). CT immunocytochemistry, ×115

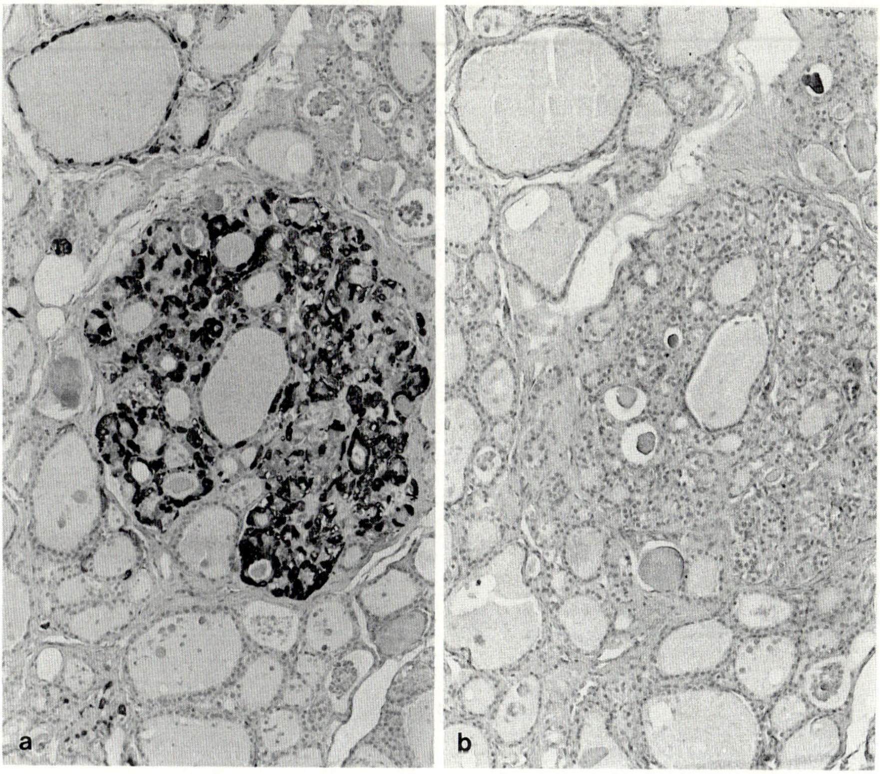

Fig. 7a,b. Serial sections of (not yet neoplastically transformed) diffuse CCH in a MEN 2A patient showing positivity for CT (**a**) but negativity for CEA (**b**), ×90

also be detected adjacent to benign and malignant follicle cell tumours of the thyroid (Albores-Saavedra et al. 1988) and in Hashimoto's thyroiditis (Libbey et al. 1989; Biddinger et al. 1991). C-cell nodules with the appearance of nodular CCH are supposed to represent a normal finding in otherwise disease-free thyroids of elderly patients (Gibson et al. 1982). Interestingly, such "physiological" non-MEN-2-associated nodular CCH may upon provocative testing be associated with pathologically increased plasma CT levels (Lips et al. 1987). Hence, the differential diagnostic value of the detection of CCH can by no means be regarded as dependable, but demands to be checked by, among others, the above-named immuncytochemical techniques. It has, furthermore, to be mentioned in this context that – with regard to the strictly bilateral occurrence of CCH in MEN 2 patients – more than 90% of hereditary MTC present themselves as bilateral neoplasms (Ljungberg 1972; Chong et al. 1975; Bigner et al. 1981; Saad et al. 1984a), yet also up to 30% of sporadic MTC can become manifest simultaneously in both thyroid lobes (Saad et al. 1984a).

It has been shown by several investigators that MEN 2A-associated C-cell carcinomas have a better prognosis, while such neoplasms occurring in the setting of MEN 2B fare worse than sporadic MTC (Carney et al. 1979; Norton et al. 1979; Jackson et al. 1983; Saad et al. 1984a). As the aggressiveness of MTC generally increases with the patients' age (Bigner et al. 1981; Schröder et al. 1988a), Samaan et al. (1989) recently supposed the more favourable behaviour of MEN 2A-associated MTC to merely reflect the lower mean age of such patients at diagnosis. Since according to Kakudo et al. (1985), the mean age at diagnosis is another 10 years lower in MEN 2B patients (23 years) as compared to MEN 2A patients (38 years, sporadic MTC: 49 years), this assumption appears, however, implausible. Rather, the differences in the malignant potential of MTC occurring as part of the MEN 2A and 2B syndromes seem to be genetically determined, thus especially in MEN 2B patients justifying thyroidectomy as soon as increased CT levels are recorded upon provocative testing (Carney et al. 1979) or, as suggested by Thompson et al. (1984), already prior to the detection of pathological hormone levels if the phenotype typical of MEN 2B is recognized.

Prognostic Criteria

The biological behaviour of MTC is generally regarded to be intermediate between the anaplastic and the differentiated thyroid carcinomas. However, patients with MTC show great variability in survival, which can vary from months to 30 years after diagnosis (Deftos 1983). Several authors therefore have examined both clinical and pathological factors which appear related to the outcome in this type of neoplasia. Although considerable discrepancies come to light when comparing the results of different investigators, certain factors emerge as important prognostic indicators.

In our studies, MTC with a spindle-cell pattern had the same prognosis as MTC composed of polygonal cells (Schröder et al. 1988a). These results contradict earlier studies claiming that spindle cells (along with increased mitoses) are unfavourable prognostic elements (Williams et al. 1966), but confirm data of other authors (Ljungberg 1972; Rougier et al. 1983; Saad et al. 1984a; El-Naggar et al. 1990) who found neither histologic structure nor cellular and nuclear polymorphism to be reliable indicators of the further course of disease. Presence of necroses (Franc et al. 1987; Kakudo 1990) and lack of amyloid (Ibanez et al. 1967; Tubiana et al. 1968; Bussolati and Monga 1979; Bergholm et al. 1989) also have been considered as bad prognostic indicators. However, in the light of our findings as well as those of others (Ljungberg 1972; Saad et al. 1984a; Holm et al. 1985; Schröder et al. 1988a; El-Naggar et al. 1990), amyloid-free MTC do not run a more malignant clinical course than amyloid-containing tumours.

The pattern of CT immunoreactivity has been claimed to be of predictive value (Saad et al. 1984b; Bergholm et al. 1989; El-Naggar et al. 1990). CT-rich tumours appeared to have a better prognosis than CT-poor neoplasms. These findings were in keeping with earlier observations that virulent MTC cells contain less CT (and simultaneously have increased dopa decarboxylase and histaminase content; Lippman et al. 1982). Our results and those of Holm et al. (1985), however, are at variance with the abovementioned observations. Both series showed patients who had survived for less than 3 years to have tumours with an essentially identical CT immunostaining pattern to those of patients who had survived 10 years or more. In like manner, the studies of Takami et al. (1988) and Pacini et al. (1991) indicated that homogeneous (uniform) staining for CT does not guarantee a favourable outcome, and poor or heterogeneous staining does not always predict aggressive behaviour. In this context it should also be mentioned that, occasionally, CT-rich primary tumours may revert to less differentiated variants with more aggressive course, thus suggesting that the longer term prognosis must remain guarded (Saad et al. 1984b; Ruppert et al. 1986).

Mendelsohn et al. (1984) reported on an inverse relationship between CEA and CT, with the latter decreasing and CEA being retained as the tumour becomes more widely metastatic. In other series (Lloyd et al. 1983; Holm et al. 1985; Krisch et al. 1985; Schröder et al. 1988a), however, CEA immunoreactivity of MTC was not demonstrated to be related to tumour prognosis. From our experience and that of others it appears that also none of several other substances typically found in MTC (such as opioid and polypeptide hormones) either alone or in combination has any prognostic significance (Deftos 1983; Emmertsen 1985; Holm et al. 1985; Sikri et al. 1985; Uribe et al. 1985). We were, however, surprised to find a strong correlation between the degree of aberrant epithelial expression of the myelomonocytic antigen Leu-M1 in tumour tissue and the prognosis of patients with MTC (Fig. 8). Irrespective of other morphological and clinical features, local recurrences occurred 2.9 times more frequently and death resulting from tumour occurred 4.3 times more frequently among MTC with marked Leu-M1 positivity compared to tumours with only slight or absent immunoreactivity (Schröder et al. 1988b).

It has, in addition, to be mentioned in this context that Pacini et al. (1991) recently reported on a significantly better outcome of somatostatin-positive as compared to somatostatin-negative MTCs. A plausible explanation for this phenomenon is as yet lacking, since Reubi et al. (1991) failed to demonstrate a correlation between the clinical course or the survival of MTC patients and their tumoral somatostatin receptor content.

Clinical factors that have been shown to influence the behaviour of MTC are age and sex of the patients and stage and type of the disease. Older patients (≥40 years) have significantly impaired prognosis compared to younger patients (Simpson et al. 1982; Rasmusson 1984; Saad et al. 1984a; Schröder et al. 1988a). From our study we also can confirm a worse prognosis for men than for women (Rasmusson 1984; Saad et al. 1984a; Tennvall et al. 1985). Post-menopausal women continue to have a better survival rate

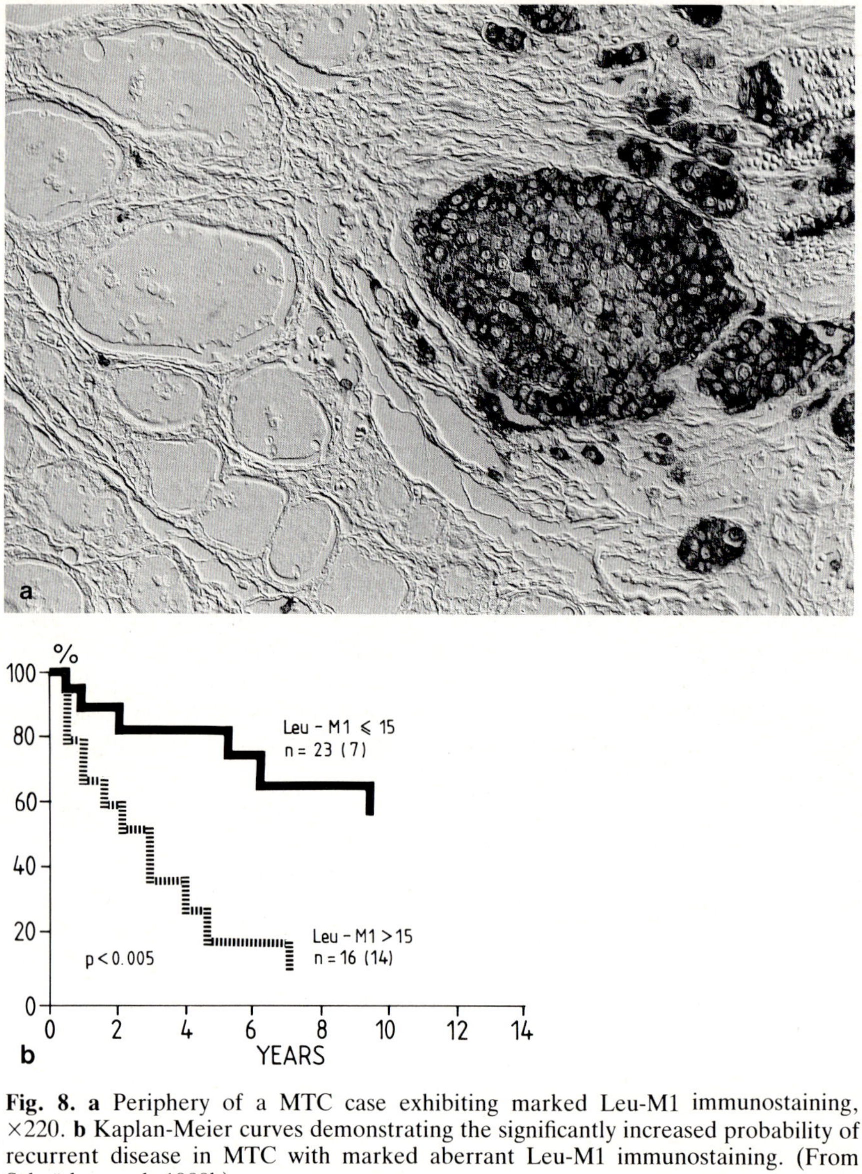

Fig. 8. a Periphery of a MTC case exhibiting marked Leu-M1 immunostaining, ×220. **b** Kaplan-Meier curves demonstrating the significantly increased probability of recurrent disease in MTC with marked aberrant Leu-M1 immunostaining. (From Schröder et al. 1988b)

than men of similar ages, indicating that sex hormones by themselves are not the causative agent (Saad et al. 1984a). The stage of the disease at presentation is of major importance. Patients having tumours extending through the thyroid capsule (pT4) show a significantly shorter survival than those with localized disease (Tennvall et al. 1985; Schröder et al. 1988a). In accordance with several other authors (Rossi et al. 1980; Holm et al. 1985; Kakudo et al. 1985; Rasmussom 1984), we found early tumour spread to cervical lymph nodes also adversely affected survival. The well-established differences in the biological behaviour of sporadic and hereditary MTC have already been described above.

Mitotic activity has been shown to be correlated with distant metastases or death from tumour in a series of hereditary MTC (Bigner et al. 1981). We refrained from counting mitoses, because estimates of mitotic activity might be significantly influenced by several factors such as variations in staining and sampling methods, thickness of the microscopic sections, and fixation time (Lee et al. 1985). Instead, we analyzed the DNA content on Feulgen-stained histological sections and on cell suspensions obtained by disaggregation of paraffin-embedded specimens. Our results (Schröder et al. 1988a) compare well with data obtained by Bäckdahl et al. (1985), Ekman et al. (1990) and El-Naggar et al. (1990). In all four studies, a benign course of disease was twice as frequent among patients with tumours of normal diploid DNA value compared to MTC of higher DNA content.

As recently described by Hay et al. (1990) and Haak et al. (1991), patients with MEN 2A syndrome have no or limited ploidy aberrations in their tumours, which correlates well with the favourable prognosis of these familial MTCs.

It should, however, be noted that the strong prognostic capacity of the nuclear DNA content found in univariate analyses may become considerably weaker when other morphological and clinical characteristics are considered (Bergholm et al. 1989).

In summary, if treatment for MTC can be differentiated in the future, the following parameters could be of value for the identification of cases with impaired prognosis which demand aggressive adjuvant therapeutic procedures: occurrence in the setting of MEN 2B, older age (≥40 years) and male sex of patients, advanced stage of disease, increased mitotic activity, aneuploid DNA content and immunoreactivity of tumours for dopa decarboxylase, histaminase and Leu-M1 antigen.

Differential Diagnosis

The majority of MTC cases are macroscopically and histologically circumscribed; however, free infiltration may also be observed microscopically in macroscopically well-demarcated neoplasms (Fig. 9). On rare occasions, encapsulated C-cell tumours occur, in which the gross encapsulation is recapitulated microscopically. Some of these lesions have been diagnosed and reported as C-cell adenomas (Beskid 1979; Kodama et al. 1988). However, as has been pointed out by Carney (1988), and as was recently reemphasized by Driman et al. (1991), it is probably best to classify such lesions as encapsulated MTC since on occasion such tumours may meta-

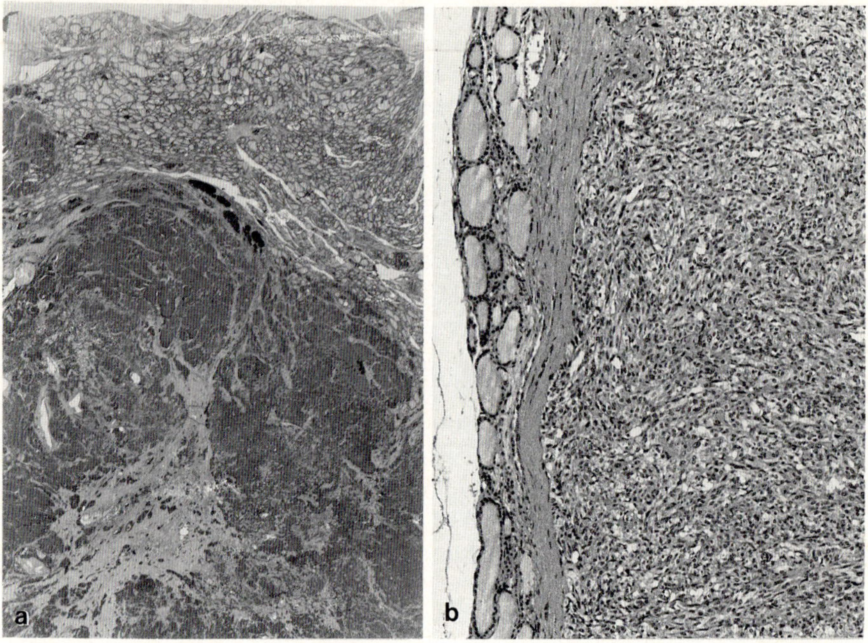

Fig. 9. a Low-power magnification of a macroscopically well demarcated yet histologically freely infiltrating MTC. CT immunocytochemistry, ×4. **b** Periphery of a macroscopically and histologically well-encapsulated C-cell neoplasm (encapsulated MTC/C-cell adenoma?). H&E, ×70

stasize, although often after many years of disease-free follow-up. The more benign course of encapsulated than of usual MTC also has been described by Mendelsohn and Oertel (1981). Some of the encapsulated MTC have fibrous stroma and contain amyloid; however, others do not (LiVolsi 1990). These lesions may be mistaken for intrathyroidal paragangliomas which immunocytochemically react for pan-neuroendocrine markers but are negative for CT and TG. A particularly useful feature is the presence of S-100 protein-positive sustentacular cells at the periphery of the zellballen (Rosai 1989), which regularly also can be detected in (parasympathetic and sympathetic) paragangliomas of other sites (Achilles et al. 1991). Differential diagnostic problems also may occur when discriminating encapsulated MTC from the recently described follicular-derived hyalinizing trabecular adenoma of the thyroid (Carney et al. 1986). Immunostaining may be critical to define this curious benign lesion, since all cases communicated so far were reported to be TG positive, although argyrophilia and reactivity for chromogranin A may also occasionally be observed with this condition (Katoh et al. 1989). As has been noted by LiVolsi (1990) it is possible that malignant variants of this tumour will be described in the future.

As far as non-encapsulated neoplasms are concerned, the above-mentioned broad spectrum of histological variants of MTC infers that C-cell carcinoma may not only resemble all other types of primary thyroid cancer, but can also mimic carcinoma metastatic to the thyroid. It is thus essential that whenever a pathologist is faced with a thyroid lesion which is atypical in appearance or when not all the criteria for a particular diagnosis are present, immunostaining for both TG and CT be performed to help arrive at a definitive diagnosis (LiVolsi 1990).

References

Achilles E, Padberg BC, Holl K, Klöppel G, Schröder S (1991) Immunocytochemistry of paragangliomas – value of staining for S-100 protein and glial fibrillary acid protein in diagnosis and prognosis. Histopathology 18:453–458

Albores-Saavedra J, LiVolsi VA, Williams ED (1985) Medullary carcinoma. Semin Diagn Pathol 2:137–146

Albores-Saavedra J, Monforte H, Nadji M, Morales AR (1988) C-cell hyperplasia in thyroid tissue adjacent to follicular cell tumors. Hum Pathol 19:795–799

Albores-Saavedra J, de la Mora TG, de la Torre-Rendon F, Gould E (1990) Mixed medullary-papillary carcinoma of the thyroid: a previously unrecognized variant of thyroid carcinoma. Hum Pathol 21:1151–1155

Bäckdahl M, Tallroth E, Auer G, Forsslund G, Granberg PO, Lundell G, Löwhagen T (1985) Prognostic value of nuclear DNA content in medullary thyroid carcinoma. World J Surg 9:980–987

Baylin SB, Mendelsohn G, Weisburger WR, Gann DS, Eggleston JC (1979) Levels of histaminase and L-dopa decarboxylase activity in the transition from C-cell hyperplasia to familial medullary thyroid carcinoma. Cancer 44:1315–1321

Berger G, Berger N, Guillaud MH, Trouillas J, Vauzelle JL (1988) Calcitonin-like immunoreactivity of amyloid fibrils in medullary thyroid carcinomas. Virchows Arch [A] 412:543–551

Bergholm U, Adami HO, Auer G, Bergström R, Bäckdahl M, Grimelius L, Hansson G, Ljungberg O, Wilander E (1989) Histopathologic characteristics and nuclear DNA content as prognostic factors in medullary thyroid carcinoma. A nationwide study in Sweden. Cancer 64:135–142

Beskid M (1979) C cell adenoma of the thyroid gland. Oncology 36:19–22

Biddinger PW, Brennan MF, Rosen PP (1991) Symptomatic C-cell hyperplasia associated with chronic lymphocytic thyroiditis. Am J Surg Pathol 15:599–604

Bigner SH, Mendelsohn G, Wells SA, Cox EB, Baylin SB, Eggleston JE (1981) Medullary carcinoma of the thyroid in the multiple endocrine neoplasia IIA syndrome. Am J Surg Pathol 5:459–472

Burk (1901) Über einen Amyloidtumor mit Metastasen. Dissertation, University of Tübingen

Bussolati G, Monga G (1979) Medullary carcinoma of the thyroid with atypical pattern. Cancer 44:1769–1777

Capella C, Bordi C, Monga G, Buffa R, Fontana P, Bonfanti S, Bussolati G, Solcia E (1978) Multiple endocrine cell types in thyroid medullary carcinoma. Evidence for calcitonin, somatostatin, ACTH, 5HT and small granule cells. Virchows Arch [A] 377:111–128

Carney JA (1988) Commentary following Kodama T, Okamoto T, Fujimoto Y, Obara T, Ito Y, Aiba M, Hirayama A (1988) C cell adenoma of the thyroid: a rare but distinct clinical entity. Surgery 104:997–1003

Carney JA, Sizemore GW, Hayles AB (1979) C-cell disease of the thyroid gland in multiple endocrine neoplasia, type 2b. Cancer 44:2173–2183
Carney JA, Ryan J, Goellner JR (1986) Hyalinizing trabecular adenoma of the thyroid gland. Am J Surg Pathol 10:672–679
Chong GC, Beahrs OH, Sizemore GW, Woolner LH (1975) Medullary carcinoma of the thyroid gland. Cancer 35:695–704
Cunliffe WJ, Black MM, Hall R, Johnston IDA, Hudgson P, Shuster S, Gudmundsson TV, Joplin GF, Williams ED, Woodhouse NJY, Galante L, MacIntyre I (1968) A calcitonin-secreting thyroid carcinoma. Lancet ii:63–66
Deftos LJ (1983) Medullary thyroid carcinoma. Karger, Basel DeLellis RA, Balogh K (1973) Histochemical characteristics of parafollicular cells and medullary thyroid carcinoma. Am J Pathol 72:119–128
DeLellis RA, Nunnemacher G, Wolfe HJ (1977) C-cell hyperplasia. An ultrastructural analysis. Lab Invest 36:237–248
DeLellis RA, Rule AH, spiler I, Nathanson L, Tashijan AT, Wolfe HJ (1978) Calcitonin and carcinoembryonic antigen as tumor markers in medullary thyroid carcinoma. Am J Clin Pathol 70:587–594
Didolkar MS, Moore GE (1974) Hormone-dependent medullary carcinoma of the thyroid. Am J Surg 128:100–103
Dominguez-Malagon H, Delgado-Chavez R, Torres-Najera M, Gould E, Albores-Saavedra J (1989) Oxyphil and squamous variants of medullary thyroid carcinoma. Cancer 63:1183–1188
Driman D, Murray D, Kovacs K, Stefaneanu L, Higgins HP (1991) Encapsulated medullary carcinoma of the thyroid. A morphologic study including immunocytochemistry, electron microscopy, and in situ hybridization. Am J Surg Pathol 15:1089–1095
Ekman T, Bergholm U, Bäckdahl M, Adami HO, Bergström R, Grimelius L, Auer G, Swedish Medullary Thyroid Cancer Study Group (1990) Nuclear DNA content and survival in medullary thyroid carcinoma. Cancer 65:511–517
El-Naggar AK, Ordonez NG, McLemore D, Schultz P, Hickey RC, Samaan N (1990) Clinicopathologic and flow cytometric DNA study of medullary thyroid carcinoma. Surgery 108:981–985
Emmertsen K (1985) Medullary thyroid carcinoma and calcitonin. Dan Med Bull 32:1–28
Eusebi V, Damiani S, Riva C, Lloyd RV, Capella C (1990) Calcitonin free oat-cell carcinoma of the thyroid gland. Virchows Arch [A] 417:267–271
Fernandes BJ, Bedard YC, Rosen I (1982) Mucus-producing medullary cell carcinoma of the thyroid gland. Am J Clin Pathol 78:536–540
Franc B, Caillou B, Carrier AM, Dutrieux-Berger N, Floquet J, Houcke M, Justrabo E, Lange F, Pages A, Rigaud C, Schwartz A, Viennet M, Lebodic MF (1987) Immunohistochemistry in medullary thyroid carcinoma: prognosis and distinction between hereditary and sporadic tumors. Henry Ford Hosp Med J 35:139–142
Gibson WGH, Peng T, Croker BP (1982) Age-associated C-cell hyperplasia in the human thyroid. Am J Pathol 106:388–393
Grün R, Eberle F (1981) Multiple endocrine neoplasia, type II (MEN II). Ergeb Inn Med Kinderheilkel 46:151–201
Haak HR, Cornelisse CJ, Goslings BM, Fleuren GJ (1991) Nuclear DNA content of medullary thyroid carcinoma in a large family with the MEN-2A syndrome. J Endocrinol Invest 14:261–264
Hales M, Rosenau W, Okerlund MD, Galante M (1982) Carcinoma of the thyroid with a mixed medullary and follicular pattern. Morphologic, immunohistochemical and clinical laboratory study. Cancer 50:1352–1359
Harach HR, Bergholm U (1988) Medullary (C-cell) carcinoma of the thyroid with features of follicular oxyphilic cell tumours. Histopathology 13:645–656

Harach HR, Williams ED (1983) Glandular (tubular and follicular) variants of medullary carcinoma of the thyroid. Histopathology 7:83–97
Hazard JB, Hawk WA, Crile G (1959) Medullary (solid) carcinoma of the thyroid – a clinicopathologic entity. J Clin Endocrinol Metab 19:152–161
Hay ID, Ryan JJ, Grant CS, Bergstrahl EJ, van Heerden JA, Goellner JR (1990) Prognostic significance of nondiploid DNA determined by flow cytometry in sporadic and familial medullary thyroid carcinoma. Surgery 108:972–980
Hedinger C, Williams ED, Sobin LH (1988) Histological typing of thyroid tumours. Springer, Berlin Heidelberg New York (international histological classification of tumours, no. 11, 2nd edn)
Heitz PU, Steiner H (1981) Pluriglanduläre endokrine Regulationsstörungen. In: Doerr W, Seifert G (eds) Pathologie der endokrinen Organe. Springer, Berlin Heidelberg New York, pp 1137–1203 (Spezielle pathologische Anatomie, vol 14/2)
Hill CS, Ibanez ML, Samaan NA, Ahearn MJ, Clark PL (1973) Medullary (solid) carcinoma of the thyroid gland. An analysis of the M.D. Anderson Hospital experience with patients with the tumor, its special features, and its histogenesis. Medicine (Baltimore) 52:141–171
Holm R, Sobrinho-Simoes M, Nesland JM, Gould VE, Johannessen JV (1985) Medullary carcinoma of the thyroid gland; an immunocytochemical study. Ultrastruct Pathol 8:25–41
Holm R, Sobrinho-Simoes M, Nesland JM, Johannessen JV (1986) Concurrent production of calcitonin and thyroglobulin by the same neoplastic cells. Ultrastruct Pathol 10:241–248
Holm R, Sobrinho-Simoes M, Nesland JM, Sambade C, Johannessen JV (1987) Medullary thyroid carcinoma with thyroglobulin immunoreactivity. A special entity? Lab Invest 57:258–268
Holm R, Farrants GW, Nesland JM, Sobrinho-Simoes M, Jorgensen OG, Johannessen JV (1989) Ultrastructural and electron immunohistochemical features of medullary thyroid carcinoma. Virchows Arch [A] 414:375–384
Ibanez ML, Cole VW, Russell WO, Clark RL (1967) Solid carcinoma of the thyroid gland. Analysis of 53 cases. Cancer 20:706–723
Jackson CE, Talpos GB, Kambouris A, Yott JB, Tashjian AH, Block MA (1983) The clinical course after definitive operation for medullary thyroid carcinoma. Surgery 94:995–1001
Jaquet J (1906) Ein Fall von metastasierenden Amyloidtumoren (Lymphosarkoma). Virchows Arch [A] 185:251–267
Kakudo K (1990) Subclassification and prognostic factors of medullary (C cell) carcinoma of the thyroid. In: Lechago J, Kameya T (eds) Endocrine pathology update, vol 1. Field and Wood, New York, pp 85–97
Kakudo K, Miyauchi A, Ogihara T, Takai SI, Kitamura H, Kosaki G, Kumahara Y (1978) Medullary carcinoma of the thyroid. Giant cell type. Arch Pathol Lab Med 102:445–447
Kakudo K, Miyauchi A, Takai S, Katayama S, Kuma K, Kitamura H (1979) C cell carcinoma of the thyroid – papillary type. Acta Pathol Jpn 29:653–659
Kakudo K, Carney JA, Sizemore GW (1985) Medullary carcinoma of thyroid. Biologic behavior of the sporadic and familial neoplasms. Cancer 55:2818–2821
Katoh R, Jasani B, Williams ED (1989) Hyalinizing trabecular adenoma of the thyroid. A report of three cases with immunohistochemical and ultrastructural studies. Histopathology 15:211–224
Khairi MRA, Dexter RN, Burzynski NJ, Johnston CC (1975) Mucosal neuroma, pheochromocytoma and medullary thyroid carcinoma: multiple endocrine neoplasia type 3. Medicine (Baltimore) 54:89–112
Kimura N, Sasano N, Yamada R, Satoh J (1988) Immunohistochemical study of chromogranin in 100 cases of pheochromocytoma, carotid body tumour,

medullary thyroid carcinoma and carcinoid tumour. Virchows Arch [A] 413: 33–38
Kini SR, Miller M, Hamburger JI, Smith MJ (1984) Cytopathologic features of medullary carcinoma of the thyroid. Arch Pathol Lab Med 108:156–159
Kodama T, Okamoto T, Fujimoto Y, Obara T, Ito Y, Aiba M, Hirayama A (1988) C cell adenoma of the thyroid: a rare but distinct clinical entity. Surgery 104: 997–1003
Krisch K, Krisch I, Horvat G, Neuhold N, Ulrich W (1985) The value of immunohistochemistry in medullary thyroid carcinomas: a systematic study of 30 cases. Histopathology 9:1077–1089
Lamberg BA, Reissel P, Stenman S, Koivuniemi A, Ekbolm M, Mäkinen J, Franssila K (1981) concurrent medullary and papillary thyroid carcinoma in the same thyroid lobe and in siblings. Acta Med Scand 209:421–424
Landon G, Ordonez NG (1985) Clear cell variant of medullary carcinoma of the thyroid. Hum Pathol 16:844–847
Lee TK, Myers RT, Marshall RB, Bond MG, Kardon B (1985) The significance of mitotic rate: a retrospective study of 127 thyroid carcinomas. Hum Pathol 16:1042–1046
Libbey NP, Nowakowski KJ, Tucci JR (1989) C-cell hyperplasia of the thyroid in a patient with goitrous hypothyroidism and Hashimoto's thyroiditis. Am J Surg Pathol 13:71–77
Lippman SM, Mendelsohn G, Trump D, Wells SA, Baylin SB (1982) The prognostic and biological significance of celluar heterogeneity in medullary thyroid carcinoma: a study of calcitonin, L-dopa decarboxylase, and histaminase. J Clin Endocrinol Metab 54:233–240
Lips CJM, Leo JR, Berends MJH, Minder WH, Blok APR, Geerdink RA, Hackeng WHL, Roelofs JMM, Vasen HFA, Vette JK (1987) Thyroid C-cell hyperplasia and micronodules in close relatives of MEN-2A patients: pitfalls in early diagnosis and reevaluation of criteria for surgery. Henry Ford Hosp Med J 35:133–138
LiVolsi VA (1990) Surgical pathology of the thyroid. Saunders, Philadelphia (Major problems in pathology, vol 22)
Ljungberg O (1972) On medullary carcinoma of the thyroid. Acta Pathol Microbiol Scand [A] Suppl 231
Ljungberg O, Bondeson L, Bondeson AG (1984) Differentiated thyroid carcinoma, intermediate type: a new tumor entity with features of follicular and parafollicular cell carcinoma. Hum Pathol 15:218–228
Lloyd RV, Sisson JC, Marangos PJ (1983) Calcitonin, carcinoembryonic antigen and neuron-specific enolase in medullary thyroid carcinoma. An immunohistochemical study. Cancer 51:2234–2239
Marcus JN, Dise CA, LiVolsi VA (1982) Melanin production in a medullary thyroid carcinoma. Cancer 49:2518–2526
Martinelli G, Bazzocchi F, Govoni E, Santini D (1983) Anaplastic type of medullary thyroid carcinoma. An ultrastructural and immunohistochemical study. Virchows Arch [A] 400:61–67
Mendelsohn G, Oertel JE (1981) Encapsulated medullary thyroid carcinoma. Lab Invest 44:43A
Mendelsohn G, Bigner SH, Egleston JC, Baylin SB, Wells SA (1980) Anaplastic variants of medullary thyroid carcinoma. Am J Surg Pathol 4:333–341
Mendelsohn G, Wells SA, Baylin SB (1984) Relationship of tissue carcinoembryonic antigen and calcitonin to tumor virulence in medullary thyroid carcinoma. An immunohistochemical study in early, localized and virulent disseminated stages of disease. Cancer 54:657–662
Meyer JS, Hutton WE, Kenny AD (1973) Medullary carcinoma of thyroid gland. Subcellular distribution of calcitonin and relationship between granules and amyloid. Cancer 31:433–441

Miettinen M (1987) Synaptophysin and neurofilament proteins as markers for neuroendocrine tumors. Arch Pathol Lab Med 111:813–818

Milhaud G, Tubiana M, Parmentier C, Coutris G (1968) Epithelioma de la thyroide secretant de la thyrocalcitonine. C R Acad Sci [D] 266:608–610

Mills SE, Stallings RG, Austin MB (1986) Angiomatoid carcinoma of the thyroid gland. Anaplastic carcinoma with follicular and medullary features mimicking angiosarcoma. Am J Clin Pathol 86:674–678

Norman T, Johannessen JV, Gautvik KM, Olsen BR, Brennhovd IO (1976) Medullary carcinoma of the thyroid. Diagnostic problems. Cancer 38:366–377

Norton JA, Froome LC, Farrell RE, Wells SA (1979) Multiple endocrine neoplasia type IIb. The most aggressive form of medullary thyroid carcinoma. Surg Clin North Am 59:109–118

Pacini F, Basolo F, Elisei R, Fugazzola L, Cola A, Pinchera A (1991) Medullary thyroid cancer. An immunohistochemical and humoral study using six separate antigens. Am J Clin Pathol 95:300–308

Parker LN, Kollin J, Wu SY, Rypins EB, Juler GL (1985) Carcinoma of the thyroid with a mixed medullary, papillary, follicular, and undifferentiated pattern. Arch Intern Med 145:1507–1509

Pfaltz M, Hedinger CE, Mühlethaler JP (1983) Mixed medullary and follicular carcinoma of the thyroid. Virchows Arch [A] 400:53–59

Rasmusson B (1984) Clinical traits in medullary carcinoma of the thyroid. Dan Med Bull 31:159–164

Reubi JC, Chayvialle JA, Franc B, Cohen R, Calmettes C, Modigliani E (1991) Somatostatin receptors and somatostatin content in medullary thyroid carcinomas. Lab Invest 64:567–573

Rosai J (1989) Thyroid gland. In: Rosai J (ed) Ackerman's surgical pathology, vol 1, 7th edn. Mosby, St Louis, pp 391–447

Rosenberg-Bourgin M, Gardet P, de Sahb R, Schlumberger M, Caillou B, Guilloud-Bataille M, Travagli JP, Feingold N, Parmentier C (1989) Comparison of sporadic and hereditary forms of medullary thyroid carcinoma. Henry Ford Hosp Med J 37:141–143

Rossi RL, Cady B, Meissner WA, Wool MS, Sedgwixck CE, Werber J (1980) Nonfamilial medullary thyroid carcinoma. Am J Surg 139:554–560

Rougier P, Parmentier C, Laplanche A, Lefevre M, Travagli JP, Caillou B, Schlumberger M, Lacour J, Tubiana M (1983) Medullary thyroid carcinoma: prognostic factors and treatment. Int J Radiat Oncol Biol Phys 9:161–169

Ruppert JM, Eggleston JC, des Bustros A, Baylin SB (1986) Disseminated calcitonin-poor medullary thyroid carcinoma in a patient with calcitonin-rich primary tumor. Am J Surg Pathol 10:513–518

Saad MF, Ordonez NG, Rashid RK, Guido JJ, Hill CS, Hickey RC, Samaan NA (1984a) Medullary carcinoma of the thyroid. A study of the clinical features and prognostic factors in 161 patients. Medicine (Baltimore) 63:319–342

Saad MF, Ordonez NG, Guido JJ, Samaan NA (1984b) The prognostic value of calcitonin immunostaining in medullary carcinoma of the thyroid. J Clin Endocrinol Metab 59:850–856

Samaan NA, Schultz PN, Hickey RC (1989) Medullary thyroid carcinoma: prognosis of familial versus nonfamilial disease and the role of radiotherapy. Horm Metab Res Suppl 21:21–25

Schimke RN, Hartmann WH, Prout TE, Rimoin DL (1968) Syndrome of bilateral pheochromocytoma, medullary thyroid carcinoma, and multiple neuromas. N Engl J Med 279:1–7

Schröder S (1988) Pathologie und Klinik maligner Schilddrüsen-tumoren. Fischer, Stuttgart (Veröffentlichungen aus der Pathologie, vol 130)

Schröder S, Klöppel G (1987a) Carcinoembryonic antigen and nonspecific cross-reacting antigen in thyroid cancer. An immunocytochemical study using polyclonal and monoclonal antibodies. Am J Surg Pathol 11:100–108
Schröder S, Klöppel G (1987b) Thyroid antibodies (Letter). Am J Surg Pathol 11:823–824
Schröder S, Dockhorn-Dworniczak B, Kastendieck H, Böcker W, Franke WW (1986) Intermediate-filament expression in thyroid gland carcinomas. Virchows Arch [A] 409:751–766
Schröder S, Böcker W, Baisch H, Bürk CG, Arps H, Meiners I, Kastendieck H, Heitz PU, Klöppel G (1988a) Prognostic factors in medullary thyroid carcinomas: survival in relation to age, sex, stage, histology, immunocytochemistry and DNA content. Cancer 62:806–816
Schröder S, Schwarz W, Rehpenning W, Dralle H, Bay V, Böcker W (1988b) Leu-M1 immunoreactivity and prognosis in medullary carcinomas of the thyroid gland. J Cancer Res Clin Oncol 114:291–296
Schröder S, Bätge B, Padberg B, von Herbay B, Dralle H (1991) Predictive value of histology and immunocytochemistry for radioiodine uptake (RIU) of metastatic and recurrent differentiated thyroid cancer. Acta Endocrinol (Copenh) 124 Suppl 1:3
Sikri Kl, Varnell IM, Hamid QA, Wilson BS, Kameya T, Ponder BAJ, Lloyd RV, Bloom SR, Polak JM (1985) Medullary carcinoma of the thyroid. An immunocytochemical and histochemical study of 25 cases using eight separate markers. Cancer 56:2481–2491
Simpson WJ, Palmer JA, Rosen IB, Mustard RA (1982) Management of medullary carcinoma of the thyroid. Am J Surg 144:420–422
Sobrinbo-Simoes M, Nesland JM, Johannessen JV (1985) Farewell to the dual histogenesis of thyroid tumors? Ultrastruct Pathol 8:iii–iv
Sobrinho-Simoes M, Sambade C, Nesland JM, Holm R, Damjanov I (1990) Lectin histochemistry and ultrastructure of medullary carcinoma of the thyroid. Arch Pathol Lab Med 114:369–375
Steiner AL, Goodman AD, Powers SR (1968) Study of a kindred with pheochromocytoma, medullary thyroid carcinoma, hyperparathyroidism, and Cushing's disease: MEN, type II. Medicine (Baltimore) 47:371–409
Stoffel E (1910) Lokales Amyloid der Schilddrüse. Virchows Arch Pathol Anat Physiol 201:245–252
Takami H, Bessho T, Kameya T, Mimura T, Ito K, Abe O, Hosoda Y, Shikata JI (1988) Immunohistochemical study of medullary thyroid carcinoma: relationship of clinical features to prognostic factors in 36 patients. World J Surg 12:572–579
Talerman A, Lindeman J, Kievit-Tyson PA, Dröge-Droppert C (1979) Demonstration of calcitonin and carcinoembryonic antigen (CEA) in medullary carcinoma of the thyroid (MCT) by immunoperoxidase technique. Histopathology 3:503–510
Tanaka T, Yoshimi N, Kanai N, Mori H, Nagai K, Fujii A, Sakata S, Tokimitsu N (1989) Simultaneous occurrence of medullary and follicular carcinoma in the same thyroid lobe. Hum Pathol 20:83–86
Tennvall J, Björklund A, Möller T, Ranstam J, Akerman M (1985) Prognostic factors of papillary, follicular and medullary carcinomas of the thyroid gland. Retrospective multivariate analysis of 216 patients with a median follow-up of 11 years. Acta Radiol [Oncol] 24:17–24
Thompson NW (1984) Commentary following Jackson CE, Talpos GB, Block MA, Norum RA, Lloyd RV, Tashjian AH (1984) Clinical value of tumor doubling estimations in multiple endocrine neoplasia type II. Surgery 96:981–987
Tubiana M, Milhaud G, Coutris G, Lacour J, Parmentier C, Bok B (1968) Medullary carcinoma and thyrocalcitonin. Br Med J 4:87–89

Ulbright TM, Kraus FT, O'Neal LW (1981) C-cell hyperplasia developing in residual thyroid following resection of sporadic medullary carcinoma. Cancer 48: 2076–2079

Uribe M, Fenoglio-Preiser CM, Grimes M, Feind C (1985) Medullary carcinoma of the thyroid gland. Clinical, pathological and immunohistochemical features with review of the literature. Am J Surg Pathol 9:577–594

Westermark P, Johnson KH (1988) The polypeptide hormone derived amyloid forms. Acta Pathol Microbiol Immunol Scand 96:475–483

Williams ED (1965) A review of 17 cases of carcinoma of the thyroid and phaeochromocytoma. J Clin Pathol 18:288–292

Williams ED (1966) Histogenesis of medullary carcinoma of the thyroid. J Clin Pathol 19:114–118

Williams ED (1985) Medullary carcinoma of the thyroid. In: Polak JM, Bloom SR (eds) Endocrine tumours. Churchill Livingstone, Edinburgh, pp 229–240

Williams ED (1986) Immunocytochemistry in the diagnosis of thyroid disease. In: Polak JM, van Noorden S (eds) Immunocytochemistry. Modern methods and applications, 2nd edn. Wright, Bristol, pp 533–546

Williams ED, Pollock DJ (1966) Multiple mucosal neuromata with endocrine tumours. A syndrome allied to von Recklinghausen's disease. J Pathol Bacteriol 91:71–80

Williams ED, Brown CL, Doniach I (1966) Pathological and clinical findings in a series of 67 cases of medullary carcinoma of the thyroid. J Clin Pathol 19:103–113

Wilson NW, Pambakian H, Richardson TC, Stokoe MR, Makin CA, Heyderman E (1986) Epithelial markers in thyroid carcinoma: an immunoperoxidase study. Histopathology 10:815–829

Wolfe HJ, Melvin KEW, Cervi-Skinner SJ, Al Saadi AA, Juliar JF, Jackson CE, Tashjian AH (1973) C-cell hyperplasia preceding medullary thyroid carcinoma. N Engl J Med 289:437–441

Wolfe HJ, DeLellis RA, Jackson CE, Greenawald KA, Block MA, Tashjian AH (1980) Immunocytochemical distinction of hereditary from sporadic medullary thyroid carcinoma. Lab Invest 42:161–162

*Epidemiology of Medullary Thyroid Carcinoma**

F. Raue

Abteilung für Innere Medizin I – Endokrinologie und Stoffwechsel,
Universität Heidelberg, Luisenstraße 5, W-6900 Heidelberg 1, FRG

Introduction

Medullary thyroid carcinoma (MTC) was first recognized as a distinct pathological entity by Hazard et al. (1959), who, out of 600 cases of thyroid cancer, identified 21 cases of this tumor from its histopathological appearance. MTC originates from the thyroid parafollicular C-cells first suggested by Williams (1967) and secretes large amounts of calcitonin, a feature which has been used for diagnosis since 1970. MTC is a rare disease which occurs in a sporadic and a familial form; the familial variant is inherited in an autosomal dominant trait associated with other endocrine tumors (multiple endocrine neoplasia, MEN). The combination of MTC with adrenal medullary tumor and parathyroid tumor (MEN 2A) was first described in 1961 by Sipple. A second variant, MEN 2B, consists of MTC, pheochromocytoma, neural tumors, and a marfanoid habitus. The third variety of MTC is the non-MEN familial MTC, a hereditary MTC without any other endocrinopathies.

Thirty-one years after the first description of MTC, pathological and biochemical techniques allow a clear discrimination of MTC from other thyroid cancers. Family screening with the tumor marker calcitonin and genetic linkage studies have led to an increase in diagnosis of early cases (Calmettes et al. 1989; Ponder et al. 1988). These cases will represent an increasing fraction of patients with MTC. The overall incidence of MTC has increased within the last three decades due to better diagnostic criteria; the distribution of different varieties of MTC has changed to an increased number of hereditary cases.

---

* This study was supported in part by a grant from the Baden-Württembergischer Krebsverband project *Prävention durch Screening*.

Table 1. Incidence of medullary thyroid carcinoma

Author	Number of cases	Frequency of MTC among all thyroid cancers (%)	Types of MTC		Sex ratio (male : female)	Mean age at diagnosis (years)
			Sporadic (%)	Familial (%)		
Hill et al. (1973)	73	9	86	14	1:1.4	47
Chong et al. (1975)	139	8	79	21	1:1.3	51
Norman (1977)	54	3.4	70	30	1:1.6	56
Rougier et al. (1983)	75	6	91	9	1:1.1	42
Saad et al. (1984)	161	8.7	76	24	1:1.6	44
Bergholm et al. (1989)	249	4.2	75	25	1:1.4	56
Raue et al. (1990)	600		75	25	1:1.3	48

Incidence

MTC is a relatively uncommon malignancy. The estimated proportion of MTC among all malignant tumors of the thyroid varies between 3% and 9% (Chong et al. 1975; Hill et al. 1973; Norman 1977; Saad et al. 1984; Bergholm et al. 1990; Fletcher 1970; Rossi et al. 1980) (Table 1). The difference in incidence may be related to geographic factors or the variation among pathologists in their criteria for the diagnosis of MTC. Calculated from the Saarländische Cancer Register with an incidence of 2.0 per 10^5 male inhabitants and 4.8 per 10^5 female inhabitants, approximately 2300 new cases of thyroid cancer occur annually in the Federal Republic of Germany (not including the former East Germany States) the majority of which are papillary and follicular. As MTC accounts for about 4.8% of all thyroid cancer in a recently performed study of 1116 patients from the area of Essen (Reinwein et al. 1989), each year about 115 newly diagnosed patients with MTC can be expected in the Federal Republic of Germany (not including the former East Germany States).

There have been only a few investigations of the incidence rate of MTC in a defined population (Norman 1977; Bergholm et al. 1990). A population-based study of MTC in Sweden based on annual obligatory reports given by physicians and pathologists to the National Cancer Registry revealed that MTC constituted 5.2% of all reported thyroid carcinomas with an overall age-standardized incidence rate per 10^5 inhabitants of 0.21. As MTC has been recognized as a distinct clinical entity only since 1967, earlier studies have either missed or underestimated by retrospective analysis the real incidence. This might be the cause of lower incidence of MTC (0.1 per 10^5) in Norway based on notification to the Norwegian Cancer Registry during 1960–1974 (Normann 1977). Differences in the geographical distribution of MTC have been found in Norway to relate to familial cases; inbreeding might explain the aggregation of cases in special areas. Recording familial distribution and establishing screening procedure for detection of the tumor at early stage will undoubtly lead to a continual increase in diagnosis especially of familial cases.

Distribution of Sporadic and Familial Disease

The majority of cases of MTC reported in the literature are sporadic with a range of 95%–75% (Chong et al. 1975; Hill et al. 1973; Saad et al. 1984; Bergholm et al. 1990). However a family history is often inadequate in establishing familial disease and more thorough evaluation by biochemical and genetic screening often reveals the presence of familial tumor in a case originally diagnosed as sporadic (Ponder et al. 1988). During the decade after familial screening started at Mayo Clinic, the average percentage of hereditary tumors among MTC increased from 7% to 21% annually

(Sizemore 1987). Efforts made by the national MTC study groups have led to increased reporting of familial cases of MTC by up to 25% (Calmettes et al. 1989; Raue et al. 1990). Among the hereditary MTC, MEN 2A is the most frequent syndrome followed by familial MTC without other endocrinopathies – the "only MTC" syndrome. A rare minority of patients suffered from the MEN 2B syndrome.

Distribution by Sex and Age

The ratio of female-to-male involvement seems to be closer to unity than in other thyroid tumors when most large series are considered – between 1.4 to 1 (Hill et al. 1973) and 1.06 to 1 (Saad et al. 1984). Concerning the familial cases there is an equal sex distribution depending on the autosomal dominant trait with high penetrance and variable expression.

The age of all patients at diagnosis of MTC varies from 9 months to 83 years with an average in the fifth decade. The age at diagnosis of familial MTC is earlier than at diagnosis of sporadic with highest incidence in the third decade for MEN 2A and only MTC and a peak incidence for MEN 2B in the second decade. The youngest-reported patient with MTC was 9 months of age (Levin et al. 1973). The occurrence of MTC in a familial pattern and at early age emphasizes the need for early diagnosis and screening procedure for the relatives of affected patients.

Register of MTC in the Federal Republic of Germany

A national register for MTC was set up by the German MTC Study Group in 1988, mainly focussing on the hereditary forms of MTC (i.e., MEN 2A, MEN 2B and only MTC) (Raue et al. 1990). For these hereditary varieties reliable screening tests exist, and if the disease is detected by family screening in an early stage curative surgery is possible. Up to December 1990 617 patients with MTC had been reported by the 27 cooperative centers. The first cases were diagnosed in 1967; from 1983 an average of 40 cases per year were registered. A total of 262 males and 338 females corresponded to a male-to-female ratio of 1:1.29. Mean age for all patients was 48.0 years; 25% had the hereditary variety of MTC, most of them MEN 2A (15%); 6% belonged to the hereditary form without other endocrinopathies (only MTC); and 3% to the MEN 2B syndrome (Fig. 1). The mean age at diagnosis for sporadic cases was 50.1 years; the familial form was diagnosed 15 years earlier (34.0 years), the younger patients belonging to the MEN 2B syndrome (mean: 27.3 years); followed by the only MTC syndrome (mean: 32.3 years); and the MEN 2A (mean: 36.0 years) (Fig. 2). The regional distribution within the Federal Republic of Germany corresponds to the catchment area of the bigger centers (Fig. 3). Calculated from the incidence

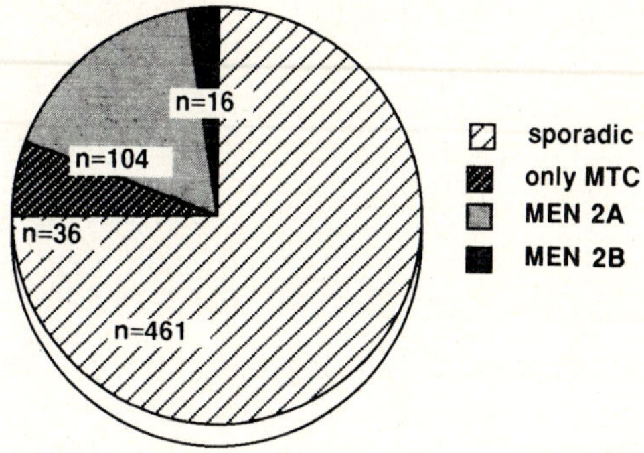

Fig. 1. Distribution of the different varieties of MTC from the German MTC Register (December 1990, 617 cases)

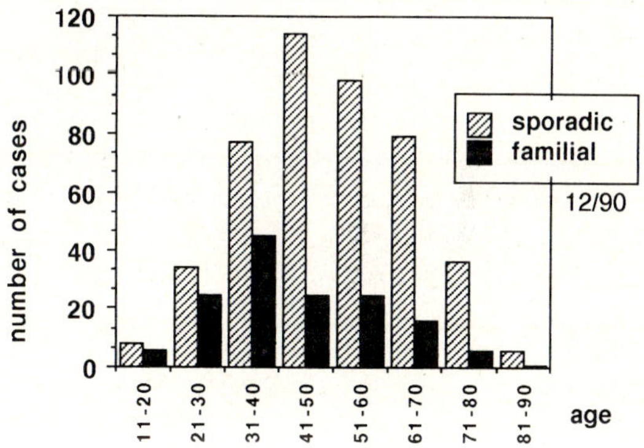

Fig. 2. Age distribution of familial and sporadic MTC from the German MTC Register (December 1990, 617 cases)

data nearly 30% of all expected cases of MTC in the Federal Republic of Germany have been registered.

Conclusion

Pathological and biochemical techniques developed within the last two decades allow a clear discrimination of MTC as a clinicopathologic entity distinct from other thyroid cancers. MTC occurs in sporadic and familial forms. The overall incidence of MTC cases has increased within the last 30 years – especially familial cases due to systematic screening procedures. Nowadays MTC accounts for approximately 8% of all thyroid cancers with an incidence rate of 0.21 (per 10^5 inhabitants). In contrast to other types of thyroid disease, MTC occurs almost equally in both sexes, patients of all ages can be affected by MTC, and patients with familial forms can be detected by screening at a younger age than those with sporadic MTC. The availability of accurate biochemical and genetic markers for MEN 2 has increased the percentage of hereditary tumor among MTC to 25% and introduced the possibility of providing preclinical diagnosis of MTC.

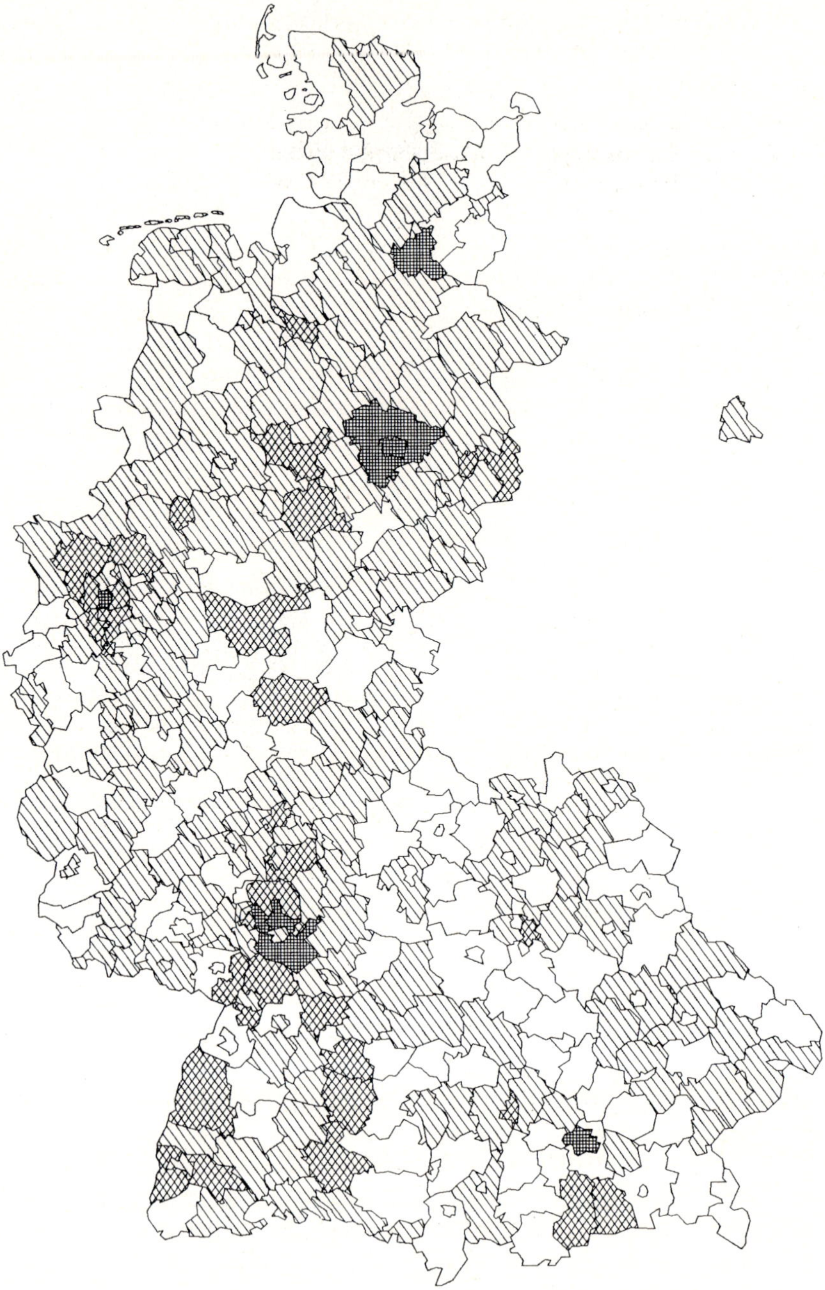

Fig. 3. Distribution of 617 patients with MTC in the Federal Republic of Germany (not including the former East German States)

Acknowledgements. The author wishes to express his gratitude to the members of the German Medullary Thyroid Carcinoma Study Group who collected the information about patients with MTC which has been the basis for the epidemiologic data (Figs. 1–3): V. Bay, Hamburg; W. Becker, Erlangen; H. Buhr, Heidelberg; R. Dorn, Munich; H. Dralle, Hanover; A. Frilling, Düsseldorf; H.G. Heinze, Karlsruhe; E. Heissen, Mülheim; J. Herrmann, Bielefeld; R. Höfer, Vienna; I. Hörnig, Münster; F. Kallinowski, Heidelberg; F.S. Keck, Ulm; I. Klempa, Bremen; J. Kotzerke, Hanover; H.-J. Langer, Homburg; H. Neumann, Freiburg; A. Passath, Graz; P. Pfannenstiel, Wiesbaden/Mainz Kastel; D. Reinwein, Essen; M. Ritter, Munich; H. Röher, Düsseldorf; O. Schober, Münster; S. Schröder, Hamburg; F. Seif, Tübingen; M. Späth-Röger, Mannheim; H. Stracke, Gießen; M. Trede, Mannheim; H. Vogt, Augsburg; R. Wahl, Frankfurt; K.F. Weinges, Homburg; J. Winter, Mannheim; S. Zabransky, Homburg; R. Ziegler, Heidelberg.

References

Bergholm U, Adami HO, Bergström R, Johansson H, Lundell G, Telenius-Berg M, Akerström G (1989) Clinical characteristics in sporadic and familial medullary thyroid carcinoma, a nationwide study of 249 patients in Sweden from 1959 through 1981. Cancer 63:1196–1204

Bergholm U, Adami HO, Telenius-Berg M, Johansson H, Wilander E (1990) Incidence of sporadic and familial medullary thyroid carcinoma in Sweden 1959 through 1981. Acta Oncol 29:9–15

Calmettes C, Chaventre A, Feingold N, Franc B, Guliana JM (1989) Screening for medullary thyroid cancer in France: a national effort. Henry Ford Hosp Med J 37:120–121

Chong GC, Beahrs OH, Sizemore GW, Woolner LH (1975) Medullary carcinoma of the thyroid gland. Cancer 35:695–704

Fletcher JR (1970) Medullary (solid) carcinoma of the thyroid gland. Arch Surg 100:257–262

Hazard JB, Hawk WA, Crile G (1959) Medullary (solid) carcinoma of the thyroid: a clinicopathologic entity. J Clin Endocrinol 19:152–161

Hill CS, Ibanez ML, Samaan NA, Ahearn MJ, Clark RL (1973) Medullary (solid) carcinoma of the thyroid gland. An analysis of the M.D. Anderson Hospital experience with patients with the tumor, its special feature, and its histogenesis. Medicine (Baltimore) 52:141–171

Levin DL, Perlia C, Tashjian AH (1973) Medullary carcinoma of the thyroid gland: the complete syndrome in a child. Pediatrics 52:192–196

Normann T (1977) Medullary thyroid carcinoma in Norway. Epidemiological and genetic data. Acta Pathol Microbiol Scand [A] 85:775–786

Ponder BAJ, Finer N, Coffey R, Harmer CL, Maisey M, Ormerod MG, Pembrey ME, Ponder MA, Rossick P, Shalet S (1988) Family screening in medullary thyroid carcinoma presenting without a family history. Oncol J Med 67:299–308

Raue F, Späth-Röger M, Winter J, Benker G, Buhr P, Dorn R, Dralle H, Frilling A, Herrmann J, Hörnig I, Meybier H, Klempa I, Kotzerke J, Pfannenstiel P, Reinwein D, Ritter M, Röher HD, Schober O, Schröder S, Seif F, Trede M, Vogt H, Wahl R, Ziegler R (1990). Register für das medulläre Schilddrüsencarcinom in der Bundesrepublik Deutschland. Med Klin 85:113–117

Reinwein D, Benker G, Windeck R, Eigler FW, Leder LD, Mlynek ML, Creutzig H, Reiners C (1989) Erstsymptome bei Schilddrüsenmalignomen: Einfluß von Alter und Geschlecht in einem Jodmangelgebiet, Erfahrungen an 1116 Patienten. Dtsch Med Wochenschr 114:775–782

Rossi RL, Cady B, Meissner WA, Wool MS, Sedgwick CE, Werber J (1980) Nonfamilial medullary thyroid carcinoma. Am J Surg 139:554–560

Rougier P, Parmentier C, Laplanche A, Lefevre M, Travagli JP, Caillou B, Schlumberger M, Lacour J, Tubiana M (1983) Medullary thyroid carcinoma: prognostic factors and treatment. Int J Radiol Oncol Biol Phys 9:161–169

Saad MF, Ordonez NG, Rashid RK, Guido JJ, Hill CS, Hickey RC, Samaan NA (1984) Medullary carcinoma of the thyroid, a study of the clinical feature and prognostic factors in 161 patients. Medicine (Baltimore) 63:319–342

Sipple JH (1961) The association of pheochromocytoma with carcinoma of the thyroid gland. Am J Med 31:163–166

Sizemore GW (1987) Medullary carcinoma of the thyroid gland. Semin Oncol 14:306–314

Williams ED (1967) Medullary carcinoma of the thyroid gland. J Clin Pathol 20:395–398

Clinical and Diagnostic Aspects of Medullary Thyroid Carcinoma

Tumor Markers for the Medullary Thyroid Carcinoma

A. Grauer and E. Blind

Abteilung für Innere Medizin I – Endokrinologie und Stoffwechsel,
Universität Heidelberg, Luisenstraße 5, W-6900 Heidelberg 1, FRG

Introduction

The medullary thyroid carcinoma (MTC) is a malignancy of the C-cell, which originates from the neural crest. In avian or teleost species, the C-cells form a separate organ, the ultimobranchial body. In mammals, however, the C-cells migrate into the thyroid during embryonic life. Within the thyroid the C-cells are located adjacent to but outside the thyroid follicle (parafollicular cells). Their neuroendocrine origin implies several features which differentiate them from follicular epithelium. These features include an uptake mechanism for biogenic amines and the production of several small polypeptide hormones, including products of the calcitonin gene like calcitonin (CT), calcitonin gene-related peptide (CGRP) and others (Bussolati and Pearse 1967; Pearse 1968). Despite their proximity there is little information as to whether hormonal or cellular interactions between the follicular epithelium and the C-cell exist.

The value of the various secretory products of the C-cell as tumor markers for the medullary thyroid carcinoma will be discussed in this chapter.

CT Gene Products

The CT gene was cloned in 1981 (Jacobs et al. 1981) It is a six-exon gene and has been subsequently shown to contain the genetic information for a whole family of peptide hormones (Fig. 1). In addition to the coding information for CT on exon 4, the CT gene, located on the short arm of chromosome 11, contains the genomic information for a peptide called CGRP on exons 5 and 6 (Rosenfeld et al. 1983), which is processed by alternative splicing. Several years later, a second CT gene was identified. This CT (II) gene, localized on the same chromosome (Hoppener et al. 1985; Steenbergh et al. 1985), codes only for CGRP (II); the region encoding a CT-like structure seems not to be expressed (Steenbergh et al. 1986).

Recent Results in Cancer Research, Vol. 125

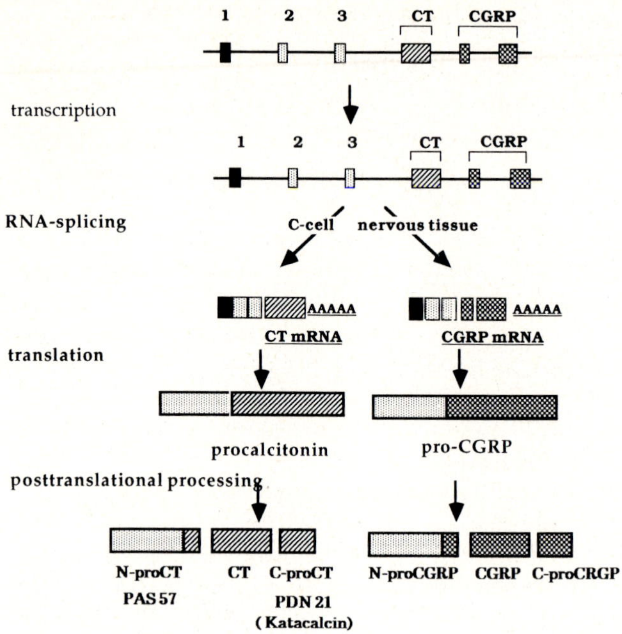

Fig. 1. Calcitonin (*CT*) gene expression. The six-exon CT gene has three common exons (1–3), an exon 4, encoding for CT and PDN 21, and two calcitonin gene-related peptide (*CGRP*)-specific exons. The maturation of the primary RNA transcript is a tissue-specific phenomenon with a predominant CT-specific splice (including oxons 1–4) in the C-cells of the thyroid, and a predominant CGRP-specific splice (exons 1–3,5 and 6) in neural tissue. The resulting precursor peptides are subjected to further cleaving into the secretory peptides in a posttranslational process. The different *shadings* indicate the exonic source of the amino acid sequences

The process of alternative splicing appears to be tissue specific (Fig. 1). The thyroid C-cell will splice the primary transcript of the CT gene to produce predominantly CT messenger ribonucleic acid (mRNA), whereas neural tissue will splice the identical primary RNA transcript to CGRP. The mechanism of the phenomenon of tissue-specific splicing of the CT gene is not fully understood. It is interesting, however, that for the rat CT/CGRP gene the *cis*-acting enhancer elements on the 5′-flanking region appear to be identical in neural and C-cell tissue. In the rat model, the tissue specificity is therefore likely to be induced by *trans*-acting factors. (Stolarsky-Fredman et al. 1990). In a human C-cell carcinoma cell line, however, an enhancer element was identified in the 5′-flanking region, whose deletion was accompanied by a loss of 70%–80% of the enhancing activity in C-cells, but did not affect transcription in a glioma cell line (Peleg et al. 1990). In normal C-cells the CT/CGRP alternative splicing ratio will be 99:1, whereas malignant C-cells reveal a different splicing behavior and may produce predominantly CT or CGRP or most commonly both (Raue et al. 1987d). In the TT cell line, which represents a well-studied in-vitro model of neoplastic C-cells a CT/CGRP ratio of 50:50 is found (Cote et al. 1987; Raue et al. 1987d). An alternative splice of the CT/CGRP gene towards CT requires sequences within exon 4, which codes for CT (Cote et al. 1990); in a human C-cell carcinoma cell line (TT) a splice into this direction is favored by dexamethasone (Cote and Gagel 1986).

Both primary mRNA transcripts – CTmRNA and CGRPmRNA – are translated into pre-prohormones. After proteolytic cleavage each prohormone will give rise to three distinct peptides. In the case of a CT splice, the mature RNA of exons 3 and 4 will be translated into pre-proCT, which consists of 141 amino acids, and cleaved to proCT (116 amino acids), containing PAS 57 or N-proCT (aminoterminal site) (Burns et al. 1989a), CT (central region) and PDN-21 or C-proCT (carboxyterminal site) (Raue et al. 1987a; Conlon et al. 1988a) (Fig. 1). PDN-21 was originally termed katacalcin because of a suspected calcium-lowering activity (MacIntyre et al. 1982), which could not be confirmed in later studies (MacIntyre et al. 1984).

In the case of a CGRP-directed splice of the primary transcript of CT gene exons 3,5, and 6, proteolytic cleavage of the primary translation product will lead to N-proCGRP, proCGRP and C-proCGRP. As the carboxy-terminal region of the common exon 3 is translated into N-proCT and N-proCGRP, both peptides reveal an identical aminoterminal amino acid sequence (Fig. 1).

Calcitonin

CT is the primary secretory product of the C-cell. It is a peptide hormone of 32 amino acids. Its existence was first postulated by Copp et al. (1962) as a calcium-lowering hormone. The discovery of the ultimobranchial origin of CT in fish led to the determination of the amino acid composition and structure of salmon CT. For the characterization of human CT, the hormone had to be extracted from an MTC (Neher 1968). The CT of various species are 32-amino acid peptides with molecular weights around 3500. They share several well-conserved features including a disulfide bridge between the cysteine residues in positions 1 and 7, forming a ring structure at the N terminal end carrying a free amino group, and a proline amide group at the C terminal.

Measurement of CT

Bioassay

The first CT measurements relied on the hypocalcemic effect produced by injection of CT into young rats. The fall in serum calcium was in a linear relation to the logarithm of the dose of CT (Cooper et al. 1967; Kumar et al. 1965). Adaptations of this rat in vivo bioassay were able to improve the sensitivity of these assays to yield a detection limit as low as 200–300 pg (60–90 fmol) of human CT. This sensitivity is still too low to allow detection of CT in human serum, unless the CT levels are grossly elevated by MTC. Recent developments introducing a new in vitro bioassay utilizing the CT-mediated cyclic adenosine monophosphate (cAMP) generation of a human breast cancer cell line (T 47 D) have improved the practicability and precision of the bioassays, without lowering the detection limit to a point where it could be of diagnostic value (Grauer et al. 1992). Other bioassays, although revealing a very high sensitivity, like the single-cell osteoclast bioassay are too arduous to perform on a routine basis and are limited to research use (Chambers et al. 1985; Chambers and Moore 1983). These ultrasensitive bioassays monitor the motility and resorptive activity of single osteoclasts and detect bioactive CT in concentrations as low as $10^{-15} M$. They offer the possibility to determine bioactive instead of immunoreactive CT. Recent reports further support the concept that the immunoreactive CT (iCT) measured in patients with MTC by classical radioimmunoassay (RIA) does not necessarily reflect its biological activity, which was found ten to 100-fold lower in osteoclast bioassays (Zaidi et al. 1990).

Immunoassays

Radioimmunoassay

The determination of iCT by means of an RIA (Clark et al. 1969) was a major step forward in the measurement of CT in terms of sensitivity, ease, and precision (Raue et al. 1987b). The detection of elevated iCT levels in manifest MCT is possible with all commercially available CT immunoassays. Several problems, however, impairing the diagnostic use of the CT RIA have prompted the search for alternatives.

Detection Limit. As the concentration of iCT in human serum appears to be very low, it has so far been impossible to define a lower limit of the normal range for the serum CT concentration. In many normal subjects, it is still impossible to detect iCT; important physiological changes can therefore be missed below the detection limits of the RIAs. This is also of concern in early cases of familial MTC, where circulating basal levels of iCT may not be raised above normal (Grauer et al. 1990; Raue et al. 1990).

Immunoheterogeneity of Circulating CT. The upper limit of the normal range varies from 10 to 300 ng/l (Heath and Sizemore 1982) and there are several explanations why the normal levels for CT reveal such a variability in different assays (Austin and Heath 1981). Impurities of the human CT (hCT) standard might have caused some problems in the past (Raue et al. 1982) as well as a variation of regional specificity for the CT molecule of different antisera (Ziegler and Raue 1984). The most important problem, however is undoubtedly the immunoheterogeneity of circulating CT (Body and Heath 1983). Although the antisera used in conventional RIA are raised against monomeric CT (mCT), they nonetheless detect other forms of iCT with higher molecular weights, including CT precursors, polymeric CT, and chemically altered CT (Snider et al. 1977). Different elution profiles of iCT were not only found in different patients with MTC, but also in normal subjects and in patients bearing other neuroendocrine tumors (Baylin et al. 1981; Dermody et al. 1981). Approaches to overcome these limitations including affinity chromatography and immunoextraction require extensive procedures for sample preparation and are therefore primarily limited to research purposes (Body and Heath 1984).

Two international quality surveys prove the fact that absolute CT values, obtained through different assays cannot be compared directly (Raue 1982). The interpretation of RIA results has to be based on normal values, validated for the individual assay applied.

Two-Site Immunometric Assays

Two-site immunoradiometric assays (IRMA) might represent a major step forward in the determination of serum CT levels. These techniques use two antibody preparations with specific immunoreactivity directed towards distinct regions of the peptide, preferably widely separated. They are often constructed as sandwich assays with one antibody preparation immobilized on a solid phase like polystyrene beads or multiwell plates. The second antibody can be theoretically labeled with radioactive ^{125}I as well as chemiluminometric or enzyme amplification markers.

In theory these two-site assays should offer several advantages: First, sensitivity could be improved, since every molecule of CT in the sample should be detected. Second, specificity should be enhanced, as the full complement of the mCT structure would be required for binding. If, however, large circulating heterogeneous forms of CT include the entire 32 amino acid sequence of mCT, they too might be detected (Carter and Heath 1990).

The results obtained with the two-site CT assays published so far reveal that this new technique is promising, but can not solve all methodological problems of iCT determination. The lower limit of detection in these assays ranges from 10 pg/ml in an overnight IRMA (Motté et al. 1988) to 2.5 pg/ml employing basically the same assay under different incubation conditions (24-h incubation at 56°C instead of overnight incubation at room temperature) (Perdrisot et al. 1990). With a different detection method, using an alkaline phosphatase conjugate coupled to one of the two monoclonal antibodies used, this enzyme immunometric assay (EIA) managed to detect iCT in concentrations as low as 6 pg/ml (overnight incubation at room temperature) (Seth et al. 1988). Although the sensitivity of the EIA is therefore somewhat lower than in the comparable IRMA, the higher stability of the detecting enzyme-antibody complex (more than 1 year) and the abdication of radioactivity represents an advantage of the EIA over the IRMA in terms of ease of performance.

The results obtained with two-site assays are somewhat disappointing, as the sensitivity of these two-site assays is therefore only marginally higher than in conventional RIAs and still does not allow the detection of a lower normal limit. Physiological studies investigating the impact of a lowered endogenous CT production are still unable to be performed in unextracted plasma.

A distinct advantage of these assays is, however, their specificity for mature CT. As the monoclonal antibody CT07 used in the assays mentioned above recognizes the 26–32 amino acid region of the hCT molecule and requires the presence of an amidated proline residue, proCT and other cleavage products are unlikely to be detected. This higher specificity for mature CT probably explains why the levels for iCT detected with the two-site assays are generally considerably lower than the CT values determined by RIA. The increased specificity improves the signal-to-noise ratio of these assays, which is far better than in conventional RIAs (Motté et al. 1988; Perdrisot et al. 1990). Higher specificity contributes probably more than higher sensitivity to the increased likelihood of detecting early MTC or C-cell hyperplasia with the new two-site assays (Motté et al. 1988; Perdrisot et al. 1990).

Another new interesting perspective has been brought to light by the two-site assays. A recent report describes an assay based on two monoclonal antibodies against the 1–11 region of PDN-21 and against the 11–17 region of CT. The assay therefore crossreacted only with precursors possessing both epitopes, but not PDN-21 or CT alone (Ghillani et al. 1988). The proCT levels were found to be correlated with the mature hCT levels in patients with MTC, but were frequently found to be elevated in patients with other neuroendocrine tumors (60%) or hepatocellular carcinomas (62%) in the presence of normal levels for mature CT.

Provocative Testing

As stated above, basal plasma iCT levels in patients with C-cell hyperplasia, or early MTC are often normal. Fortunately, the abnormal C-cell will increase CT secretion after an appropriate stimulus. Provocative testing is therefore crucial for early diagnosis of hereditary forms of MTC and recurrence after surgery of manifest MTC. As calcium is the major physiological stimulus of CT secretion of the C-cell, it was the obvious secretagogue to use in the first reports (Tashjian et al. 1970). In the following years the pentagastrin test was introduced as a provocative test for CT in the diagnosis and follow-up of MTC (Hennessy et al. 1973). For physicians taking care of patients with MTC, these two secretagogues are still the most important stimulatory agents, although there have been a number of reports about additional stimuli of CT secretion, including glucagon, cholecystokinin-pancreozymin, secretin, and ethanol (Cohen et al. 1973). None of them could prevail, because they were either as unreliable as the famous whisky test or even more unpleasant than the already uncomfortable pentagastrin test. (Telenius-Berg et al. 1977; Ziegler et al. 1985). In recent years, thyrotropin-releasing hormone (TRH) was suggested as another alternative provocative agent, after CT monolayer cultures in vitro responded to TRH in concentrations of 10^{-5}–10^{-6} M with an increase of CT secretion. In two patients with MTC, reported in the same paper, 500 µg TRH i.v. resulted in a similar stimulation of CT secretion (Nakamura et al. 1987b). A comparative study of a combined calcium-pentagastrin (C-Pg) test with the TRH test revealed, however, that the stimulation of CT secretion evoked by TRH was considerably lower than with the C-Pg test and was only present in patients with clearly elevated basal CT levels. TRH was not able to stimulate CT secretion in a first-degree relative of a patient with MTC with normal basal CT levels but a positive C-Pg test (O'Connell et al. 1990). These data lead to the conclusion that the experience with the TRH test as a provocative test for CT secretion are very limited and that the data so far available in the literature should discourage its use.

Over the years three standard stimulation tests have found wide acceptance:

1. *Pentagastrin Test*: 0.5 µg pentagastrin/kg body weight, via rapid i.v. injection with blood sampling at 0,2, and 5 min; sampling at 10,20,30 min has to be considered optional.
2. *Calcium Infusion*: 3 mg calcium^{2+}/kg body weight in 50 ml isotonic saline over 10 min i.v. with blood sampling at the end of the infusion (t = 10 min), at 20 and 30 min.
3. *Combination Calcium-Pentagstrin Test (C-Pg)*: Various reports in the literature use different protocols; one feasible method is the i.v. injection of 2 mg/kg body weight calcium over 1 min, followed by a rapid pentagastrin injection (0.5 µg/kg body weight) with blood sampling at t = 2,5,10,20, and 30 min (O'Connell et al. 1990).

The provocative tests are not dangerous but very often unpleasant. A clear description of the side effects to be expected should be provided before a pentagastrin injection. The patient has to be aware of the onset of severe abdominal discomfort and nausea, generally without vomiting, approximately 20 s after the injection. The discomfort will last for about 30–60 s; after 5 min the patients usually feel fine again. During the calcium infusion, the side effects are generally milder, including nausea and perioral or digital paresthesias.

Whether or not calcium, pentagastrin, or C-Pg testing should be applied in routine use has always raised controversy. Data suggest that a short calcium stimulus (5 min) may be a better stimulus in normal subjects than pentagastrin, whereas the latter appears to be the superior secretagogue in MTC patients (Gharib et al. 1987). Early reports claim higher increases of CT secretion and therefore a higher diagnostic sensitivity in the combination C-Pg test (Wells et al. 1978) An elaborate study, designed to evaluate the diagnostic specificity of those three standard tests revealed that basically all of the three test forms were able to provoke a supranormal increase of CT secretion. The problem in this study was, however, a considerable overlap between pathological responses of each of the three tests in patients with normal basal CT values and C-cell hyperplasia, and normal subjects with an exaggerated CT stimulation without apparent C-cell disease (McLean et al. 1984). There is evidence that either extraction of the serum prior to the analysis (Body and Heath 1984; Gharib et al. 1987) or the new two-site immunometric assays will eliminate a considerable portion of the overlap between normal subjects and patients with early MTC or C-cell hyperplasia, as these reports find a clear discrimination between those groups when performing a standard pentagastrin test (Guilloteau et al. 1990).

CT Secretion in Normal Subjects and Patients Without Malignant Tumors

Measurement of CT levels in normal subjects or patients with diseases unrelated to the human C-cell is problematic as stated above, because circulating CT levels in physiologic conditions are low, and even with advanced CT immunoassays often undetectable (Fig. 2a).

Newborns and premature babies have significantly higher CT levels, which followed over 6 years were shown to decrease constantly (Klein et al. 1984). This decrease continues until adult age is reached (Samaan et al. 1975). This issue requires special attention, as it should influence the interpretation of high CT levels in children of multiple endocrine neoplasià (MEN) 2 kindreds.

Age-dependent normal ranges for sensitive CT assays are therefore required to establish new sensitive CT assays. Among adults, age does not have an important influence on circulating CT levels (Tiegs et al. 1986; Body and Heath 1983).

Men have, on average, higher basal and stimulated CT levels than women (Heath and Sizemore 1977; Body and Health 1983; McLean et al. 1984; Gharib et al. 1987; Seth et al. 1988), which is apparently due to a decreased production rate rather than an increase in metabolic clearance rate (Tiegs et al. 1986). This finding prompted research into whether the differences in CT levels between men and women might be due to sex hormones, and could be related to the development of post-menopausal

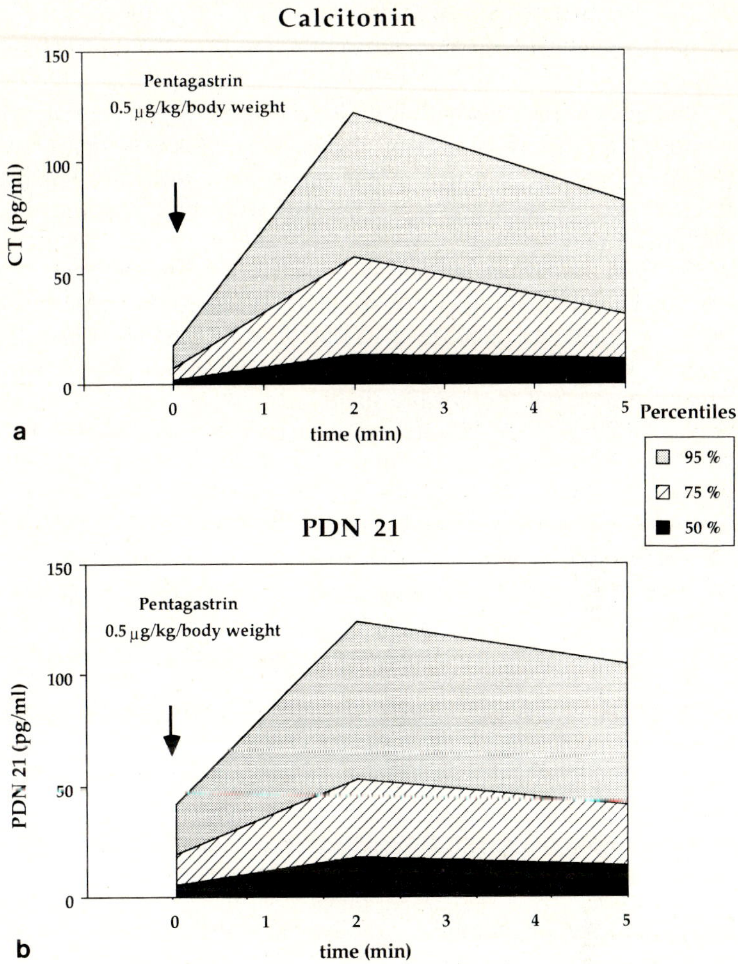

Fig. 2 a,b. Plasma levels of calcitonin and PDN-21 in normal subjects as measured by a two-site assay for hCT (**a** Zink, unpublished observation) and by RIA for PDN-21 (**b** Blind et al. 1992a). Values before and after stimulation with pentagastrin (0.5 µg/kg body weight i.v.) in 30 and 27 healthy persons, respectively. The *black area* represents the median plasma level after 0,2 and 5 min; the other areas indicate the 75th and 95th percentiles. Concentrations of PDN-21 below 10 ng/l (detection limit) were also used for the calculations

osteoporosis (PMO). This hypothesis was nourished by findings that women in early menopause had a diminished CT reserve after calcium stimulation (Perez Cano et al. 1989; Stevenson et al. 1982) and that elevations of midday CT secretion after application of either oral or percutaneous estrogens were found (Stevenson et al. 1981). A recent study finds a striking impairment of the CT production rate in postmenopausal women compared to healthy controls matched for age and estrone levels, concluding a possible role of CT production rate in the development of PMO, which is not likely to be associated with endogenous estrogen (E2) levels (Reginster et al. 1989).

The question as to whether endogenous CT plays a significant role in the pathogenesis of PMO is very controversial. CT levels measured in immuno-extracted plasma of postmenopausal women were not significantly lower than in age-matched controls This was true for basal levels under fasting conditions (Prince et al. 1989), after stimulation with calcium (Tiegs et al. 1985), and under maintenance of stabile ionized calcium levels by the calcium clamp technique (Sjoberg et al. 1989). Measurements of extractable mCT revealed no increase of basal or stimulated CT in postmenopausal women during a 4-week treatment cycle with either E2, E2 and calcium, or calcium alone, but there was a slight decrease in the E2-treated group (Body et al. 1989b). These results are in accordance with other recent studies, where neither oral contraceptives in young women, nor E2 therapy in postmenopausal women enhanced basal or stimulated CT secretion. On the contrary, the E2-treated group revealed a decrease in basal and stimulated extractable CT levels, parallel to a documented fall in serum calcium (Hurley et al. 1989). The magnitude of CT reserve in patients with PMO failed also to predict the rate of bone loss in a placebo-controlled study with women taking synthetic estrogens (Leggate et al. 1984).

In summary, it seems to be proven that women have lower CT levels than men; the data collected suggest, however, that E2 plays no major role in CT secretion, which is also consistent with recent in-vitro data (Lazaretti-Castro et al. 1991). E2 deficiency, although being a major contributing factor for PMO has no major influence on CT metabolism.

Racial differences in CT secretion have been suggested with British white women having lower CT levels than black women in Gambia (Stevenson et al. 1984).

Patients with renal failure may have moderately elevated basal iCT levels (up to five times higher than the upper normal limit), as demonstrated with two-site IRMAs (Guilloteau et al. 1990; Motté et al. 1988).

Expression of CT Gene Products Outside the Thyroid Gland

For a specific diagnostic tumor marker, rather than a screening parameter or a marker valuable in the follow-up of a tumor patient, it would be desirable that the secretion of the marker was limited to a single tumor. As regards CT, this specificity for the thyroidal C-cell is very high; certain normal cell types outside the thyroid gland, however, can also generate the peptide. Isolated cells within the pituitary (Catherwood and Deftos 1980; Gagel et al. 1983), adrenal, and prostate gland; thymus; and the Kulchitsky cells of the lung (Linnoila et al. 1984) produce CT in their normal state.

The presence of iCT in larger molecular forms in milk of thyroidectomized women also suggests an extrathyroidal production site, maybe the mammary gland itself (Bucht et al. 1986). Other cell types, predominantly of neuroendocrine origin gain the capacity to express the CT gene after neoplastic transformation. The small cell carcinoma of the lung is the most prominent example in a group of tumors, including breast cancer, hepatoma, pheochromocytoma, vipoma, and others (Becker et al. 1982; Heath and Edis 1979). In most cases, the secretory product of these cells appears to be a proCT (Conlon et al. 1988a), rather than fully processed CT, which can be identified by two-site immunoassays specific for a proCT spanning the CT and PND-21 part of the prohormone (Ghillani et al. 1988). Provocative testing can be used to differentiate between hypercalcitoninemia from C-cell and non-C-cell origin, as in many of these cell types CT release appears not to be regulated by the same factors as in the MTC. Calcium or pentagastrin stimulation may therefore not further stimulate elevated CT levels, other than those of C-cell origin (Samaan et al. 1980).

Calcitonin Gene-Related Peptide

The strange name "calcitonin gene-related peptide" has historical rather than functional origins. The existence of CGRP was predicted from the analysis of the nucleotide sequence of the CT gene as an alternative splicing product, predominantly present in neural tissues. There are two distinct forms of human CGRP, termed CGRP I and II, or α and β, both 37 amino acids long, produced by two different genes, and both located on chromosome 11. CGRP exerts a variety of biological functions, primarily as a neurotransmitter in the central and peripheral nervous system (O'Halloran and Bloom 1991). It may also regulate the number of acetylcholine receptors at the neuromuscular junction (New and Mudge 1986). Outside the nervous system, the peptide plays an important part in the control of regional blood flow. It is the most powerful vasodilator yet identified, probably exerting its biological function at the arterioles (Brain et al. 1985). So far it is unclear, however, what promotes its release from the perivascular neural network. There is a reported interaction of CGRP with the CT receptor, whereby CGRP reveals a lower affinity to the CT receptor and exerts a biological response several orders of magnitude lower than that of CT. (Goltzman and Mitchell 1985; Raue et al. 1987c). It is likely that mild anti-bone-resorbing (D'Souza et al. 1986) and calcium-lowering actions (Roos et al. 1986) of CGRP are caused by interaction with the CT receptor.

CGRP was isolated from human MTC tissue; the amino acid sequence was subsequently determined by mass spectrometry and it matched the sequence predicted from the nucleotide analysis of the CT gene. First measurements of iCGRP in normals revealed no age or sex dependency, with plasma levels ranging from 9.7 to 71 pM (mean 25 ± 1.2). They are about fivefold higher than CT levels, but not correlated to the CT levels (Girgis et al. 1985). This has been confirmed by other groups using different assays (Kim et al. 1989; Schifter 1991). The data about CGRP in the serum of patients with MTC differ considerably. Early studies reported elevated plasma levels in patients with MTC (Morris et al. 1984). In recent years some studies have revealed a high number of MTC patients with elevated CGRP levels (Mason et al. 1986; Schifter et al. 1986; Takami et al. 1990b); others do not (Schifter 1989b; Kim et al. 1989; Born et al. 1991). The response of CGRP to standard provocative tests for CT secretion like calcium or pentagastrin is also the subject of controversy. One study reports an increase of CGRP secretion with provocative testing in all six patients studied (Mason et al. 1986); another study finds an increase of CGRP release only in two of five patients with MTC after calcium, and in three of five after tetragastrin stimulation (Kim et al. 1989). In normal subjects, calcium stimulation was not able to significantly enhance CGRP secretion (Born et al. 1991). Elevated CGRP levels have been eported in some other endocrine tumors, including parathyroid adenoma, insulinoma and carcinoid (Takami et al. 1990). Controversial findings concerning the presence of CGRP in pheochromocytomas have been reported. One study showed three patients with pheochromocytoma with normal CGRP levels. In another study in situ hybridization was performed and revealed no evidence of CGRP (Zajac et al. 1986), whereas in a third investigation evidence of CGRP mRNA in such a tumor was found (Hoppener et al. 1986). In several small cell lung cancer cell lines CGRP could be demonstrated (Nelkin et al. 1984); this could not be confirmed for several primary tumors (Zajac et al. 1986).

In MTC tumors, CGRP is detectable by immunocytochemistry and in situ hybridization in most cases (Schifter et al. 1986; Boultwood et al. 1990; Noel et al. 1990) and the question has often been raised whether a relative increase in CGRP over CT expression is a marker for dedifferentiation and poor prognosis (Lippman et al. 1982). Recent data find a distinct elevation of CGRP mRNA in neoplastic over normal C-cells via in-situ hybridization and a concomitant decrease in CT expression. In addition a decrease in the ratio of CT peptide to mRNA suggesting a defective posttranscriptional processing has been reported (Boultwood et al. 1990). A new methodological approach using polymerase chain reaction (PCR) amplification of the CGRP II gene revealed that CGRP I was easily detectable in normal and neoplastic C-cells, whereas CGRP II was present in neoplastic C-cells, but only barely detectable in normal thyroid tissue (Lasmoles et al. 1990). The question as to whether the CT/CGRP ratio of expression is a reliable marker of tumor differentiation certainly needs more detailed studies on all levels of regulation before it can be definitively answered. At present, CGRP certainly plays no major role as a *serum* tumor marker in diagnosis and follow-up of MTC.

PDN-21 (Katacalcin)

Another peptide derived from the CT precursor peptide is a 21-amino acid C-terminal flanking peptide, PDN-21 (Fig. 1) (Fischer and Born 1985; Hillyard et al. 1983; MacIntyre et al. 1982; Raue et al. 1987a). The name PDN-21 was derived from its chemical structure and indicates the first and last amino acids (P = peptide, D = amino acid 1, N = amino acid 21) (Tatemoto and Mutt 1980). It is also known as katacalcin, suggesting an initially assumed calcium-lowering function of the peptide (MacIntyre et al. 1982), although this has not been confirmed subsequently (MacIntyre et al. 1984). In fact, there is at present no known biological function of the peptide.

Numerous studies have shown the presence of PDN-21 in thyroid and metastatic MTC tissue (Ali-Rachedi et al. 1983; Conlon 1989; Conlon et al. 1988c; Raue et al. 1987; Sikri et al. 1985) (see also Schröder et al., this volume). PDN-21 is cosecreted equimolarly with CT in health and disease and both peptides reach comparable levels in plasma (Hurley et al. 1988; Ittner et al. 1985; Takami et al. 1990a; Tobler et al. 1984; Woloszczuk et al. 1986). Theoretically, PDN-21 should be a tumor marker for MTC equal to CT, which is regarded as the classic marker and "gold standard." Probably for historical reasons, PDN-21 is, however, far less often used in diagnosing MTC than CT.

Measurement of PDN-21 and CT in a large number of patients with MTC, either sporadic or familial, showed an excellent comparability of both parameters (Ittner et al. 1985; Takami et al. 1990). In 65 patients with MTC, PDN-21 levels were highly correlated with CT levels as determined by RIA ($r = 0.99$); the mean ratio of CT/PDN-21, on a molar base, was 0.96 ± 0.33 over the entire range (Blind et al. 1992a). The close correlation of plasma levels of both peptides is also maintained at different tumor stages as shown in long-term follow-up studies of MTC patients (Fig. 3). The diagnostic value of PDN-21 determination is equal to that of CT and PDN-21 determination can be used instead of a CT RIA without any limitations. In the case of borderline results obtained with CT assays, the additional determination of PDN-21 may help to clarify the diagnostic problem.

In a recent study, i.v. pentagastrin as a secretagogue of thyroid C-cells gave a significant increase of PDN-21 levels in plasma in 12 out of 27 healthy persons tested. (Blind et al. 1992a) (Fig. 2b). This is usually not the case for CT levels measured with conventional RIAs. It has therefore been suggested that PDN-21 is measured as a supplement of CT measurements in stimulation tests for screening for MTC (Schifter 1989a).

PDN-21 has also been suggested as a tumor marker for lung cancer (Body et al. 1989a), since both CT and PDN-21 can be secreted ectopically by lung cancer cells. PDN-21 in plasma was more often increased (44%) than CT (only in 19%). High levels of PDN-21, however, were found only in patients with concomitantly elevated CT plasma levels.

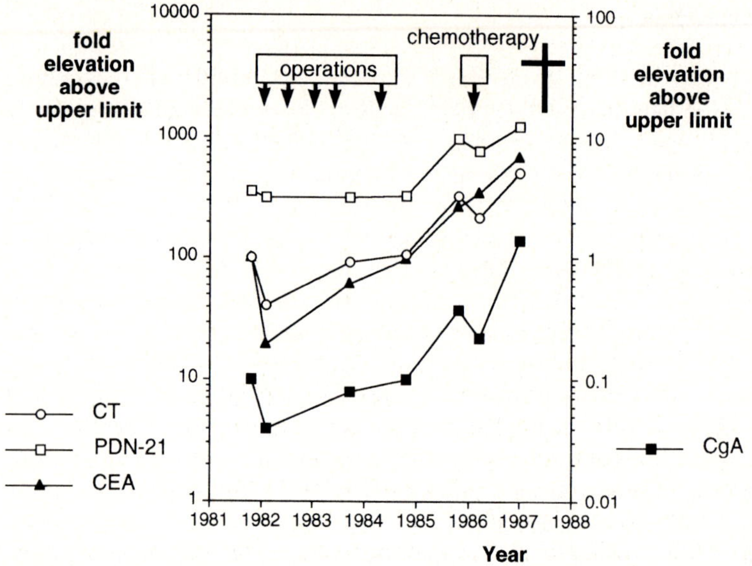

Fig. 3. Plasma concentrations of calcitonin (*CT*), PDN-21, carcinoembryonic antigen (*CEA*), and chromogranin A (*CgA*) in a patient with sporadic MTC suffering from progressive disease during a follow-up period of 7 years. CT, PDN-21, and CEA were highly abnormal whereas CgA remained initially within the normal range. The subsequent relapse was accompanied by a further increase in CT, PDN-21, and CEA levels and CgA levels became elevated. Values on the y axis are represented as elevation above the upper limit of normal of the assays (200 ng/l for CT, 40 ng/l for PDN-21, 2.5 μg/l for CEA, and 50 μg/l for CgA. (From Blind et al. 1992a,b)

In a recent evaluation of a commercially available PDN-21 kit, Takami et al. found in only 4 out of 15 normal persons detectable amounts of PDN-21 (Takami et al. 1990a). In contrast, PDN-21 was measureable in 74 of 80 normal subjects with the very sensitive RIA of Ittner et al. (1985), and in 73% with the RIA of Blind et al. (1992a). PDN-21 could be determined in all normal subjects by extracting plasma samples with columns prior to measurement in an RIA (Hurley et al. 1988; Woloszczuk et al. 1986); this was, however, a laborious procedure and required a sample volume of 10 ml (Hurley et al. 1988). The relative ease of measuring PDN-21 directly in normal subjects (compared with CT) has already been described by Ittner et al. (1985) and may be related to the problem of different circulating forms of CT in plasma. Little is known about circulating forms of PDN-21 in plasma. In extracts from MTC tissue, PDN-21-like material was predominantly the "intact" peptide and only minor quantities of PDN-21 fragments(1–20), (1–19), (1–15), and (1–13) were found (Conlon et al. 1988c). To its disadvantage, PDN-21, containing only 21 amino acid residues, is a small peptide and more might be difficult to detect by sensitive and specific two-site assays than CT.

In addition to hCT assays, the determination of PDN-21 serves as an important tool in diagnosis and follow-up of patients with MTC. As a second independent assay, it can help to clarify borderline cases. Specific advantages in sensitivity, however, that were present compared to the conventional hCT assays are not longer of importance after the introduction of the new two-site assays for hCT.

N-Procalcitonin (PAS 57 or N-CAP)

According to the amino acid sequence derived from the proCT mRNA, two other peptides beside CT have been predicted, PAS 57 (57 amino acids) on the N-terminal site of the prohormone and PDN-21 (katacalcin, 21 amino acids) on the C-terminal site. The identification and isolation of PAS 57 from MTC tissue has confirmed the amino acid sequence predicted from the DNA structure (Conlon et al. 1988; Burns et al. 1989) The functional properties of this substance are not completely understood. There have been reports that PAS 57 may act as a growth factor with a mitogenic activity in normal and neoplastic human osteoblasts (Burns et al. 1989b), although recent data could not confirm these findings for normal human osteoblast-like cells (Hassager et al. 1991). The first evidence about the diagnostic relevance of PAS 57 has recently become available (Born et al. 1991). After immunoextraction PAS 57 is measurable in normal human subjects; levels are higher in men than in women, they increase significantly after calcium infusion, and are markedly elevated in the serum of patients with MTC. In normal subjects PAS 57 levels have been found to be, on a molar basis 10.7-fold higher in men and 7.4-fold higher in women than CT levels; in MTC patients this ratio was even higher with 21 times higher in male and 26 times higher in female patients. As for PDN-21, the other flanking peptide, equimolar serum levels have been reported. The reasons for this obvious difference between PAS 57 and CT are not quite clear; they might involve secretion and/or metabolism of the peptides (Born et al. 1991). Considering the fact that PAS 57 levels are markedly higher than CT levels, PAS 57 might have the potential to become a valuable additional tumor marker in the diagnosis and follow-up of MTC.

Other Secretory Products

MTC tissue releases several biologically active substances into the circulation, and many of them are hormones since thyroid C-cells are of neuroendocrine origin. The search for new tumor markers for this disease has led to the evaluation of several of these substances. The classical plasma marker peptides released by MTC are peptide products from the CT gene. CT is the prototype of these peptides and its usefulness as a plasma marker of MTC is

Table 1. Substances produced or released by MTC

Peptides from the calcitonin gene	
	Calcitonin (CT)
	PDN-21 (katacalcin, C-terminal flanking peptide)
	PAS-57 (N-terminal flanking peptide)
	Calcitonin gene-related peptide (CGRP)
Neuroendocrine markers	
	Chromogranin A (CgA)
	Neuron-specific enolase (NSE)
	Synaptophysin
	7B2
	HISL-19
Peptide hormones and releasing factors	
	Somatostatin (SRIF)
	Gastrin-releasing peptide (GRP)
	Adrenocorticotropic hormone (ACTH)
	Parathyroid hormone-related protein (PTHrP)
Others	
	Carcinoembryonic antigen (CEA)
	Histaminase
	L-dopa decarboxylase
	Helodermin
	Prostaglandins
	Tissue polypeptide antigen (TPA)

unique, since it is not only sensitive but also highly specific, which is rarely the case with any other tumor marker. In general, other bioactive secretory products have revealed interesting insights into some biological features of MTC (explaining some signs and symptoms, etc.), but were not able to add any information, exceeding that gained by CT, as far as the genesis of the tumor (sporadic or familial), the time of outbreak in familial disease (as screening test), the relapse of MTC, and the prognosis are concerned.

Many substances produced by MTC have been demonstrated immunohistochemically in MTC tissue (see Schröder et al., this volume). Several of them are summarized in Table 1. Only some of these substances appear in plasma in measurable circulating levels, allowing an evaluation of their clinical usefulness as plasma tumor markers. Some substances of possible relevance will be discussed subsequently.

Carcinoembryonic Antigen

Since the recognition of carcinoembryon antigen (CEA) as a marker of MTC 15 years ago (Ishikawa and Hamada 1976), many investigations have evaluated the usefulness of CEA immunohistochemistry in MTC tissue

(Krisch et al. 1985; Lloyd et al. 1983; Mendelsohn et al. 1984; Schröder et al. 1988; Schröder and Kloppel 1987) or, additionally, CEA determinations in plasma from MTC patients (Busnardo et al. 1984; Miyauchi et al. 1986; Pacini et al. 1991; Palmer et al. 1984; Raue et al. 1983; Rougier et al. 1983; Saad et al. 1984; Samaan and Hickey 1987; Samaan et al. 1989a).

An immunohistochemical study in 200 primary thyroid carcinomas showed that monoclonal antibodies against CEA-specific epitopes stained exclusively MTCs (in 77%) but not other thyroid tumors (Schröder and Kloppel 1987). Since CEA plasma levels are elevated in many conditions, elevated plasma CEA lacks, however, specificity to diagnose MTC, and plasma levels of CEA and CT are only loosely correlated.

A remaining role for plasma CEA determinations in MTC might be, therefore, its possible prognostic usefulness. It has been suggested that plasma CEA might be a better prognostic marker than CT (Saad et al. 1984; Samaan and Hickey 1987), since it discriminated better between patients with and without metastasis, and highest CEA values were found in patients with bone metastasis (Samaan et al. 1989a). Immunohistochemical positivity or negativity for CEA, however, is of no prognostic value (Schröder et al. 1988). Additionally, in some patients with progressive disease, an increase of CEA levels in the absence of a parallel increase of CT levels was sometimes observed (Busnardo et al. 1984), suggesting that in advanced disease CEA may be sometimes a more useful marker of poor prognosis.

CEA is, however, often less sensitive than CT in many patients, because (a) postoperative CT levels often remain persistently above normal limits due to the persistence of small tissue quantities, whereas CEA levels become completely normal, and (b) during follow-up, doubling times of CEA levels are longer in most patients than doubling times of CT levels (Miyauchi et al. 1986).

CEA measurements are not useful in stimulation tests and selective venous catheterizations: In vitro and in vivo, CEA release from MTC tissue cannot be stimulated measurably by pentagastrin or calcium (Oosterom et al. 1987; Raue et al. 1985). In selective venous catheterization, the value of CEA determination was found to be inferior to that of CT (Raue et al. 1983).

Chromogranin A

Chromogranin A (CgA) is a 431-amino acid protein and was originally described as the major soluble protein in catecholamine storage vesicles, where it is costored and coreleased with catecholamines (Smith and Winkler 1967; Smith and Kirshner 1967). A proposed physiological function of the peptide is its involvement in intracellular packaging and processing of peptide hormones and neuropeptides (Huttner et al. 1991). CgA is found in many neuroendocrine tissues, and circulating levels in plasma can be elevated in patients with endocrine hormone-producing tumors, such as pheochromocytoma, parathyroid adenoma, insulinoma, and intestinal carcinoid (O'Connor et al. 1983; O'Connor and Deftos 1986; Simon and Aunis 1989). Consequently, CgA is considered to be a useful additional parameter in evaluating such tumors (Hsiao et al. 1990b; O'Connor and Deftos 1987).

CgA has been detected in both normal and neoplastic C-cells of the thyroid (O'Connor et al. 1983; Simon and Aunis 1989). In MTC, plasma levels of CgA and CT are moderately correlated ($r = 0.87$) (Blind et al. 1992b), but CgA becomes elevated in most patients only in advanced disease: 13 patients with MTC studied by O'Connor and Deftos (1986) all had elevated basal CgA levels in plasma with a mean elevation of fivefold above the upper limit of normal and a mean CT value of 13.2 µg/l indicating advanced disease. In another study (Blind et al. 1991b) only 14 out of 61 patients had elevated CgA levels, but patients with CT > 10 µg/l also had elevated CgA in 83% of cases. Patients with advanced stages of the disease (indicated by high plasma levels of CT) had much higher CgA levels than patients with localized disease. This suggests that CgA levels in plasma correspond to tumor burden, but fail to detect early cases of MTC, despite the fact that CgA can be regularly detected imunohistochemically: In metastatic tissue from eight patients with MTC, CgA and CT were detectable immunohistologically in all cases, but plasma CgA was elevated only in two and CT in seven of them (Blind et al. 1992b).

MTC tissue is probably the major source of circulating CgA (Blind et al. 1992b) if patients have the sporadic form of the disease (thus excluding the adrenal medulla as a source), and renal or hepatic dysfunction can also be ruled out as another cause of elevated plasma CgA (O'Connor et al. 1989). In MEN, however, CgA plasma levels should be interpreted with caution, since CgA may be released from two different sources, i.e., adrenal medulla or thyroid C-cells in these patients.

CgA immunoreactivity in plasma was found to have an apparent initial half-life of approximately 18 min (O'Connor and Bernstein 1984). In their two-compartment model derived from studies during removal of pheochromocytomas, Hsiao et al. suggested two different half-lives: an initial rapid half-life of 16 min followed by a longer half-life of 520 min, which might correspond to a large extravascular CgA pool (Hsiao et al. 1990a).

In contrast to measurement of CT, which is extremely helpful in stimulation tests or venous localization studies, measuring CgA is not useful in this setting: Pentagastrin (as a secretagogue of thyroid C-cells) does not measurably stimulate the release of CgA from C-cells in MTC patients, at least in cases with only moderately elevated CT (Fig. 4) (Blind et al. 1992b). The release of small quantities of CgA from C-cells might, however, not be detectable, because all changes of CgA levels in plasma have to be detected against the high circulating plasma pool of CgA, with concentrations 2–3

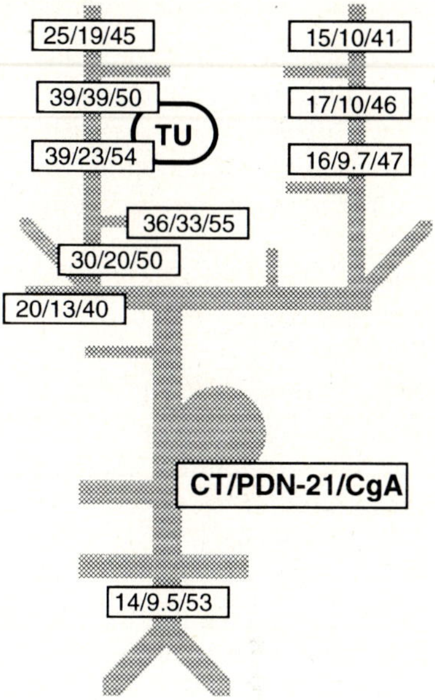

Fig. 4. Concentrations of calcitonin (*CT*) PDN-21, and chromoganin A, (*CgA*) in samples obtained by selective venous catheterization of a patient with multiple endocrine neoplasia (MEN), type 2A. The three values in each box are concentrations (in µg/l) of CT (*left*) PDN-21 (*middle*) and CgA (*right*). The highest concentrations of CT were found in the upper part of the right jugular vein. An MTC was confirmed surgically in the right thyroid lobe (indicated by *TU*). Peak (sample of the right jugular vein, C4) to peripheral (inferior vena cava) ratios were 4.1-fold for PDN-21 and 2.8-fold for CT, whereas no venous gradient of CgA was detected. The average molar ratio for CT/PDN-21 in the samples obtained was 1.04. (From Blind et al. 1992a,b)

orders of magnitude higher than CT plasma levels (O'Connor and Deftos 1986). The same is true for detecting venous gradients of CgA for localization studies in patients with MTC; a similar situation occurs with adrenal medullary venous sampling (Takiyyuddin et al. 1990).

Neuron-Specific Enolase

Neuron-specific enolase (NSE) is a dimeric enzyme widely distributed in central and peripheral neuronal tissue and "neuroendocrine" tissue, such as pheochromocytoma, pulmonary small cell carcinoma, pancreatic islet cell tumor, carcinoid tumors, and MTC (Seshi et al. 1988). NSE can be demonstrated immunohistochemically in normal and neoplastic thyroid C-cells (Lloyd et al. 1983). It is found in 75%–100% of thyroid MTC tissue (Grauer et al. 1987; Pacini et al. 1991b; Schröder et al. 1988). Results with NSE as a plasma tumor marker are discrepant: Elevated levels in MTC patients were found in none of 6 or 7 patients (Oishi and Sato 1988; Touitou and Heshmati 1988), in 5 of 35 (Grauer et al. 1987), 7 of 15 (Pacini et al. 1991b), and in up to 20 of 25 patients (Pacini et al. 1986). In the latter study by Pacini et al., only 3 of 13 patients with no evidence of disease (but elevated CT in 10 of them) had elevated levels, compared to 9 of 12 patients with metastasis. Raised plasma NSE seems, therefore, to indicate a large tumor mass and metastatic disease (Pacini et al. 1986, 1991b). Apart from different patient characteristics, different results with NSE immunoassay are probably caused by different specificities of antibodies used, since it has been shown that monoclonal antibodies against distinct epitopes of NSE give differing staining patterns in a spectrum of neuroendocrine tissues (Seshi et al. 1988). As with many other additional MTC markers, NSE is not useful in stimulation tests or localization studies by selective venous catheterization (Grauer et al. 1987).

Somatostatin

Somatostatin (SRIF) is a tetradecapeptide, which was originally isolated from the hypothalamus. SRIF is released from primary MTC cell culture or cell lines of rat or human origin (Aron et al. 1986; Gagel et al. 1986; Nakamura et al. 1987a). In immunohistochemical studies, SRIF can be found in primary MTC in 30%–65% of cases (Deftos et al. 1980; Ekblom et al. 1987; Franc et al. 1987; Henninger et al. 1988; Holm et al. 1985; Modigliani et al. 1990a; Pacini et al. 1989, 1991b; Sikri et al. 1985). Positivity is, however, usually restricted to a few scattered cells, and metastatic tissue is SRIF positive less frequently than primary tumors are. The presence of SRIF in MTC tissue may be of biological relevance, since MTC cells possess high-affinity SRIF receptors (Reubi et al. 1990), and SRIF is able to inhibit hormone release of various endocrine tissues originating from the APUD system. In patients with MTC, i.v. SRIF is able to inhibit CT release from tumor tissue and has improved symptoms in some studies (Gordin et al. 1978; Libroia et al. 1989; Mahler et al. 1990; Pacini et al. 1989; Samaan et al. 1989b), though not in others (Geelhoed et al. 1986) – through mechanisms not yet known exactly. It might, therefore, be a regulatory peptide with negative control on C-cells. Plasma levels of SRIF in MTC patients have been found to be elevated in various degrees: Elevated levels were found in up to 50% of patients (Pacini et al. 1991b), or in as few as 2 of 55 patients (Neradilova et al. 1989). One study reports that a low frequency of elevated plasma SRIF of 20% was found, despite the fact that SRIF was detectable in the tumor itself in high concentrations in 71% of patients (Modigliani et al. 1990a). The authors speculated that this might be either caused by intermittent SRIF release together with a short plasma half-life or by low plasma levels resulting from nonsecretion of the peptide. Quantitated tumoral SRIF is usually not related to tumor size or epidemiologic type (Modigliani et al. 1990a). The most useful but still controversial aspect might be that, as stated in one report (Pacini et al. 1991b), SRIF positive immunostaining is linked to a longer survival rate; a limitation of this report was, however, the fact that the groups studied were not identical in the frequency of the presence of distant metastasis.

Gastrin-Releasing Peptide

Gastrin-releasing peptide (GRP) is another peptide of the APUD system and the mammalian homologue of the amphibian peptide bombesin. It has been demonstrated regularly in MTC tissue (Conlon et al. 1988b; Matsubayashi et al. 1984; Modigliani et al. 1990b; Yamaguchi et al. 1984), both as intact peptide and as the C-terminal fragment (18–27), also called neuromedin C. Concentrations of GRP in MTC tissue were found to be correlated to SRIF, but were elevated (94%) more regularly than SRIF (70%) (Modigliani et al. 1990b). Reports about circulating levels of GRP are rare; out of 5 patients GRP was elevated in 3 and could be stimulated in 1 of 2 (Yamaguchi et al. 1984). Currently, GRP has no role as a plasma tumor marker in MTC. It is hypothesized that GRP might play a role as a growth factor in both normal and neoplastic tissue (Sunday et al. 1988), but, like SRIF, its biological function in MTC remains to be established.

Adrenocorticotropic Hormone

In rare cases of MTC, adrenocorticotropic hormone (ACTH) is produced ectopically and results in Cushing's syndrome (Belsky et al. 1985; Blunt et al. 1989; Jex et al. 1985; Lind and Weitzman 1985; Tourniaire et al. 1988). Elevated plasma levels of ACTH (Raue et al. 1983) or its immunohistological presence in MTC tissue seems to be more frequent in patients with MTC, but seldom lead to Cushing's syndrome. ACTH seems, therefore, to be released either infrequently by MTC or in a biologically largely inactive form (Goltzman et al. 1979). Apart from secretion of ACTH by the tumor, Cushing's syndrome can occasionally be caused by pituitary ACTH hypersecretion due to other substances released by MTC tissue, as in the case of a bombesin-like substance (Howlett et al. 1985). Clinically, in most tumors ectopic ACTH production usually happens during rapidly progressing disease, and the course is dominated by the tumor itself. By contrast, ACTH production in MTC may be accompanied by long survival and, although rare, signs, symptoms, and complications of Cushing's syndrome may become clinically even more relevant than the MTC disease itself.

Other Neuroendocrine Markers of MTC

7B2 is a recently isolated pituitary protein of about 190 amino acids. It is often expressed in the same neuroendocrine tissues as chromogranin, with some exceptions including the parathyroid glands, where it is not found. Elevated plasma levels were demonstrated in three patients with MTC (Natori et al. 1988; Ohashi et al. 1990), whereas it was immunohistochemically localized in only 3 out of 17 MTCs (Marcinkiewicz et al. 1988). The usefulness of this secretory peptide will have to be investigated further.

The antigen recognized by monoclonal antibody *HISL-19* raised against a human islet cell preparation is another marker for neuroendocrine tissue and usually stains positive in MTC (Deftos et al. 1988).

Synaptophysin is a membrane glycoprotein and also a marker of neuroendocrine tissue (Wiedenmann et al. 1987). It is usually found immunohistochemically in MTC (Buffa et al. 1987; Miettinen 1987).

Other Factors

Out of the large number of substances produced by MTC (see Schröder et al., this volume), a few with possible relevance for the future will be mentioned: *Histaminase* is an enzyme which is able to deaminate histamine. Histaminase content is elevated in primary and metastatic tissue (Baylin et al. 1970, 1972a,b) and elevated plasma levels can be found in half of the patients with MTC – with higher levels in metastatic disease. Its sensitivity and specificity is, however, inferior to that of CT, and it does not correlate well with reduced tissue quantity after surgery (Baylin 1974). Another enzyme, *L-dopa decarboxylase* has demonstrated high activity in the TT cell line, a human MTC cell line (Berger et al. 1984). *Prostaglandins* are released by MTC tissue, and may (Hill et al. 1973) or may not Rambaud et al. 1988) have a pathogenetic role in diarrhea associated with MTC.

Helodermin is a vasoactive investiral polypeptide (VIP)/secretin-like 35-amino acid peptide originally isolated from the venom of the lizard Gila monster. Normal C-cells and seven out of eight MTC have been found to contain helodermin-like immunoreactive material (Sundler et al. 1988; Tsutsumi et al. 1990). *Parathyroid hormone-related protein* is a recently discovered factor probably causative in many instances for the syndrome of humoral hypercalcemia of malignancy. This protein is expressed in and released from the human TT cell line (Deftos et al. 1989; Ikeda et al. 1989). Whether it is detectable in plasma in MTC patients is not yet known.

Thymosin-β4 (Conlon et al. 1988a), tissue polypeptide antigen (TPA) (Martino et al. 1984; Pacini et al. 1985; Raue et al. 1983), γ-trace (Lofberg et al. 1983), and melanin are other products detectable in MTC tissue (Beerman et al. 1990; Eng and Chen 1989; Kimura et al. 1989).

Summary: Clinical Relevance of Different Tumor Markers for the MTC

Early Diagnosis. The "golden standard" as a tumor marker for MTC is still represented by hCT. hCT is valuable in early diagnosis of MTC and in the family screening of potentially affected members of MEN 2 families (Table 2). Especially after pentagastrin stimulation, the determination of hCT is a powerful tool to detect early MTC or even C-cell hyperplasia. The new two-site assays for hCT have even improved this situation, leading to a slightly

Table 2. Clinical relevance of different tumor markers for MTC

Marker	Purpose		
	Screening	Follow-up	Immunohisto-chemistry
CT	+++	++	+++
KC (PDN-21)	+++	++	+++
CgA	–	+	++
NSE	–	+	++
CEA	–	+++	+

CT, calcitonin; KC, katacalcin; CgA, chromogranin A; NSE, neuron-specific enolase; CEA, carcinoembryonic antigen.

higher sensitivity and markedly higher specificity of hCT assays. PDN-21, the C-terminal cleavage product of proCT is cosecreted with hCT in an equimolar fashion. The peptide may be too small to develop a two-site assay for PDN-21, but as the existing assays are very sensitive, PDN-21 serves as an additional tool in the screening for MTC, and is practically as valuable as hCT. We use the determination of PDN-21 in borderline cases to strengthen a suspected diagnosis by a second, independent assay system. All other tumor markers evaluated so far for the MTC do not match the diagnostic sensitivity and specificity of the two above-mentioned tumor markers in human plasma (Table 2).

Follow-up. hCT and PDN-21 are also very valuable in the follow-up of MTC. Their plasma levels reflect the tumor burden very well over a wide extent of the disease. In extensive disease, however, hCT levels sometimes fail to rise further, despite obviously progressive disease. In these cases, CEA determination may give additional information; there are also reports that CEA can discriminate better between patients with or without metastases (Table 2).

Immunohistochemistry. A variety of neuroendocrine and other markers can be detected in MTC tissue by immunohistochemistry. CT and PDN-21 again are very reliable, but are not as specific as immunohistochemical markers as they are as markers in the plasma. NSE, CgA, and CEA are other valuable markers – among others – that facilitate the diagnosis of MTC (Table 2).

Pending Problems. To date, there is no way to predict the development of MTC in potentially affected members of MEN 2 families. Currently, all of these family members have to undergo regular screening investigations, including pentagastrin tests. It is also impossible to directly identify the nature of the disease in a patient diagnosed to have MTC without any information about familial disease. In this case the presence of familial MTC can not be ruled out. First-degree relatives will have to undergo screening procedures, which could be spared if familial or sporadic MTC could be positively identified. So far there is no tumor marker available which could solve these problems; the validation of a genetic probe, predicting the gene carrier status with a sufficient degree of certainly would be a major step in this direction.

Another open question is the prognosis of an individual patient suffering from MTC. Although in extended disease CEA offers some advantages over hCT in monitoring the progress of the disease, there is, at an early stage of MTC, to date no tumor marker capable of predicting the further course of the disease.

An improved knowledge concerning the properties of C-cell differentiation might add further insight to this question and consequently influence management strategies in the case of recurrent disease.

References

Ali-Rachedi A, Varndell IM, Facer P, Hillyard CJ, Craig RK, MacIntyre I, Polak JM (1983) Immunocytochemical localisation of katacalcin, a calcium-lowering hormone cleaved from the human calcitonin precursor. J Clin Endocrinol Metab 57:680–682

Aron DC, Mendelsohn G, Roos BA (1986) Elaboration of nonsomatostatin peptides containing the amino-terminal portion of prosomatostatin in a somatostatin-secreting human medullary thyroid carcinoma cell line. J Clin Endocrinol Metab 62:1237–1242

Austin LA, Heath HI (1981) Calcitonin. Physiology and pathophysiology. N Engl J Med 304:269–278

Baylin SB (1974) Medullary carcinoma of the thyroid gland. Use of biochemical parameters in detection and surgical management of the tumor. Surg Clin North Am 54:309–323

Baylin SB, Beaven MA, Engelman K, Sjoerdsma A (1970) Elevated histaminase activity in medullary carcinoma of the thyroid gland. N Engl J Med 283:1239–1244

Baylin SB, Beaven MA, Buja LM, Keiser HR (1972a) Histaminase activity: a biochemical marker for medullary carcinoma of the thyroid. Am J Med 53:723–733

Baylin SB, Beaven MA, Keiser HR, Tashjian AH, Melvin KEW (1972b) Serum histaminase and calcitonin levels in medullary carcinoma of the thyroid. Lancet 1:455–458

Baylin SB, Wieman KC, O'Neil JA, Roos BA (1981) Multiple forms of human tumor calcitonin demonstrated by denaturing polyacrylamide gel electrophoresis and lectin affinity chromatography. J Clin Endocrinol Metab 53:489–497

Becker KL, Silva OL, Snider RH et al. (1982) The surgical implications of hypercalcitoninemia. Surg Gynecol Obstet 154:897–908

Beerman H, Rigaud C, Bogomoletz WV, Hollander H, Veldhuizen RW (1990) Melanin production in black medullary thyroid carcinoma (MTC). Histopathology 16:227–233

Belsky JL, Cuello B, Swanson LW, Simmons DM, Jarrett RM, Braza F (1985) Cushing's syndrome due to ectopic production of corticotropin-releasing factor. J Clin Endocrinol Metab 60:496–500

Berger CL, de Bustros A, Roos BA, Leong SS, Mendelsohn G, Gesell MS, Baylin SB (1984) Human medullary thyroid carcinoma in culture provides a model relating growth dynamics, endocrine cell differentiation, and tumor progression. J Clin Endocrinol Metab 59:338–343

Blind E, Raue F, Klaiber T, Zink A, Schroth J, Buhr H, Ziegler R (1992a) Evaluation of sensitive PDN-21 (katacalcin) determination as tumormarker in medullary thyroid carcinoma. J Endocrinol Invest

Blind E, Schmidt-Gayk H, Sinn HP, O'Connor DT, Raue F (1992b) Chromogranin A as tumor marker in medullary thyroid carcinoma. Thyroid

Blunt SB, Pirmohamed M, Chatterjee VK, Burrin JM, Allison DJ, Joplin GF (1989) Use of adrenal arterial embolization in severe ACTH-dependent Cushing's syndrome. Postgrad Med J 65:575–579

Body JJ, Heath H III (1983) Estimates of circulating monomeric calcitonin: physiological studies in normal and thyroidectomized man. J Clin Endocrinol Metab 57:897–903

Body JJ, Heath H III (1984) Nonspecific increases in plasma immunoreactive calcitonin in healthy individuals: discrimination from medullary thyroid carcinoma by a new extraction technique. Clin Chem 30:511–514

Body JJ, Dumon JC, Sculier JP, Dabouis G, Lacroix H, Libert P, Richez M, Bureau G, Mommen P, Raymakers N, Paesmans M, Klastersky J (1989a) A preliminary evaluation of calcitonin and PDN-21 as tumor markers for lung cancer. EORTC Lung Cancer Working Party. Henry Ford Hosp Med J 37:190–193

Body JJ, Struelens M, Borkowski A, Mandart G (1989b) Effects of estrogens and calcium on calcitonin secretion in postmenopausal women. J Clin Endocrinol Metab 68:223–226

Born W, Beglinger C, Fischer JA (1991) Diagnostic relevance of the amino-terminal cleavage peptide of procalcitonin (PAS-57), calcitonin and calcitonin gene-related peptide in medullary thyroid carcinoma patients. Regul Pept 32:311–319

Boultwood J, Wynford TD, Richards GP, Craig RK, Williams ED (1990) In-situ analysis of calcitonin and CGRP expression in medullary thyroid carcinoma. Clin Endocrinol (Oxf) 33:381–390

Brain SD, Williams TJ, Tippins JR, Morris HR, MacIntyre I (1985) Calcitonin gene related peptide is a potent vasodilator. Nature 313:54–56

Bucht E, Telenius-Berg M, Lundell G, Sjöberg HE (1986) Immunoextracted calcitonin in milk and plasma from totally thyroidectomized women. Evidence of monomeric calcitonin in plasma during pregnancy and lactation. Acta Endocrinol (Copenh) 113:529–535

Buffa R, Rindi G, Sessa F, Gini A, Capella C, Jahn R, Navone F, De CP, Solcia E (1987) Synaptophysin immunoreactivity and small clear vesicles in neuroendocrine cells and related tumours. Mol Cell Probes 1:367–381

Burns DM, Birnbaum RS, Roos BA (1989a) A neuroendocrine peptide derived from the aminoterminal half of rat procalcitonin. Mol Endocrinol 3:140–147

Burns DM, Forstrom JM, Friday KE, Howard GA, Roos BA (1989b) Procalcitonin's aminoterminal cleavage peptide (N-procalcitonin) is a bone cell mitogen. Proc Natl Acad Sci USA 86:9519–9523

Busnardo B, Girelli ME, Simioni N, Nacamulli D, Busetto E (1984) Nonparallel patterns of calcitonin and carcinoembryonic antigen levels in the follow-up of medullary thyroid carcinoma. Cancer 53:278–285

Bussolati G, Pearse AGE (1967) Immunofluorescent localization of calcitonin in the "C" cells of pig and dog thyroid. J Endocrinol37:205–209

Carter WB, Heath H III (1990) Clinically useful calcitonin assays. Trends Endocrinol Metab 288–291

Catherwood BD, Deftos LJ (1980) Presence by radioimmunoassay of a calcitonin-like substance in porcine pituitary glands. Endocrinology 106:1886–1891

Chambers T, Moore A (1983) The sensitivity of isolated osteoclasts to morphological transformation by calcitonin. J Clin Endocrinol Metab 57:819–824

Chambers T, McSheehy P, Thosom B, Fuller K (1985) The effect of calcium regulating hormones and prostaglandins on bone resorption by osteoclasts disaggregated from neonatal rabbit bones. Endocrinology 116:234–239

Clark M, Boyd G, Byfield PGH, Foster GV (1969) A radioimmunoassay for human calcitonin M. Lancet 2:74–77

Cohen SL, MacIntyre I, Grahame-Smith D, Walker JG (1973) Alcohol-stimulated calcitonin release in medullary thyroid carcinoma of the thyroid. Lancet 2:1172–1173

Conlon JM (1989) Post-translation processing of neurohormonal peptide precursors in a human medullary thyroid carcinoma. Horm Metab Res Suppl 21:12–15

Conlon JM, Grimelius L, Thim L (1988a) Structural characterization of a high-molecular-mass form of calcitonin [procalcitonin-(60–116)-peptide] and its corresponding N-terminal flanking peptide [procalcitonin-(1–57)-peptide] in a human medullary thyroid carcinoma. Biochem J 256:245–250

Conlon JM, Grimelius L, Wallin G, Thim L (1988b) Isolation and structural characterization of thymosin-beta 4 from a human medullary thyroid carcinoma. J Endocrinol 118:155–159

Conlon JM, McGregor GP, Wallin G, Grimelius L, Thim L (1988c) Molecular forms of katacalcin, calcitonin gene-related peptide and gastrin-releasing peptide, in a human medullary thyroid carcinoma. Cancer Res 48:2412–2426

Cooper C, Hirsch P, Toverud S, Munson P (1967) An improved method for the biological assay of thyrocalcitonin. Endocrinology 81:610–616

Copp DH, Cameron EC, Cheney BA, Davidson AGF, Henze KG (1962) Evidence for calcitonin-a new hormone from the parathyroid that lowers blood calcium. Endocrinology 70:638–649

Cote GJ, Gagel RF (1986) Dexamethasone differentially affects the levels of calcitonin and calcitonin gene-related peptide mRNAs expressed in a human medullary thyroid carcinoma cell line. J Biol Chem 261:15524–15528

Cote GJ, Gould JA, Huang SC, Gagel RF (1987) Studies of short-term secretion of peptides produced by alternative RNA processing. Mol Cell Endocrinol 53:211–219

Cote GJ, Nguyen IN, Berget SM, Gagel RF (1990) Calcitonin exon sequences influence alternative RNA processing. Mol Endocrinol 4:1744–1749

Deftos LJ, Bone HG, Parthemore JG (1980) Immunohistological studies of medullary thyroid carcinoma and C-cells hyperplasia. J Clin Endocrinol Metab 51:857–862

Deftos LJ, Woloszczuk W, Krisch I, Horvat G, Ulrich W, Neuhold N, Braun O, Reiner A, Srikanta S, Krisch K (1988) Medullary thyroid carcinomas express chromogranin A and a novel neuroendocrine protein recognized by monoclonal antibody HISL-19. Am J Med 85:780–784

Deftos LJ, Gazdar AF, Ikeda K, Broadus AE (1989) The parathyroid hormone-related protein associated with malignancy is secreted by neuroendocrine tumors. Mol Endocrinol 3:503–508

Dermody WC, Rosen MA, Ananthaswamy R, Levy AG, Hixson CV, Aldenderfer PH, Nelson RWA, Marangos PJ, Swanson EC (1981) Characterization of calcitonin- and adrenocorticotropin-producing human cloned cell lines. J Clin Endocrinol Metab 53:970–977

D'Souza SM, MacIntyre I, Girgis SI, Mundy GR (1986) Human synthetic calcitonin gene-related peptide inhibits bone resorption in vitro. Endocrinology 119:58–61

Ekblom M, Valimaki M, Pelkonen R, Jansson R, Sivula A, Franssila K (1987) Familial and sporadic medullary thyroid carcinoma: clinical and immunohistological findings. QJ Med 65:899–910

Eng HL, Chen WJ (1989) Melanin-producing medullary carcinoma of the thyroid gland. Arch Pathol Lab Med 113:377–380

Fischer JA, Born W (1985) Novel peptides from the calcitonin gene: expression, receptors and biological function. Peptides 3:265–271

Franc B, Chayvialle JA, Modigliani E, Calmettes C, Caillou B, Dutrieux BN, Houdent C, Kujas M (1987) Plasma and tumor levels of somatostatin (SRIF) and somatostatin immunochemistry in medullary thyroid carcinoma: apparently discrepant preliminary results. Henry Ford Hosp Med J 35:147–148

Gagel RF, O'Briain DS, Voelkel EF, Wolfe HJ, DeLellis RA, Lee AK, Tashjian AH Jr (1983) Pituitary immunoreactive calcitonin-like material: lack of evidence for cross-reactivity with proopiomelanocortin. Metabolism 32:686–696

Gagel RF, Palmer WN, Leonhart K, Chan L, Leong SS (1986) Somatostatin production by a human medullary thyroid carcinoma cell line. Endocrinology 118:1643–1651

Geelhoed GW, Bass BL, Mertz SL, Becker KL (1986) Somatostatin analog: effects on hypergastrinemia and hypercalcitoninemia. Surgery 100:962–970

Gharib H, Kao PC, Heath H III (1987) Determination of silica-purified plasma calcitonin for the detection and management of medullary thyroid carcinoma: comparison of two provocative tests. Mayo Clin Proc 62:373–378

Ghillani P, Motte P, Bohuon C, Bellet D (1988) Monoclonal antipeptide antibodies as tools to dissect closely related gene products. A model using peptides encoded by the calcitonin gene. J Immunol 141:3156–3163

Ghillani PP, Motte P, Troalen F, Jullienne A, Gardet P, Le Chevalier T, Rougier P, Schlumberger M, Bohuon C, Bellet D (1989) Identification and measurement of calcitonin precursors in serum of patients with malignant diseases. Cancer Res 49:6845–6851

Girgis SI, MacDonald DWR, Stevenson JC, Lynch C, Wimalawansa SJ, Self CH, Morris HR, MacIntyre I (1985) Calcitonin gene related peptide: potent vasodilator and major product of the calcitonin gene. Lancet 2:14–16

Goltzman D, Mitchell J (1985) Interaction of calcitonin and calcitonin gene-related peptide at receptor sites in target tissues. Science 227:1343–1345

Goltzman D, Huang SN, Browne C, Solomon S (1979) Adrenocorticotropin and calcitonin in medullary thyroid carcinoma: frequency of occurrence and localization in the same cell type by immunocytochemistry. J Clin Endocrinol Metab 49:364–369

Gordin A, Lamberg BA, Pelkonen R, Almqvist S (1978) Somatostatin inhibits the pentagastrin-induced release of serum calcitonin in medullary carcinoma of the thyroid. Clin Endocrinol (Oxf) 8:289–293

Grauer A, Raue F, Rix E, Tschahargane C, Ziegler R (1987) Neuron-specific enolase in medullary thyroid carcinoma: immunohistochemical demonstration, but no significance as serum tumor marker. J Cancer Res Clin Oncol 113:599–602

Grauer A, Raue F, Gagel RF (1990) Changing concepts in the management of hereditary and sporadic medullary thyroid carcinoma. Endocrinol Metab Clin North Am 19:613–35

Grauer A, Raue F, Reinel H, Schneider H, Schroth J, Kabay A, Brügger P, Ziegler R (1992) A new in vitro bioassay for human calcitonin: validation and comparison to the rat hypocalcemia bioassay. Bone and Mineral 17:65–74

Guilloteau D, Perdrisot R, Calmettes C, Baulieu JL, Lecomte P, Kaphan G, Milhaud G, Besnard JC, Jallet P, Bigorgne JC (1990) Diagnosis of medullary carcinoma of the thyroid (MCT) by calcitonin assay using monoclonal antibodies: criteria for the pentagestrin stimulation test in hereditary MCT. J Clin Endocrinol Metab 71:1064–1067

Hassager C, Bonde SK, Anderson MA, Rink H, Spelsberg TC, Riggs BL (1991) Procalcitonin NH2-terminal cleavage peptide has no mitogenic effect on normal human osteoblast-like cells. J Bone Miner Res 6:489–493
Heath H III, Edis AJ (1979) Pheochromocytoma associated with hypercalcemia and ectopic secretion of calcitonin. Ann Intern Med 91:208–210
Heath H III, Sizemore GW (1977) Plasma calcitonin in normal man. Differences between men and women. J Clin Invest 60:1135–1140
Heath H III, Sizemore GW (1982) Radioimmunoassay for calcitonin. Clin Chem 28:1219–1226
Hennessy JF, Gray TK, Cooper CW, Ontjes DA (1973) Stimulation of thyrocalcitonin secretion by pentagastrin and calcium infusion as provocative agents for the detection of medullary carcinoma of the thyroid. J Clin Endocrinol Metab 36:200–203
Henninger S, Schatz H, Stracke H, Wagner U, Kracht J (1988) Immunohistochemical hormone content in medullary and undifferentiated thyroid carcinoma and prognosis after surgery. Acta Histochem (Jena) 83:51–56
Hill CS, Ibanez ML, Samaan NA, Ahearn MJ, Clark RL (1973) Medullary (solid) carcinoma of the thyroid gland. An analysis of the M.D. Anderson Hospital experience with patients with the tumor, its special features, and its histogenesis. Medicine (Baltimore) 52:141–171
Hillyard CJ, Myers C, Abeyasekera G, Stevenson JC, Craig RK, MacIntyre I (1983) Katacalcin, a new plasma calcium-lowering hormone. Lancet 1:846–848
Holm R, Sobrinho SM, Nesland JM, Gould VE, Johannessen JV (1985) Medullary carcinoma of the thyroid gland: an immunocytochemical study. Ultrastruct Pathol 8:25–41
Hoppener JW, Steenbergh PH, Zanberg J, Geurts vKAH, Baylin SB, Nelkin BD, Jansz HS, Lips CJM (1985) The second human calcitonin/CGRP gene is located on chromosome 11. Hum Genet 70:259–263
Hoppener JW, Steenbergh PH, Moonen PJ, Wagenaar SS, Jansz HS, Lips CJ (1986) Detection of mRNA encoding calcitonin, calcitonin gene related peptide and proopiomelanocortin in human tumors. Mol Cell Endocrinol 47:125–130
Howlett TA, Price J, Hale AC, Doniach I, Rees LH, Wass JA, Besser GM (1985) Pituitary ACTH dependent Cushing's syndrome due to ectopic production of a bombesin-like peptide by a medullary carcinoma of the thyroid. Clin Endocrinol (Oxf) 22:91–101
Hsiao RJ, Neumann HPH, Parmer RJ, Barbosa JA, O'Connor DT (1990a) Chromogranin-A in familial pheochromocytoma: diagnostic screening value, prediction of tumor mass, and postresection kinetics indicating two-compartment distribution. Am J Med 88:607–613
Hsiao RJ, Seeger RC, Yu A, O'Connor DT (1990b) Chromogranin A in children with neuroblastoma: serum concentration parallels disease stage and predicts survival. J Clin Invest 85:1555–1559
Hurley DL, Katz HH, Tiegs RD, Calvo MS, Barta JR, Heath H III (1988) Cosecretion of calcitonin gene products: studies with a C18-cartridge extraction method for human plasma PDN-21 (katacalcin). J Clin Endocrinol Metab 66:640–644
Hurley DL, Tiegs RD, Barta J, Laakso K, Heath H III (1989) Effects of oral contraceptive and estrogen administration on plasma calcitonin in pre- and postmenopausal women. J Bone Miner Res 4:89–95
Huttner WB, Gerdes HH, Rosa P (1991) The granin (chromogranin/secretogranin) family. Trends Biochem Sci 16:27–30
Ikeda K, Lu C, Weir EC, Mangin M, Broadus AE (1989) Transcriptional regulation of the parathyroid hormone-related peptide gene by glucocorticoids and vitamin D in a human C-cell line. J Biol Chem 264:15743–15746

Ishikawa N, Hamada S (1976) Association of medullary carcinoma of the thyroid with carcinoembryonic antigen. Br J Cancer 34:111–115

Ittner J, Dambacher MA, Born W, Ketelslegers JM, Buys-Schaert M, Albert PM, Lambert AE, Fischer JA (1985) Diagnostic evaluation of measurements of carboxyl-terminal flanking peptide (PDN-21) of the human calcitonin gene in serum. J Clin Endocrinol Metab 61:1133–1137

Jacobs JW, Goodman RH, Chin WW, Dee PC, Habener JF, Bell NH, Potts JT Jr (1981) Calcitonin messenger RNA encodes multiple polypeptides in a single precursor. Science 213:457–459

Jex RK, van Heerden JA, Carpenter PC, Grant CS (1985) Ectopic ACTH syndrome. Diagnostic and therapeutic aspects. Am J Surg 149:276–282

Kim S, Morimoto S, Kawai Y, Koh E, Onishi T, Ogihara T (1989) Circulating levels of calcitonin gene-related peptide in patients with medullary thyroid carcinoma. J Clin Chem Clin Biochem 27:423–427

Kimura N, Ishioka K, Miura Y, Sasano N, Takaya K, Mouri T, Kimura T, Nakazato Y, Yamada R (1989) Melanin-producing medullary thyroid carcinoma with glandular differentiation. Acta Cytol 33:61–66 [published erratum appears in Acta Cytol (1989) 33:951]

Klein G, Wadlington E, Collins E, Catherwood B, Deftos L (1984) Calcitonin levels in sera of Infants and children: relations to age and periods of bone growth. Calcif Tissue Int 36:635–638

Krisch K, Krisch I, Horvat G, Neuhold N, Ulrich W (1985) The value of immunohistochemistry in medullary thyroid carcinoma: a systematic study of 30 cases. Histopathology 9:1077–1089

Kumar M, Slack E, Edwards A, Soliman H, Baghdiantz A, Foster G, MacIntyre I (1965) A biological assay for calcitonin. J Endocrinol 33:469–475

Lasmoles F, Minvielle S, Cohen R, Guliana JM, Delehaye MC, Segond N, Calmettes C, Milhaud G, Moukhtar MS (1990) PCR amplification of CGRP II mRNA. Variable expression in tumoral and non-tumoral human thyroid. FEBS Lett 277:243–6

Lazaretti-Castro M, Grauer A, Mekonnen Y, Raue F, Ziegler R (1991) 17-b-Estradiol effects on calcitonin secretion and content in a human medullary thyroid carcinoma cell line. J Bone Miner Res 6:1191–1195

Leggate J, Farish E, Fletcher CD, McIntosh W, Hart DM, Somerville JM (1984) Calcitonin and postmenopausal osteoporosis. Clin Endocrinol (Oxf) 20:85–92

Libroia A, Verga U, Di SG, Piolini M, Muratori F (1989) Use of somatostatin analog SMS 201–995 in medullary thyroid carcinoma. Henry Ford Hosp Med J 37:151–153

Lind SE, Weitzman SA (1985) The insidious development of symptomatic secondary hormone syndromes in patients with malignant endocrine tumors. Am J Med Sci 290:107–110

Linnoila RI, Becker LK, Silva OL, Snider RH, Moore CF (1984) Calcitonin as a marker for diethylnitrosamine-induced pulmonary endocrine cell hyperplasia in hamsters. Lab Invest 51:39–45

Lippman SM, Mendelsohn G, Trump DL, Wells SA Jr, Baylin SB (1982) The prognostic and biological significance of cellular heterogeneity in medullary thyroid carcinoma: a study of calcitonin, L-dopa decarboxylase, and histaminase. J Clin Endocrinol Metab 54:233–240

Lloyd RV, Sisson JC, Marangos PJ (1983) Calcitonin, carcinoembryonic antigen and neuronspecific enolase in medullary thyroid carcinoma. Cancer 51:2234–2239

Lofberg H, Grubb A, Davidsson L, Kjellander B, Stromblad LG, Tibblin S, Olsson SO (1983) Occurrence of gamma-trace in the calcitonin-producing C-cells of simian thyroid gland and human medullary thyroid carcinoma. Acta Endocrinol (Copenh) 104:69–76

MacIntyre I, Hillyard CJ, Murphy P, Renolds JJ, Gaines Das RE, Craig RK (1982) A second plasma-lowering peptide from the human calcitonin precursor. Nature 298:460–462

MacIntyre I, Hillyard CJ, Murphy P, Renolds JJ, Gaines Das RE, Craig RK (1984) A second plasma-lowering peptide from the human calcitonin precursor – a re-evaluation. Nature 300:84

Mahler C, Verhelst J, de Longouville M, Harris A (1990) Long-term treatment of metastatic medullary thyroid carcinoma with the somatostatin analogue octreotide. Clin Endocrinol (Oxf) 33:261–269

Marcinkiewicz M, Benjannet S, Falgueyret JP, Seidah NG, Schurch W, Verdy M, Cantin M, Chretien M (1988) Identification and localization of 7B2 protein in human, porcine, and rat thyroid gland and in human medullary carcinoma. Endocrinology 123:866–873

Martino E, Bambini G, Aghini LF, Motz E, Pacini F, Lari R, Baschieri L, Pinchera A (1984) Serum tissue polypeptide antigen (TPA) in thyroid cancer. J Endocrinol Invest 7:249–252

Mason RT, Shulkes A, Zajac JD, Fletcher AE, Hardy KJ, Martin TJ (1986) Basal and stimulated release of calcitonin gene-related peptide and calcitonin in medullary thyroid carcinoma. Clin Endocrinol (Oxf) 25:703–710

Matsubayashi S, Yanaihara C, Ohkubo M, Fukata S, Hayashi Y, Tamai H, Nakagawa T, Miyauchi A, Kuma K, Abe K et al. (1984) Gastrin-releasing peptide immunoreactivity in medullary thyroid carcinoma. Cancer 53:2472–2477

McLean GW, Rabin D, Moore L, Deftos LJ, Lorber D, McKenna TJ (1984) Evaluation of provocative tests in suspected medullary carcinoma of the thyroid: heterogeneity of calcitonin responses to calcium and pentagastrin. Metabolism 33:790–796

Mendelsohn G, Wells SJ, Baylin SB (1984) Relationship of tissue carcinoembryonic antigen and calcitonin to tumor virulence in medullary thyroid carcinoma. An immunohistochemical study in early, localized, and virulent disseminated stages of disease. Cancer 54:657–662

Miettinen M (1987) Synaptophysin and neurofilament proteins as markers for neuroendocrine tumors. Arch Pathol Lab Med 111:813–818

Miyauchi A, Onishi T, Matsuzuka F, Hirai K, Kuma K, Takai S, Nakamoto K, Nakamura K, Nanjo S, Maeda M (1986) Prognostic values of the doubling time of serum carcinoembryonic antigen and calcitonin levels in medullary thyroid carcinoma. Gan No Rinsho 32:1519–1524

Modigliani E, Alamowitch C, Cohen R, Calmettes C, Guliana JM, Franc B, Bernard C, Chayvialle JA (1990a) The intratumoral immunoassayable somatostatin concentration is frequently elevated in medullary thyroid carcinoma. Results in 34 cases. Cancer 65:224–228

Modigliani E, Casanova S, Chayvialle JA, Bernard C, Franc B, Cohen R, Calmettes C (1990b) Immunoreactive gastrin-releasing peptide in medullary thyroid carcinoma. J Clin Endocrinol Metab 71:831–835

Morris HR, Panico M, Etienne T, Tippins J, Girgis SI, MacIntyre I (1984) Isolation and characterization of human calcitonin gene-related peptide. Nature 308:746–748

Motté P, Vauzelle P, Gardet P, Ghillani P, Caillou B, Parmentier C, Bohuon C, Bellet D (1988) Construction and clinical validation of a sensitive and specific assay for serum mature calcitonin using monoclonal anti-peptide antibodies. Clin Chim Acta 174:35–54

Nakamura A, Kakudo K, Watanabe K (1987a) Establishment of a new human thyroid medullary carcinoma cell line. Morphological studies. Virchows Arch [B] 53:332–335

Nakamura H, Someda H, Mori T, Imura H (1987b) Thyrotrophin releasing hormone induced calcitonin secretion in patients with medullary carcinoma of the thyroid. Clin Endocrinol (Oxf) 27:69–74

Natori S, Iguchi H, Ohashi M, Nawata H (1988) Plasma 7B2 (a novel pituitary protein) immunoreactivity concentrations in patients with various endocrine disorders. Endocrinol Jpn 35:651–654

Neher R (1968) Human calcitonin. Nature 220:984–986

Nelkin BD, Rosenfeld KI, de Bastros A, Leong SS, Roos BA, Baylin SB (1984) Structure and expression of a gene encoding human calcitonin and calcitonin gene related peptide. Biochem Biophys Res Commun 123:648–655

Neradilova M, Nemec J, Zamrazil V, Bednar J, Pechova M, Soutorova M (1989) Plasma somatostatin activity in medullary cancer of the thyroid. Oncology 46:378–380

New HV, Mudge AW (1986) Calcitonin gene-related peptide regulates muscle acetylcholine receptor synthesis. Nature 323:809–811

Noel M, Gavoille A, Lasmoles F, Kahn E, Caillous B, Gardet P, Fragu P (1990) Quantification of intracellular calcitonin gene transcripts in human medullary thyroid carcinoma (MTC) by in situ hybridization. J Endocrinol Invest 13:567–573

O'Connell JE, Dominiczak AF, Isles CG, McLellan AR, Davidson G, Gray CE, Connell JM (1990) A comparison of calcium pentagastrin and TRH tests in screening for medullary carcinoma of the thyroid in MEN IIA. Clin Endocrinol (Oxf) 32:417–421

O'Connor DT, Bernstein KN (1984) Radioimmunoassay of chromogranin A in plasma as a measure of exocytotic sympathoadrenal activity in normal subjects and patients with pheochromocytoma. N Engl J Med 311:764–770

O'Connor DT, Deftos LJ (1986) Secretion of chromogranin A by peptide-producing endocrine neoplasms. N Engl J Med 314:1145–1151

O'Connor DT, Deftos LJ (1987) How sensitive and specific is measurement of plasma chromogranin A for the diagnosis of neuroendocrine neoplasia? Ann NY Acad Sci 493:379–386

O'Connor DT, Burton DW, Deftos LJ (1983) Immunoreactive human chromogranin A in diverse polypeptide hormone producing human tumors and normal endocrine tissues J Clin Endocrinol Metab 57:1084–1086

O'Connor DT, Pandian MR, Cariton E, Cervenka JH, Hsiao RJ (1989) Rapid radioimmunoassay of circulating chromogranin A: in vitro stability, exploration of the neuroendocrine character of neoplasia, and assessment of the effects of organ failure. Clin Chem 35:1631–1637

O'Halloran DJ, Bloom SR (1991) Calcitonin gene related peptide – a major neuropeptide and the most powerful vasodilator known. Br Med J 302:739–740

Ohashi M, Natori S, Fujio N, Iguchi H, Nawata H (1990) Secretory protein 7B2. A novel tumor marker of medullary carcinoma of the thyroid. Horm Metab Res 22:114–116

Oishi S, Sato T (1988) Elevated serum neuron-specific enolase in patients with malignant pheochromocytoma. Cancer 61:1167–1170

Oosterom R, Verleun T, Bruining HA, Hackeng WH, Lamberts SW (1987) Human medullary thyroid carcinoma in tissue culture; secretion of calcitonin and carcinoembryonic antigen. J Endocrinol Invest 10:117–121

Pacini F, Martino E, Bambini G, Aghini LF, Taddei D, Lari R, Pinchera A, Baschieri L (1985) Humoral markers for thyroid carcinoma. Cancer Detect Prev 8:17–22

Pacini F, Elisei R, Anelli S, Gasperini L, Schipani E, Pinchera A (1986) Circulating neuron-specific enolase in medullary thyroid cancer. Int J Biol Markers 1:85–88

Pacini F, Elisei R, Anelli S, Basolo F, Cola A, Pinchera A (1989) Somatostatin in medullary thyroid cancer. In vitro and in vivo studies. Cancer 63:1189–1195

Pacini F, Basolo F, Elisei R, Fugazzola L, Cola A, Pinchera A (1991) Medullary thyroid cancer. An immunohistochemical and humoral study using six separate antigens. Am J Clin Pathol 95:300–308

Palmer BV, Harmer CL, Shaw HJ (1984) Calcitonin and carcino-embryonic antigen in the follow-up of patients with medullary carcinoma of the thyroid. Br J Surg 71:101–104

Pearse AGE (1968) Common cytochemical and ultrastructural characteristics of cells producing polypeptide hormones (the APUD series) and their relevance to thyroid and ultimobranchial C cells and calcitonin. Proc R Soc Lond [Biol] 170:71–80

Peleg S, Abruzzese RV, Cote GJ, Gagel RF (1990) Transcription of the human calcitonin gene is mediated by a C cell – specific enhancer containing E-box-like elements. Mol Endocrinol 4:1750–1757

Perdrisot R, Bigorgne JC, Guilloteau D, Jallet P (1990) Monoclonal immunoradiometric assay of calcitonin improves investigation of familial medullary thyroid carcinoma. Clin Chem 36:381–383

Perez Cano R, Montoya MJ, Moruno R, Vazquez A, Galan F, Garrido M (1989) Calcitonin reserve in healthy women and patients with postmenopausal osteoporosis. Calcif Tissue Int 45:203–208

Prince RL, Dick IM, Price RI (1989) Plasma calcitonin levels are not lower than normal in osteoporotic women. J Clin Endocrinol Metab 68:684–687

Rambaud JC, Jian R, Flourie B, Hautefeuille M, Salmeron M, Thuillier F, Ruskone A, Florent C, Chaoui F, Bernier JJ (1988) Pathophysiological study of diarrhoea in a patient with medullary thyroid carcinoma. Evidence against a secretory mechanism and for the role of shortened colonic transit time. Gut 29:537–543

Raue F (1982) Interlaboratory comparison of radioimmunological calcitonin determination J Clin Chem Clin Biochem 20:157–161

Raue F, Streibl W, Ziegler R (1982) Synthetic human calcitonin (cibacalcin, Ciba-Geigy), use for radioimmunoassay and bioassay. Endokrinologie 79:118–124

Raue F, Schmidt GH, Ziegler R (1983) Tumor markers in C-cell cancer. Dtsch Med Wochenschr 108:283–287

Raue F, Boller G, Rix E, Schmidt GH, Ziegler R (1985) Secretion of calcitonin and carcinoembryonic antigen in long-term organ culture of human medullary thyroid carcinoma: biochemical and immunocytochemical studies. Klin Wochenschr 63:205–210

Raue F, Boden M, Girgis S, Rix E, Ziegler R (1987a) Katacalcin-a new tumor marker in C-cell cancer of the thyroid gland. Klin Wochenschr 65:82–86

Raue F, Minne HW, Ziegler R (1987b) Calcitonin. In: Pesce A, Kaplan L (eds) Methods in clinical chemistry. Mosby, St Louis, pp 696–701

Raue F, Schneider HG, Zink A, Ziegler R (1987c) Action of calcitonin gene-related peptide at the calcitonin receptor of the T47D cell line. Horm Metab Res 19:563–564

Raue F, Serve H, Rix E, Ziegler R (1987d) In vitro secretion of peptides of the calcitonin family: calcitonin, katacalcin, and calcitonin gene-related peptide. Henry Ford Hosp Med J 35:143–146

Raue F, Schneider H-G, Grauer A (1990) Diagnostic value of the peptides from the calcitonin gene. In: Schmidt-Gayk H, Armbruster FP, Bouillon R (eds) Calcium regulating hormones, vitamin D metabolites and cyclic AMP. Assays and their clinical application. Springer, Berlin Heidelberg New York, pp 48–59

Reginster JY, Deroisy R, Albert A, Denis D, Leart MP, Colette J, Franchimont P (1989) Relationship between whole plasma calcitonin levels, calcitonin secretory reserve, and plasma levels of estrone in healthy women and postmenopausal osteoporotics. J Clin Invest 83:1073–1077

Reubi JC, Krenning E, Lamberts SW, Kvols L (1990) Somatostatin receptors in malignant tissues. J Steroid Biochem Mol Biol 37:1073–1077
Roos BA, Fischer JA, Pignat W, Alander CB, Raisz LG (1986) Evaluation of the in vivo and in vitro calcium-regulating actions of noncalcitonin peptides produced via calcitonin gene expression. Endocrinology 118:46–51
Rosenfeld MG, Mermod JJ, Amara SG, Swanson LW, Sawchenko PE, Rivier J, Vale WW, Evans RM (1983) Production of a novel neuropeptide encoded by the calcitonin gene via tissue-specific RNA processing. Nature 304:129–135
Rougier P, Calmettes C, Laplanche A, Travagli JP, Lefevre M, Parmentier C, Milhaud G, Tubiana M (1983) The values of calcitonin and carcinoembryonic antigen in the treatment and management of nonfamilial medullary thyroid carcinoma. Cancer 51:855–862
Saad MF, Fritsche HJ, Samaan NA (1984) Diagnostic and prognostic values of carcinoembryonic antigen in medullary carcinoma of the thyroid. J Clin Endocrinol Metab 58:889–894
Samaan NA, Hickey RC (1987) Medullary carcinoma of the thyroid: differentiating the types and current management. Oncology (Williston Park) 1:21–28
Samaan NA, Anderson CD, Adam-Mayne ME (1975) Immunoreactive calcitonin in the mother, neonate, child and adult. Am J Obstet Gynecol 121:622–625
Samaan NA, Castillo S, Schultz PN, Khalil K-G, Johnston DA (1980) Serum calcitonin after pentagastrin stimulation in patients with bronchogenic and breast cancer compared to that in patients with medullary thyroid carcinoma. J Clin Endocrinol Metab 51:237–241
Samaan NA, Schultz PN, Hickey RC (1989a) Medullary thyroid carcinoma: prognosis of familial versus nonfamilial disease and the role of radiotherapy. Horm Metab Res Suppl 21:21–25
Samaan NA, Yang KP, Schultz P, Hickey RC (1989b) Diagnosis, management, and pathogenetic studies in medullary thyroid carcinoma syndrome. Henry Ford Hosp Med J 37:132–137
Schifter S (1989a) Calcitonin and PND-21 as tumor markers in MEN2 family screening (Abstr). 7th Meeting of the International Society of Oncodevelopmental Biology and Medicine, Freiburg
Schifter S (1989b) Calcitonin gene-related peptide and calcitonin as tumor markers in MEN 2 family screening. Clin Endocrinol (Oxf) 30:263–270
Schifter S (1991) Circulating concentrations of calcitonin gene-related peptide (CGRP) in normal man determined with a new, highly sensitive radioimmunoassay. Peptides 12:365–369
Schifter S, Williams ED, Craig RK, Hansen HH (1986) Calcitonin gene-related peptide and calcitonin in medullary thyroid carcinoma. Clin Endocrinol (Oxf) 25:703–710
Schröder S, Kloppel G (1987) Carcinoembryonic antigen and nonspecific cross-reacting antigen in thyroid cancer. An immunocytochemical study using polyclonal and monoclonal antibodies. Am J Surg Pathol 11:100–108
Schröder S, Bocker W, Baisch H, Burk CG, Arps H, Meiners I, Kastendieck H, Heitz PU, Kloppel G (1988) Prognostic factors in medullary thyroid carcinomas. Survival in relation to age, sex, stage, histology, immunocytochemistry, and DNA content. Cancer 61:806–816
Seshi B, True L, Carter D, Rosai J (1988) Immunohistochemical characterization of a set of monoclonal antibodies to human neuron-specific enolase. Am J Pathol 131:258–269
Seth R, Motté P, Kehely A, Wimalawansa SJ, Self CH, Bellet D, Bohuon C, MacIntyre I (1988) A sensitive and specific two-site enzyme-immunoassay for human calcitonin using monoclonal antibodies. J Endocrinol 119:351–357
Sikri KL, Varndell IM, Hamid QA, Wilson BS, Kameya T, Ponder BA, Lloyd RV, Bloom SR, Polak JM (1985) Medullary carcinoma of the thyroid. An

immunocytochemical and histochemical study of 25 cases using eight separate markers. Cancer 56:2481–1491
Simon JP, Aunis D (1989) Biochemistry of the chromogranin A protein family (Review). Biochem J 262:1–13
Sjoberg HE, Torring O, Granberg B, Ehrensten U, Bucht E (1989) Postmenopausal osteoporosis: response of immunoextracted calcitonin to a calcitonin clamp. Bone 10:15–18
Smith AD, Winkler H (1967) Purification and properties of an acidic protein from chromaffin granules of bovine adrenal medulla. Biochem J 103:483–492
Smith WJ, Kirshner N (1967) A specific soluble protein from the catecholamine storage vesicles of bovine adrenal medulla. I. Purification and chemical characterization. Mol Pharmacol 3:52–62
Snider HR, Silva OL, Becker KL, Moore CF (1977) Immunochemical heterogeneity of calcitonin on man: effect on radioimmunoassy. Clin Chim Acta 76:1–14
Steenbergh PH, Hoppener JW, Zandberg J, Lips CJM, Jansz HS (1985) A second human calcitonin/CGRP gene. FEBS Lett 183:403–407
Steenbergh PH, Hoppener JW, Zandberg J, Visser A, Lips CJ, Jansz HS (1986) Structure and expression of the human calcitonin/CGRP genes. FEBS Lett 209:97–103
Stevenson JC, Hillyard CJ, Abeyasekera G, Phang KG, MacIntyre I (1981) Calcitonin and the calcium-regulating hormones in postmenopausal women: effect of oestrogens. Lancet 1:693–695
Stevenson JC, White MC, Joplin GF, MacIntyre I (1982) Osteoporosis and calcitonin deficiency. Br Med J 285:1010–1011
Stevenson JC, Myers CH, Ajdukiewicz AB (1984) Racial differences in calcitonin and katacalcin. Calcif Tissue Int 36:725–728
Stolarsky-Fredman L, Leff SE, Klein ES, Crenshaw EB III, Yeakley J, Rosenfeld MG (1990) A tissue-specific enhancer in the rat-calcitonin/CGRP gene is active in both neural and endocrine cell types. Mol Endocrinol 4:497–504
Sunday ME, Wolfe HJ, Roos BA, Chin WW, Spindel ER (1988) Gastrin-releasing peptide gene expression in developing, hyperplastic, and neoplastic human thyroid C-cells. Endocrinology 122:1551–1558
Sundler F, Christophe J, Robberecht P, Yanaihara N, Yanaihara C, Grunditz T, Hakanson R (1988) Is helodermin produced by medullary thyroid carcinoma cells and normal C-cells? Immunocytochemical evidence. Regul Pept 20:83–89
Takami H, Shikata J, Horie H, Sekine K, Ito K (1990a) PDN-21: possible tumor marker for medullary thyroid carcinoma. J Surg Oncol 44:205–207
Takami H, Shikata J, Kakudo K, Ito K (1990b) Calcitonin gene-related peptide in patients with endocrine tumors. J Surg Oncol 43:28–32
Takiyyuddin MA, Cervenka JH, Sullivan PA, Pandian MR, Parmer RJ, Barbosa JA, O'Connor DT (1990) Is physiologic sympathoadrenal catecholamine release exocytotic in humans? Circulation 81:185–195
Tashjian AH, Howland BG, Kenneth BA, Melvin KEW, Hill CS (1970) Immunoassay of human calcitonin – clinical measurement. Relation to serum calcium in patients with medullary carcinoma. N Engl J Med 283:890–895
Tatemoto K, Mutt V (1980) Isolation of two novel candidate hormones using a chemical method for finding naturally occurring polypeptides. Nature 285:417–418
Telenius-Berg M, Almquist S, Berg B, Hedner P, Ingemensson S, Tibblin S, Wasthed B (1977) Screening for medullary carcinoma of the thyroid in families with Sipple's syndrome: evaluation of new stimulation tests. Eur J Clin Invest 7:7–16
Tiegs RD, Body JJ, Wahner HW, Barta J, Riggs BL, Heath H III (1985) Calcitonin secretion in postmenopausal osteoporosis. N Engl J Med 312:1097–1100

Tiegs RD, Body JD, Barta JM, Heath H III (1986) Secretion and metabolism of monomeric human calcitonin: effect of age, sex and thyroid damage. J Bone Miner Res 1:339–349
Tobler PH, Tschopp FA, Dambacher MA, Fischer JA (1984) Salmon and human calcitonin-like peptides in man. Clin Endocrinol (Oxf) 20:253–259
Touitou Y, Heshmati HM (1988) Neuron-specific enolase in medullary thyroid carcinoma. Clin Chem 34:2375–2376
Tourniaire J, Rebattu B, Conte DB, Trouillas J, Grino M, Berger DN, Peix JL, Pugeat M (1988) Cushing's syndrome caused by ectopic production of CRF by a medullary carcinoma of the thyroid body. Ann Endocrinol (Paris) 49:61–67
Tsutsumi Y, Kamoshida S, Iguchi K, Mochizuki T, Yanaihara N (1990) Is helodermin-like immunoreactivity in human thyroid C cells due to a salmon calcitonin-like substance? Regul Pept 31:11–21
Wells SA Jr, Baylin SB, Linehan WM, Farrell RE, Cox EB, Cooper CW (1978) Provocative agents and the diagnosis of medullary carcinoma of the thyroid gland. Ann Surg 188:139–141
Wiedenmann B, Kuhn C, Schwechheimer K, Waldherr R, Raue F, Brandeis WE, Kommerell B, Franke WW (1987) Synaptophysin identified in metastases of neuroendocrine tumors by immunocytochemistry and immunoblotting. Am J Clin Pathol 88:560–569
Woloszczuk W, Schuh H, Kovarik J (1986) Determination of circulating monomeric katacalcin and calcitonin: physiological studies in normal subjects. J Clin Chem Clin Biochem 24:451–455
Yamaguchi K, Abe K, Adachi I, Suzuki M, Kimura S, Kameya T, Yanaihara N (1984) Concomitant production of immunoreactive gastrin-releasing peptide and calcitonin in medullary carcinoma of the thyroid. Metabolism 33:724–727
Zaidi M, Chambers TJ, Moonga BS, Oldoni T, Passarella E, Soncini R, MacIntyre I (1990) A new approach for calcitonin determination based on target cell responsiveness. J Endocrinol Invest 13:119–126
Zajac JD, Penschow J, Mason RT, Tregear G, Coghlan J, Martin TJ (1986) Identification of calcitonin and calcitonin gene-related peptide messenger ribonucleic acid in medullary thyroid carcinomas by hybridization histochemistry. J Clin Endocrinol Metab 62:1037–1043
Ziegler R, Raue F (1984) Variations of plasma calcitonin levels measured by radioimmunoassay systems for human calcitonin. Biomed Pharmacother 38:245–251
Ziegler R, Beck C, Raue F (1985) Calcitonin response to provocative stimuli. In: Pecile A (ed) Calcitonin. Elsevier, Amsterdam, pp 71–79

Sporadic Medullary Thyroid Carcinoma: Clinical Features and Diagnosis

R. Ziegler

Abteilung für Innere Medizin I – Endokrinologie und Stoffwechsel, Universität Heidelberg, Luisenstraße 5, W-6900 Heidelberg 1, FRG

Introduction

Medullary thyroid carcinoma (MTC) or C-cell carcinoma is a rather young endocrinopathy, i.e., its rareness in combination with its discrete clinical symptoms explains why it was only realized as a clinical entity about 30 years ago. Hazard et al. (1959) recognized the typical amyloid pattern and differentiated MTC from the melting pot of thyroid cancer. A few years later, calcitonin was discovered by Copp et al. (1962) and Hirsch et al. (1963) – however, some years passed before the ultimobranchial origin of calcitonin was demonstrated in 1967 (Bussolati and Pearse 1967). One year later it became evident that MTC exerts endocrine activity by secreting calcitonin in excessive amounts (Meyer and Abdel Bari 1968). Since then MTC has been handled as a specific disease quite different from the malignancies of the thyrocytes.

Statistics state that MTC comprises about 5% of thyroid malignancies; the data range from 0.7% to 11.0% (Winter 1991) depending on geographical factors, the local frequency of affected families and the availability of diagnostic tools.

In addition to sporadic cases the familial forms of MTC were discovered very soon afterwards: "pure" MTC, multiple endocrine neoplasia (MEN) 2A and MEN 2B (see Gagel et al. this volume for details of these special genetic variants).

According to the first MTC statistics, about 80% of cases belonged to the sporadic type and 20% to the hereditary types (Baylin 1974); however, as screening for MTC in siblings of affected patients became more frequent, the incidence of the inherited types also rose. From 161 MTC cases reported between 1944 and 1983 in Houston, Texas, 125 (77.6%) were sporadic, and 36 (22.4%) were MEN cases (Saad et al. 1984). In a nationwide survey in Japan, a total of 242 MTC patients were reported; of these, 160 cases (66.1%) belonged to the sporadic, and 82 (33.9%) to the hereditary type

Recent Results in Cancer Research, Vol. 125

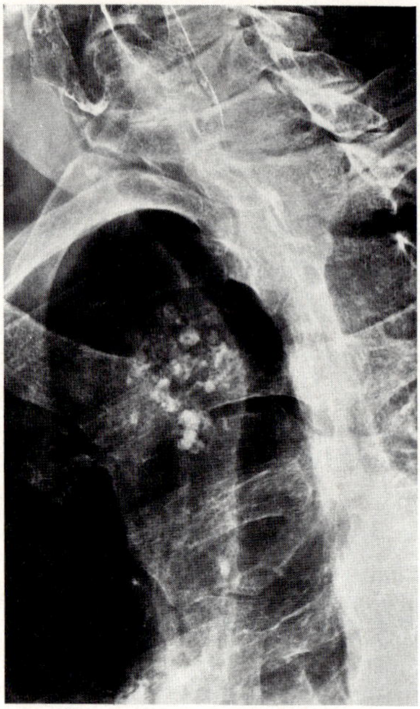

Fig. 1. Ossified substernal metastasis of MTC

(Takai et al. 1984). The Swedish Cancer Registry contained diagnosed cases of 249 MTC from 1959 through 1981; 186 of these (75%) were considered to be sporadic, and 63 (25%) belonged to the familial type (Bergholm et al. 1989). Our own series of 61 MTC patients shows 53 sporadic and 8 familial cases (Winter 1991).

Between about 1970 and 1980, many partially treated cases of MTC were discovered among the bulk of thyroid cancer patients. The systematic measurement of calcitonin in blood samples from thyroid carcinoma patients with a somehow not fully typical histology revealed several cases of MTC in our own thyroid cancer care unit. Nowadays, MTC has been included in medical text books and is taught in the curricula; nevertheless, delayed diagnosis may still occur.

The following case history illustrates typical clinical traits of MTC as well as the recognition of a new disease: In 1971, a 50-year-old physician developed a sciatic nerve syndrome on his left side. The pains were severe, and walking was impaired. He was X-rayed including tomography of the pelvic bones leading to the diagnosis of an osteolytic tumor (metastasis?) of the os sacrum. The tumor was removed, and histology was "malignant epithelial tumor of unknown origin". Two years later, the patient realized a slowly progressive swelling of his thyroid. Scintigraphy revealed that it was a "cold" nodule, which was afterwards removed. Histology was now declared as MTC, and 1 year later a calcitonin determination was performed. The elevated calcitonin level of 4–6 ng/ml signalized that tumor tissue was still present. Upon chest X-ray, a calcified mass of walnut size was seen in the upper mediastinum (Fig. 1). The surgeons suggested the mass to be a calcified hematoma, but the patient remembered reading in a paper on MTC that its metastases could calcify or ossify. He insisted on reoperation, and indeed a substernal partially ossified MTC metastasis was removed. Afterwards, calcitonin levels fell to about half of the preoperative level. From then on the patient was seen in our institution about once per year, and 6 years after the pelvic operation, at a calcitonin concentration of around 10 ng/ml, diarrhea slowly started. At a staging examination, bone scintigraphy showed two hot spots in the calvarium (Fig. 2) which obviously were osteolytic metastases (Fig. 3). These spots were removed by the surgeon and the defects filled with palakos. Postoperatively calcitonin levels again fell, but did not normalize. The following years were complicated by increases in stool frequency; tinctura opii was needed for symptomatic relief. Other trials including prostaglandin synthesis inhibitors, cyproheptadine and others were not sufficient. Finally, after 10 years, multiple metastases including those of the skin were discovered, and the patient died due to tumor cachexia.

The following paragraphs describe the appearance of the tumor in its original organ, the thyroid gland, and in the regional lymph nodes or distant tissues. Symptoms include diarrhea as a sign of later disease state. Sometimes, a paraneoplastic Cushing's syndrome accompanies MTC. Prognosis depends on early diagnosis and treatment.

General Appearance

There is no specific or characteristic clinical feature of sporadic MTC, at least not during the first few years. Elevated calcitonin itself does not lead to symptoms; therefore, symptomatology depends on local tumor growth (goiter, thyroid nodule), and the appearance of local (lymph node), or distant metastases (see above-mentioned case report). Diarrhea and weight loss are also unspecific. Therefore, in contrast to the MEN 2 where accompanying endocrinopathies or morphological abnormalities point towards the disease, sporadic MTC is diagnosed rather late and even occasionally misdiagnosed.

The data on sex distribution are somewhat divergent. The statistics from Saad et al. (1984), Houston, do not show a preference; both sexes were equally affected (female : male, 1.06 : 1). Also in a national survey from France which evaluated 1031 MTC cases, including 226 familial cases, no sex differences were seen (Calmettes 1989). In contrast, more female MTC patients were diagnosed in Sweden (female : male, 1.35 : 1) (Bergholm et al. 1989). This is in agreement with our own patient series, where female patients were seen slightly more frequently than male patients (female : male 1.26 : 1).

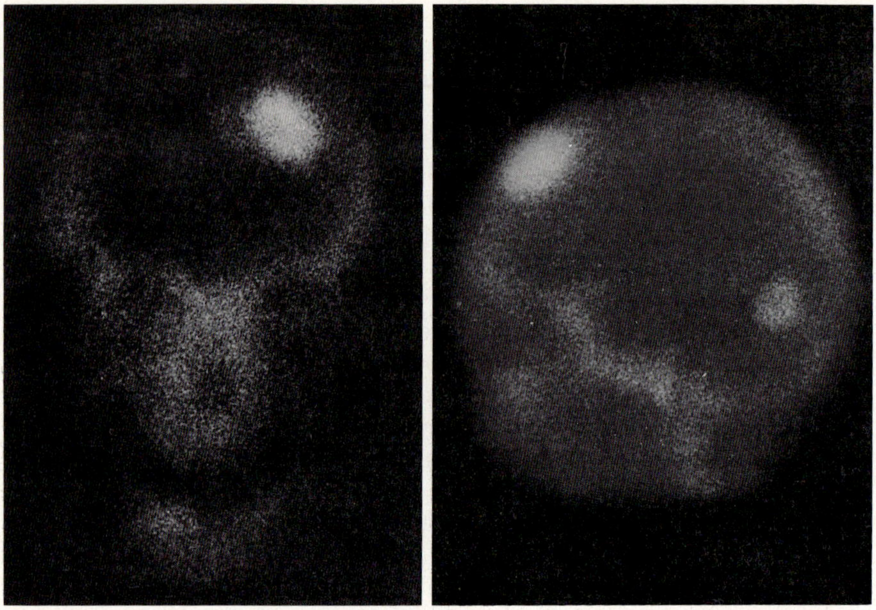

Fig. 2. Bone scintigraphy showing increased tracer uptake ("hot spots"), suggesting metastases of MTC

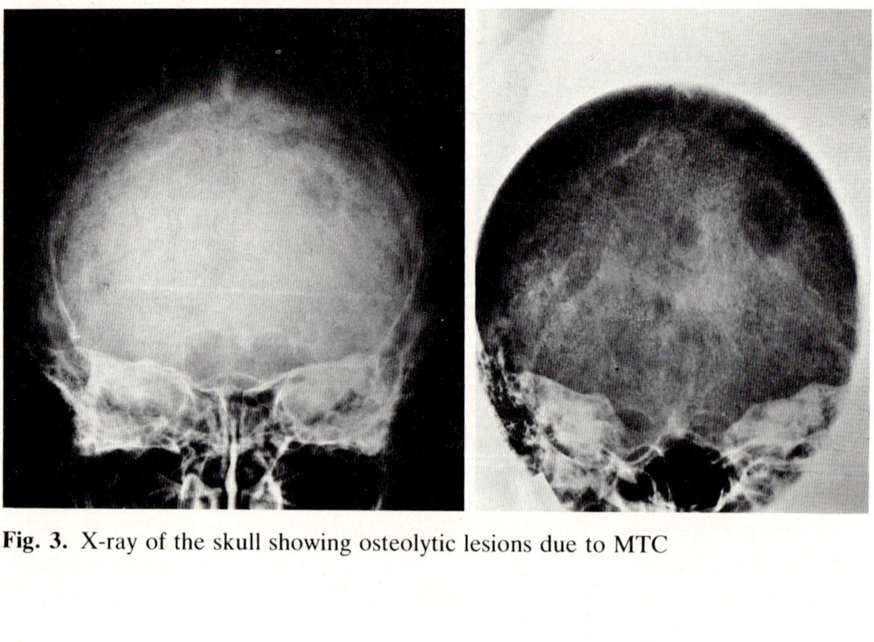

Fig. 3. X-ray of the skull showing osteolytic lesions due to MTC

In Japan, the unfavorable sex ratio for women was even more pronounced (female: male, 2.6:1) (Takai et al. 1984).

The mean age at diagnosis was 46.1 years in the case of sporadic MTC in our Heidelberg series (Winter 1991); the statistics from Japan showed a somewhat lower age of 43.4 years (Takai et al. 1984). For France, a sex difference was observed for the age of discovery, being 43 years for women, but 52 for men (Calmettes 1989).

In most sporadic cases, diagnosis is made by histology after thyroid surgery – the subsequent measurement of calcitonin shows whether the tumor has been totally removed or whether there is persistence, which is more often the case. As a rule, sporadic MTC has already metastasized at the time of diagnosis. As long as only local lymph node metastases have developed, extensive second-look surgery, according to Tisell et al. (1986), is promising.

With respect to common hypercalcitoninemia in MTC patients pre- as well as postoperatively, it is still surprising that no clinical symptoms are produced by the, in part, excessively elevated calcitonin levels in blood although the circulating hormone is biologically active. Due to the escape phenomenon, all organs and cell systems which are definitely influenced by calcitonin upon *acute* administration, do not react any more when they are chronically exposed to the hormone. Whereas calcitonin injection or infusion causes an impairment of glucose assimilation and insulin secretion or an inhibition of gastric and pancreatic enzyme secretion in normocalcitoninemic subjects, such effects are absent in individuals with permanently elevated calcitonin concentrations in blood such as MTC patients (Hotz et al. 1978; Ziegler et al. 1984). There is no hypocalcemia in MTC patients, and they do not suffer from tetany. In bone tissue, the inhibitory effect of calcitonin on osteoclast activity is not long lasting either. The resorbing cells also escape a calcitonin reaction. Bone biopsies from MTC patients with high calcitonin levels in the blood do not show low turnover or diminished osteoclast counts (Delling 1975); sometimes, even increased trabecular bone remodeling has been described (Emmertsen et al. 1984).

In agreement with these findings, hypercalcitoninemic MTC patients do not present with increased bone mass although it has been theoretically discussed that osteoclast blockade could lead to a positive bone balance. In 21 cases, Hurley et al. (1987) found even slightly lower bone mineral density at the spine whereas the radius was unaffected. In our own series of 39 MTC patients no bone mineral density differences were seen in comparison with the healthy control collective (Wüster et al. 1992). Therefore, bone mass measurements in MTC do not support the expectation of increased bone mass when calcitonin is chronically elevated e.g., for the treatment of osteoporosis. Presumably the latter purpose requires intermittent treatment schedules and high turnover as a pretreatment condition (McDermott and Kidd 1987).

Tumor Markers

Calcitonin is the classical tumor marker of MTC; the concomitant measurement of PDN-21 may be a useful second marker (Raue et al. 1989a). Carcinoembryonic antigen (CEA) rises later, is less specific for MTC, but may be of prognostic value; calcium gene-related peptide (CGRP) may be elevated, too.

In every newly diagnosed case of MTC without positive family history, it should be considered that the patient could be the index case of a new family. Therefore, calcitonin should be determined in all accessible kindreds once in order not to overlook additional MTC cases. If no elevated calcitonin concentrations are found in any of the investigated kindreds, further screening can be stopped in this family, and the patient may be regarded as a sporadic case.

The wisdom of this general screening is illustrated by a recent study by Simpson et al. (1990). In 51 cases of "first-case" MTC, the families were tested (altogether 200 people). Abnormal results were found in 15 families; C-cell disease was proven in 13 families. The authors concluded that in their studies 25% of patients with primarily apparently sporadic MTC had relatives with MTC, and should, therefore be regarded as familial cases.

Thyroid Nodules

MTC develops within the thyroid; ectopic primary tumors are not known. A superficial nodule in an otherwise normal thyroid gland is somewhat suspicious; however, there are no statistics (due to the rareness of the tumor) on whether the diagnosis of MTC takes place earlier in a non-goiter area than in regions with endemic goiter. Germany (the former states of West Germany) is still an "under-developed" country with respect to goiter prophylaxis by the use of iodinated salt. Therefore, on the basis of an incidence of MTC of 0.15 per 10^5 inhabitants per year, *one* new case of MTC *has* to be discovered in a population of 660000 including about 20% with goiters and corresponding nodules! When comparing the mean age of our own sporadic cases in Heidelberg (46.1 years; Winter 1991) with the Japanese series (43.4 years; Takai et al. 1984), a later diagnosis is apparent in Germany, perhaps because of a more complicated anatomical situation of the thyroid (endemic goiter area with many nodules inside the thyroid gland) where the tumor growth is to be found. The French data (Calmettes 1989) regarding sex differences illustrate the complexity of the problem.

The MTC nodule grows without pain; sensations of a lump in the throat are so frequent that reports of occasional pressure are to be judged with reservation. Among our series of 53 sporadic MTC patients, 38 (76%) had a goiter which had been known for 7.5 years on average; this illustrates the problems discussed above. Thirty-one (62%) had goiter nodules, known for a mean of 2.3 years (Table 1). Thus, MTC must be considered when

Table 1. Signs and symptoms at the time of diagnosis of MTC

Signs and symptoms	Houston, USA[a] Sporadic MTC (n = 125) (%)	Houston, USA[a] Familial MTC (n = 36) (%)	Houston, USA[a] All cases (n = 161) (%)	Uppsala, Sweden[b] Sporadic MTC (n = 186) (%)	Uppsala, Sweden[b] Familial MTC (n = 63) (%)	Uppsala, Sweden[b] All cases (n = 249) (%)	Heidelberg, Germany[c] Signs and symptoms	Heidelberg, Germany[c] Sporadic MTC (n = 53) (%)	Sporadic MTC Mean time before diagnosis (years)	Familial MTC (n = 8) (%)	Familial MTC Mean time before diagnosis (years)	All cases (n = 61) (%)	All cases Mean time before diagnosis (years)
Thyroid swelling (Houston) or palpaple thyroid mass (Uppsala)	93.6	55.6	91.3	82.7	63.4	77.9	Goiter	76	7.5	75	2.5	75.9	7
							Thyroid nodule	62	2.3	75	2.3	63.8	2.3
Enlarged cervical lymph node	52	16.6	44	44	23.8	34.5	Enlarged cervical lymph node	40	2.1	25		37.7	2.1
Diarrhea	28.8	5.5	23.5	20	15.8	18.8	Diarrhea	17	7.8	28	8.6	18.3	7.9
							Weight loss (3.5–20 kg)	12	2.1	13	0.25	11.8	1.8

[a] Saad et al. 1984.
[b] Bergholm et al. 1989.
[c] Winter 1991.

examining endemic goiters plus nodules in regions poor in iodine. Of course, in countries with sufficient iodine supply, goiters and especially thyroid nodules are still more suggestive of malignancies, although the absolute frequency does not seem to differ too much.

The *ultrasound procedure* depicts MTC nodules as hypoechogenic. Ultrasound has proved to be very useful for the follow-up of MTC patients after surgical treatment with respect to local recurrence and lymph node appearance (Raue et al. 1989b). However, the ultrasound pattern is not pathognomonic or specific as other thyropathies such as local inflammation or thyrocyte tumors may be hypoechogenic, too. Nevertheless, 92% of our patients showed an indicative hypoechogenic pattern (Winter 1991).

Upon thyrocyte *scintigraphy*, the MTC presents as a "cold" nodule (73% in our series). Efforts are being made to detect positive MTC with scintigraphy using metaiodobenzyl guanidine (MIBG) or dimercaptosuccinic acid (DMSA) (Udelsman et al. 1989).

If the nodules are large enough and/or superficially situated in such a way as to guarantee a reliable evaluation, *fine needle aspiration* (FNA) and cytology may yield a specific diagnosis, especially if immunohistology or immunocytology is also included (Geddie et al. 1984; Kini et al. 1984). The relevant patient series are rather small to permit a statistical evaluation of the method; however, the correct diagnosis was made in 13 out of 15 patients (87%) (Söderström et al. 1975). Cytologists stress the point that the morphological pattern is rather variable; thus, the characteristic pleomorphism may on the one hand lead to overdiagnosis of MTC, but, on the other hand, be suggestive of MTC (Zeppa et al. 1990).

In sporadic MTC, the tumor is mostly unilateral, and without treatment it may infiltrate the adjacent tissue. Symptoms may then include laryngeal nerve paresis, obstruction of the trachea, or erosion of the passing vessels. Final stages of the disease may show this pattern.

As a variant, benign *C-cell adenoma* has been described (Beskid et al. 1971). After the first description further hidden cases were expected, but further studies in which, for example, screening with calcitonin measurements and routine ultrasound examinations of the thyroid were included did not confirm this assumption. Further reports are still episodic (Kodama et al. 1988), and the first report in 1971 may be overlooked by later authors.

It must be mentioned that calcitonin screening is not recommended, for example, in all patients with scintigraphically "cold" thyroid nodules, since this type of procedure detected only one case of MTC among 400 screened patients (Schmidt-Gayk 1980, personal communication).

Lymph Nodes

MTC is a malignant tumor which from on early stage spreads along the lymph vessels – hematogenic spreading is also common (see below). In our own series, 40% of cases had enlarged cervical lymph nodes at the time of diagnosis (Winter 1991; Table 1). When assessing the symptoms leading to the examination of the patient, another 9 patients (14.8%) were investigated because of their lymph nodes (Table 2). At the time of operation, involved lymph nodes were found in two-thirds of patients (Williams et al. 1966). Systematic autopsy in 20 MTC patients revealed lymph node metastases (including mediastinum) in 13 of them (Williams et al. 1966). Therefore, deliberate and extensive lymph node exploration at MTC surgery is decisive for the patients' prognosis (Tisell et al. 1986).

Distant Metastases

In larger studies, distant metastases were found in 15 of 125 patients with sporadic MTC (12%) and in 2 of 35 MEN II cases (5.7%) (Saad et al. 1984). In Sweden, 19% of sporadic and 22% of familial MTC patients had distant metastases (Bergholm et al. 1989). The above-mentioned autopsy study (Williams et al. 1966) showed the following frequency and distribution of distant metastases in 20 MTC patients: lungs, 9; liver, 5; skeleton, 4; adrenals, 4; pleura, 2; heart, pancreas, ovary, 1 each; only 4 patients had neither lymph node nor distant metastases. Bone metastases in particular may be also osteoblastic, although calcifications or ossifications may also occur outside the bone (see Fig. 1). The osteolytic type of skeletal metastasis is shown in Figs. 2 and 3. In the case of vertebral involvement, paralysis due to cord compression may take place.

With respect to single metastases, surgical resection should be performed even if a larger number of operations becomes necessary over the years (see case history). There is no indication that any other kind of treatment would yield better results than the strategy of removing all accessible metastases.

Diarrhea

Frequent, watery stools are a complication of advanced MTC. At the time of diagnosis, 9 out of 53 sporadic cases (17%) already suffered from diarrhea (Winter 1991; Table 1). Most of them also presented with weight loss which was evident in 6 patients (12%) from our series. In 3 patients (4.9%), diarrhea was even a leading symptom (Table 2), and such patients mostly have a history of extensive gastrointestinal examinations including therapeutic trials (pancreatic enzyme substitution, glucocorticoids, etc.). It is quite typical for MTC diarrhea to respond only badly to classical antidiarrheic drugs such as loperamide; use of tinctura opii cannot then be avoided.

The responsible tumor factor leading to diarrhea has not yet been definitely identified. Calcitonin itself is not a candidate because most systems

Table 2. Leading signs and symptoms initiating the examination of 61 MTC patients (53 sporadic, 8 familial cases). (According to Winter, 1991)

Signs and symptoms	Perentage of patients
Goiter	31.2
Thyroid nodule	29.5
Enlarged cervical lymph node	14.8
Diarrhea	4.9
Distant metastases	1.6
Flush	1.6
Others or no comment	16.4

of the organism escape a reaction to chronically elevated calcitonin levels (Ziegler et al. 1984). As the C-cell carcinoma paraneoplastically secretes a lot of hormones and biogenic amines, there are a lot of candidates which could induce diarrhea (Williams 1989) such as serotonin, histaminase, prostaglandins, vasoactive intestinal peptide (VIP), substance P, neurotensin, bombesin, and corticotropin-releasing hormone (CRH); adrenocorticotropic hormone (ACTH) and CGRP have already been mentioned. There is no definite correlation between such factors and the severity of diarrhea, although mapping of the factors is mostly incomplete in the respective patients. With respect to the pathogenesis of MTC diarrhea, colonic transit time was seen to be shortened, presumably due to increased motor activity of the colon (Ramband et al. 1988).

As expected, diarrhea in MTC is a factor of impaired prognosis. Five years survival is seen in only 62% of diarrheal patients compared to a rate of 83% in patients with normal stool. Nevertheless, survival with MTC and diarrhea is possible for many years. Flushes are a rarely seen event (see Table 2).

Cushing's Syndrome

As early as 1970, Melvin et al. described a woman with mild cushingoid appearance in whom they documented paraneoplastic ACTH secretion by MTC leading to adrenal hyperplasia. Since then, not only ACTH- but also corticotropin-releasing factor (CRF)-induced paraneoplastic Cushing's syndrome has been discovered (Tourniaire et al. 1988). The same tumor may contain ACTH and CRF and even prolactin production-stimulating activity leading to galactorrhea (Birkenhäger et al. 1976). On the basis of the suggested common precursor for calcitonin *and* ACTH (Lips et al. 1978), the combination of MTC and Cushing's syndrome is no longer any great surprise; however, the clinical manifestation of hypercortisolism in MTC is restricted to about 5% of those affected (Melvin et al. 1972).

Table 3. Survival rates of 61 German MTC patients. (From Winter 1991)

Criterion	Number of patients	Survival rate (%)			Death rate during time of observation	
		3 years	5 years	7 years[a]	Number of patients	Percentage of patients
Total	61 (161)	93	84 (78.2)	77 (61.4)	12 (54)	19.7 (33.8)
Sex						
Male	27	92	88 (62.9)	72 (46.0)		
Female	34	93	80 (87.8)	80 (77.1)		
Tumor stage						
I	30		100 (93)	(80)	1	3.3
II	13		70 (90)	(88)	3	23
III	15		64 (57)	(22)	6	40
IV	3	66	(40)	(23)	2	66.7
Types						
Sporadic	53		84 (72)	(54)		
Familial (MEN 2A)	8		85 (100)	(94)		
Age						
<40 years	26		86 (93.2)	86 (73.3)		
>40 years	35		82 (67.3)	68 (52.7)		
Diarrhea	11	80	62 (80.3)	(30.9)		
No diarrhea			(71.6)	(73.9)		

For comparison, values from the USA according to Saad et al. 1984 are given in parentheses.
[a] Values in parentheses are 10-year survival rates from Saad et al. 1984.

Prognosis

When first calculations of life expectancy were done a few years after recognition of MTC as a separate entity, prognosis was rather poor; after 5 years only 48% of patients were alive; after 10 years, 12% (Fletcher 1970). These data reflect a history of inadequate treatment of an unknown disease.

Nowadays, the situation has distinctly improved due to strategies of faster detection, adequate surgery, and more efficient follow-up examination including markers, localization techniques such as ultrasound, computerized axial tomography (CAT) scan, magnetic resonance imaging (MRI), specific scintigraphy, and venous catheterization for calcitonin measurements. Evaluating 161 patients, Saad et al. (1984) found a 5-year adjusted survival rate of 78.2% for all of them; for 10 and 15 years the percentages were 61.4% and 57.5%, respectively. A recent evaluation of our own patients revealed that patients with sporadic MTC had a somewhat worse prognosis than those with familial types. However, for both, the stage of the disease was decisive, stressing the importance of early diagnosis. Table 3 summarizes the results (Winter 1991). As only a few patients were observed for longer than 10 years, the table contains survival rates at 5 and 7 years. Even our sporadic cases had a 5-year survival rate of 84%. Further improvement is to be expected with still more intensive knowledge of the disease and early transfer of the affected patients to centers with appropriate diagnostic and surgical experience.

References

Baylin SB (1974) Medullary carcinoma of the thyroid gland: use of biochemical parameters in detection and surgical management of the tumor. Surg Clin North Am 54:309–315

Bergholm U, Adami H-O, Bergström R, Johansson H, Lundell G, Telenius-Berg M, Åkerström G, Swedish MTC Study Group (1989) Clinical characteristics in sporadic and familial medullary thyroid carcinoma. Cancer 63:1196–1204

Beskid M, Lorenc A, Rosciszewska A (1971) A thyroid C-cell adenoma in man. J Pathol 103:343–346

Birkenhäger JC, Upton GV, Seldenrath HJ, Krieger DT, Tashjian AH Jr (1976) Medullary thyroid carcinoma: ectopic production of peptides with ACTH-like, corticotrophin releasing factor-like and prolactin production-stimulating activities. Acta Encocrinol (Copenh) 83:280–292

Bussolati G, Pearse AGE (1967) Immunofluorescent localization of calcitonin in the "C" cells of pig and dog thyroid. J Endocrinol 37:205–209

Calmettes C (1989) Screening for medullary cancer of the thyroid in France. Horm Metab Res Suppl 21:1–2

Copp DH, Cameron EC, Cheney BA, Davidson AGF, Henze KG (1962) Evidence for calcitonin – a new hormone from the parathyroid that lowers blood calcium. Endocrinology 70:638–649

Delling G (1975) Endokrine Osteopathien. Fischer, Stuttgart, pp 65–68

Emmertsen K, Melsen F, Mosekilde L, Lund B, Lund B, Sørensen OH, Charles P, Møller J (1984) Vitamin D levels and trabecular bone remodelling before and after surgery for medullary thyroid carcinoma. Acta Endocrinol (Copenh) 106:346–349

Fletcher JR (1970) Medullary (solid) carcinoma of the thyroid gland, a review of 249 cases. Arch Surg 100:257–262

Geddie WR, Bedard YC, Strawbridge HTG (1984) Medullary carcinoma of the thyroid in fine-needle aspiration biopsies. Am J Clin Pathol 82:552–558

Hazard JB, Hawk WA, Crile G Jr (1959) Medullary (solid) carcinoma of the thyroid – a clinicopathologic entity. J Clin Endocrinol 19:152–161

Hirsch PF, Gauthier GF, Munson PL (1963) Thyroid hypocalcemic principle and recurrent laryngeal nerve injury as factors affecting the response to parathyroidectomy in rats. Endocrinology 73:244–252

Hotz J, Goebell H, Ziegler R (1978) Magensekretion und exokrine Pankreasfunktion bei Patienten mit medullärem Schilddrüsencarcinom sowie mit Morbus Paget unter Therapie mit Calcitonin. Z Gastroneterol 16:547–552

Hurley DL, Tiegs RD, Wahner HW, Heath H III (1987) Axial and appendicular bone mineral density in patients with long-term deficiency or excess of calcitonin. N Engl J Med 317:537–541

Kini SR, Miller JM, Hamburger JI, Smith MJ (1984) Cytopathologic features of medullary carcinoma of the thyroid. Arch Pathol Lab Med 108:156–159

Kodama T, Okamoto T, Fujimoto Y, Obara T, Ito Y, Aiba M, Hirayama A (1988) C cell adenoma of the thyroid: a rare but distinct clinical entity. Surgery 104:997–1003

Lips CJ, van der Sluys Veer J, ven der Donk JA, van Dam RH, Hackeng WH (1978) Common precursor molecule as origin for the ectopic hormone producing tumour syndrome. Lancet 1:16–18

McDermott MT, Kidd GS (1987) The role of calcitonin in the development and treatment of osteoporosis. Endocr Rev 8:377–390

Melvin KEW, Tashjian AH Jr, Cassidy CE, Givens JR (1970) Cushing's syndrome caused by ACTH- and calcitonin-secreting medullary carcinoma of the thyroid. Metabolism 19:831–838

Melvin KEW, Tashjian AH Jr, Miller HH (1972) Studies in familial (medullary) thyroid carcinoma. Recent Prog Horm Res 28:399–407

Meyer JS, Abdel Bari W (1968) Granules and thyrocalcitonin-like activity in medullary carcinoma of the thyroid gland. N Engl J Med 278:523–529

Rambaud JC, Jian R, Flourie B, Hautefeuille M, Salmeron M, Thuillier F, Ruskone A, Florent C, Chaoui F, Bernier JJ (1988) Pathophysiological study of diarrhoea in a patient with medullary thyroid carcinoma. Evidence against a secretory mechanism and for the role of shortened colonic transit time. Gut 29:537–543

Raue F, Blind E, Grauer A (1989a) Diagnostische Bedeutung der Peptide des Calcitonin-Gens: Calcitonin, Katacalcin und "Calcitonin gene-related peptide". Lab Med 13:464–469

Raue F, Winter J, Frank-Raue K, Lorenz D, Herfarth C, Ziegler R (1989b) Diagnostic procedure before reoperation in patients with medullary thyroid carcinoma. Horm Metab Res Suppl 21:31–34

Saad MF, Ordonez NG, Rashid RK, Guido JJ, Hill GS Jr, Hickey RC, Samaan NA (1984) Medullary carcinoma of the thyroid. A study of the clinical features and prognostic factors in 161 patients. Medicine (Baltimore) 63:319–342

Simpson WJ, Carruthers JS, Malkin D (1990) Results of a screening program for C-cell disease (medullary thyroid cancer and C-cell hyperplasia). Cancer 65:1570–1576

Söderström N, Telenius-Berg M, Åkerman M (1975) Diagnosis of medullary carcinoma of the thyroid by fine needle aspiration biopsy. Acta Med Scand 197:71–76

Takai S, Miyauchi, A, Matsumoto H, Ikeuchi T, Miki T, Kuma K, Kumahara Y (1984) Multiple endocrine neoplasia type 2 syndromes in Japan. Henry Ford Hosp Med J 32:246–250

Tisell LE, Hansson G, Jansson S, Salander H (1986) Reoperation in the treatment of asymptomatic metastasizing medullary thyroid carcinoma. Surgery 99:60–66

Tourniaire J, Rebattu B, Conte-Devolx B, Trouillas J, Grino M, Berger-Dutrieux N, Peix J-L, Pugeat M (1988) Syndrome de Cushing secondaire à la production ectopique de CRF par un carcinome médullaire du corps thyroïde. Ann Endocrinol (Paris) 4:61–67

Udelsman R, Mojiminiyi OA, Soper NDW, Buley ID, Shepstone BJ, Dudley NE (1989) Medullary carcinoma of the thyroid: management of persistent hypercalcitonaemia utilizing [^{99m}Tc] (v) dimercaptosuccinic acid scintigraphy. Br J Surg 76:1278–1281

Williams ED (1989) Medullary carcinoma of the thyroid. In: Degroot LJ (ed) Endocrinology, vol 2. pp 1132–1150

Williams ED, Brown CL, Doniach I (1966) Pathological and clinical findings in a series of 67 cases of medullary carcinoma of the thyroid. J Clin Pathol 19:103–113

Winter J (1991) Das medulläre Schilddrüsencarcinom – Klinik, Diagnostik und Therapie. Dissertation, University of Heidelberg

Wüster C, Raue F, Mayer C, Bergmann M, Ziegler R (1992) Long-term excess of endogenous calcitonin in patients with medullary thyroid carcinoma does not affect bone mineral density. J Endocrinology 134

Zeppa P, Vetrani A, Marino M, Fulciniti F, Boschi R, de Rosa G, Palombini L (1990) Fine needle aspiration cytology of medullary thyroid carcinoma: a review of 18 cases. Cytopathology 1:35–44

Ziegler R, Dautschle U, Raue F (1984) Calcitonin in human pathophysiology. Horm Res 20:65–73

Screening for MEN 2 with Biochemical and Genetic Markers

M.F. Robinson, R.F. Gagel, and F. Raue

Baylor College of Medicine and the M.D. Anderson Cancer Center, Box 15, 1515 Holocombe Boulevard, Houston, TX 77030, USA

Introduction

The term "multiple endocrine neoplasia type 2" (MEN 2) denotes a genetic syndrome characterized by the independent appearance of benign or malignant changes of several endocrine organs (the thyroid, parathyroid, and adrenal glands) as well as occasional changes of neuronal, muscular, and connective tissue. Despite the large number of variations of these manifestations, three different forms have been identified:

1. MEN 2A (Sipple's syndrome, Sipple 1961), characterized by medullary thyroid carcinoma (MTC) in association with pheochromocytoma and parathyroid hyperplasia.
2. MEN 2B, including MTC, pheochromocytoma and mucosal neuromas, and a marfanoid-like habitus (Williams and Pollock 1966).
3. MTC-only syndrome, a hereditary MTC without the other components of MEN 2A (Farndon et al. 1986). Whether this represents a separate syndrome or merely a variant of MEN 2A in which the genetic component is modified to delay the onset of all manifestations of the MEN 2A syndrome is not clear.

The MEN 2 syndrome is transmitted as an autosomal dominant trait with a high degree of penetrance, although not every family member affected will develop all of the polyglandular neoplasia manifestations for the particular syndrome. The changes in the individual glands appear to be causally and temporally independent of each other. A spectrum of pathologic changes exists in the affected glands which range from hyperplasia to adenoma to carcinoma. The carcinomatous state is almost always preceded by a state of hyperplasia and the pathologic process is almost always multicentric, frequently resulting in bilateral disease. The appearance of an endocrine tumor known to be associated with MEN 2 should alert the physician to the possibility of a MEN 2 syndrome. The existence of one manifestation of

Recent Results in Cancer Research, Vol. 125

MEN 2 should suggest the possibility of others. When the possibility of such a syndrome exists, screening and long-term observation should be initiated in order to diagnose a carcinoma in its earliest stages before either clinical manifestations or excessive hormone production develop. If diagnosed early, all of the serious features of MEN 2 are treatable and even curable.

Clinical Presentation of MEN 2A

The most common manifestation and the hallmark of the disease is hyperplasia of the thyroidal C-cells, which progresses through several intermediate stages to develop into MTC. About 50% of affected individuals will develop unilateral or bilateral pheochromocytoma and a lower percentage will develop parathyroid hyperplasia or multiple parathyroid adenomas.

Medullary Thyroid Carcinoma. MTC develops by malignant transformation of the parafollicular C-cells of the thyroid gland. The C-cells migrate from the neural crest during embryonic development. The most common presentation of MTC in the familial or MEN 2 setting is diffuse C-cell hyperplasia which may persist for years before the development of a multicentric carcinoma. C-cell hyperplasia or MTC has been reported in children with MEN 2A as young as 1.5 years or 2.8 years of age (Telander et al. 1989). The prolonged period of C-cell hyperplasia results in a protracted period during which the thyroidal neoplasia is clinically silent. The first clinical indication of the disease in index cases does not appear to differ from the clinical presentation in sporadic MTC (see R. Ziegler in this volume). These clinical signs include cold thyroid nodules detected by thyroid scan or the appearance of a clinical syndrome caused by hypersecretion of one or more hormones by the tumor, e.g., adrenocorticotropic hormone (ACTH) causing Cushing's syndrome. It is now possible to consistently detect MTC by prospective screening of potentially affected family members at early stages prior to the development of metastatic disease. In those patients detected by such screening, the clinical presentation is silent (Gagel et al. 1988; Vasen et al. 1987).

Hereditary MTC is usually associated with other components of the MEN 2A syndrome, but there have been some families described in which hereditary MTC was the only observed manifestation of MEN 2A (the MTC-only syndrome) (Farndon et al. 1986). In addition, eight kindreds have been identified recently in which MEN 2A has been associated with a hereditary form of localized pruritus (cutaneous lichen amyloidosis) (Gagel et al. 1989; Nunziata et al. 1989). This skin lesion, therefore, serves as a phenotypic marker of MEN 2A.

Pheochromocytoma. Approximately 50% of patients with MEN 2A will develop pheochromocytoma at some point in life (Saad et al. 1984; Chong et al. 1975). In most cases, diagnosis of adrenal medullary disease follows the identification of MTC although there are a few examples of pheochromocytoma preceding C-cell disease (Gagel et al. 1988; Jadoul et al. 1989; Raue et al. 1985). Conversely, only 5% of all pheochromocytomas appear to be familial and, of these, 20% occur within the framework of MEN 2. Typically, the pheochromocytomas are bilateral and multifocal (70%) and almost never extra-adrenal (Lips et al. 1981); the malignancy rate is lower (fewer than ten reported cases) than that of the sporadic form of pheochromocytoma (Chong et al. 1975) although invasion of the adrenal medullary capsule is commonly seen in advanced pheochromocytoma. The development of pheochromocytoma associated with MEN 2 is preceded by diffuse and nodular hyperplasia of the adrenal medulla, analogous to the hyperplasia of the C-cells seen in the thyroid gland. These pathologic changes commonly occur simultaneously in both adrenals but can be asynchronous (Carney et al. 1976a). Both the presence of adrenal medullary hyperplasia and pheochromocytoma can cause symptoms of catecholamine excess, although the incidence of clinically apparent disease is much lower in the adrenal medullary hyperplasia patients. In fact, about 50% of MEN 2A patients with pheochromocytoma are asymptomatic and normotensive (Saad et al. 1984). This may be due to the early diagnosis of the tumor in those patients who have familial disease because of the awareness of the disease. Nonetheless, it is important to note that pheochromocytoma is a dangerous condition in MEN 2 as, sometimes, patients die of hypertensive crisis during operation (Lips et al. 1981). Patients with MEN 2 must, therefore, be carefully evaluated to rule out the presence of a pheochromocytoma prior to performing thyroidectomy for MTC.

Hyperparathyroidism. Hyperparathyroidism is the third and least common of the three clinical manifestations of MEN 2A. Approximately 25% of known MEN 2A gene carriers will develop hyperparathyroidism, usually after the third decade (Cance and Wells 1985). The reported incidence of hyperparathyroidism in MEN 2A varies between 18% and 85% (Keiser et al. 1973; Gagel et al. 1988; Steiner et al. 1968). This marked difference in incidence can be attributed to the variability in MEN 2A gene expression in different families. Some families exhibit all the features of the syndrome (Keiser et al. 1973; Steiner et al. 1968) while others may show MTC with either pheochromocytoma (Schimke and Hartmann 1965; Steiner et al. 1968) or hyperparathyroidism (Markey et al. 1973) without the third component of the syndrome. The disparity in incidence also can be attributed to differences in criteria (clinical, or biochemical, or histopathologic) used by different investigators for the diagnosis of hyperparathyroidism. The etiology of hyperparathyroidism in MEN 2 is unknown, although it clearly is not caused by hypercalcitoninemia because parathyroid disease is not observed in association with sporadic MTC. The earliest functional abnormality detected is incomplete suppression of parathyroid hormone secretion as determined by calcium infusion (Heath et al. 1976). The clinical features do not differ from those seen in patients with sporadic hyperparathyroidism and include hypercalcemia, hypercalciuria, urolithiasis, and parathyroid hormone-induced bone disease. Multiglandular parathyroid hyperplasia is most commonly seen (Melvin et al. 1972) although adenomatous changes do occur in a small percentage of patients (Steiner et al. 1968; Cance et al. 1985). MEN 2 patients detected early by screening often manifest little clinical evidence of hyperparathyroidism, although hyperplasia of parathyroid glandular tissue may be observed during the removal of one or two parathyroid glands from patients undergoing thyroidectomy for the C-cell disease (Gagel et al. 1988).

Clinical Appearance of MEN 2B

The clinical syndrome of MTC, pheochromocytoma, multiple mucosal neuromas, and ganglioneuromatosis has been called MEN 2B (or MEN 3). The distinctive features of the syndrome were first convincingly described by Williams and Pollock 1966 (Williams and Pollock 1966), and include mucosal neuromas and ganglioneuromatosis throughout the gastrointestinal tract.

Mucosal Neuromas. Patients with mucosal neuromas are identified by the characteristic phenotype in which the mucosal neuromas are located in a centrofacial distribution on the tongue, oral mucosa, lips, eyelids, and the conjunctiva. These patients also have a marfanoid-like habitus (Fig. 1). The clinical spectrum of the mucosal neuroma syndrome may vary considerably from very prominent neuromas to subtle manifestations. Neuromas can usually be detected in the first year of life and generally precede the clinical presentation of the other features of the syndrome (Khairi et al. 1975; Frank et al. 1984; Raue et al. 1986). Other common presentations in early childhood, which precede the manifestation of endocrine neoplasia may be gastrointestinal disorders including colic, cramping, constipation, and diarrhea as a result of the presence of neuromas throughout the gastrointestinal tract (Griffiths et al. 1990; Williams and Pollock 1966; Khan et al. 1987; Carney et al. 1976b; Khairi et al. 1975). Besides confusion with Hirschsprung's disease (Mahaffey et al. 1990), Crohn's disease, and ulcerative colitis, ganglioneuromatosis is often mistaken for von Recklinghausen's neurofibromatosis. A rectal biopsy should be performed to establish the diagnosis.

Marfanoid Habitus. Marfanoid features include long, thin extremities, an altered upper/lower body ratio, decreased body fat, and poor muscle development. Associated skeletal abnormalities are common and include a slipped femoral epiphysis, dorsal kyphoscoliosis, pes cavus, and pectus

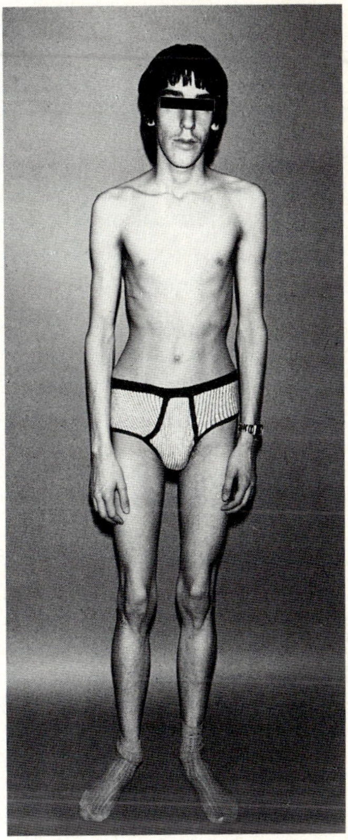

Fig. 1. The clinical features of a patient with MEN 2B. Characteristic features include a marfanoid habitus, an elongated face, and thickened lips. (From Frank et al. 1984)

excavatum (Carney et al. 1979). In contrast to the Marfan syndrome, pes cavus occurs instead of pes planus, and neither ectopia lentis nor aortic abnormalities are seen.

Hyperparathyroidism. Hyperparathyroidism is a rare occurrence in MEN 2B (Carney et al. 1978).

Pheochromocytoma. It appears that the incidence of pheochromocytoma is higher in patients with MEN 2B than in those with MEN 2A. Indeed, more than 50% of patients with MEN 2B will develop a pheochromocytoma, whereas in patients with MEN 2A the incidence ranges from 5% to 50% (Chong et al. 1975; Hill et al. 1973; Grün and Eberle 1981; Khairi et al. 1975). These patients may have minimal symptoms and signs. Laboratory findings, including provocative tests, may be normal even though a pheochromocytoma is present. The pheochromocytomas are bilateral and multicentric and have many of the same characteristics described earlier for MEN 2A.

Medullary Thyroid Carcinoma. MTC associated with MEN 2B is generally more aggressive and develops earlier in life than MTC in patients with MEN 2A (Carney et al. 1979). MEN 2B associated with C-cell hyperplasia has been reported in a patient 15 months old, with MTC in a patient 6 months old, and with MTC and subsequent metastasis in a child 5.5 years old (Telander et al. 1989). Metastatic disease generally occurs earlier, and symptomatic patients have metastases at the time of surgery and a higher rate of tumor recurrence (Vasen et al. 1987; Telander et al. 1986; Stjernholm et al. 1980; Kakuda et al. 1985). The bilateral and multicentric histologic changes associated with MTC in MEN 2A are also found in MEN 2B. MEN 2B is also transmitted as an autosomal dominant trait. Families with the syndrome have been described, but they represent a minority of the patients described in the literature (Dyck et al. 1979).

Screening for MEN 2A

Despite the fact that the MEN 2A syndrome has been characterized for at least 30 years, new families with this disorder are discovered regularly. Medical detective work will frequently demonstrate a relationship between the newly discovered family and a previously identified kindred known to carry the gene for this disorder (Ponder et al. 1988), although occasionally it is not possible to make this type of connection. As neither a negative family history nor absence of associated lesions conclusively prove a sporadic mutation of MTC, family screening should be considered for every new patient who presents with apparently sporadic MTC.

Identifying a new kindred places the physician in a difficult position. It is known that early intervention by screening and treatment results in lowered morbidity and mortality for those afflicted with this syndrome, making it important for the physician to apprise family members of the risks associated with the disease and the benefits of screening and treatment (Wells et al. 1985; Gagel et al. 1988). At the same time, however, there is concern that it may be intrusive of the physician to inform a family member, whom he does not know personally, that he or she is at risk to develop cancer. An approach to this problem that has been used with considerable success is to provide the affected family member (proband) with copies of a pamphlet describing the clinical findings and the risk for development of the syndrome[1] and ask that the patient take the responsibility for distributing this

[1] Gagel RF, Feldman ZT: Familial medullary thyroid carcinoma. A guide for affected families. This pamphlet describes the thyroid, parathyroid, and adrenal manifestations of multiple endocrine neoplasia type 2A utilizing simple diagrams and an approach to screening. A recent update includes information on genetic testing. It has been translated into the Swedish and Portuguese languages. A copy can be obtained from Robert F. Gagel, M.D., Box 15, 1515 Holcombe Blvd., Houston, TX 77030, USA.

information to other family members. In most instances, the proband is aware both of the seriousness of the syndrome and of the family social dynamics, and is willing to make this information available to family members in the least threatening manner. This initial contact usually results in the physician receiving calls from several concerned family members making it possible to organize a family meeting to discuss the disorder and organize screening efforts. In almost every family, there will be some members who, initially, will refuse counseling or screening. In most cases, this results from fear of testing or the fear of discovering a malignancy. For many of these individuals, an adjustment period is necessary for them to understand the benefits of screening procedures. In addition, family pressure to conform is sometimes a greater motivator than counsel from a physician. It is important, however, for medico-legal reasons, that the physician document efforts to apprise family members of the possibility of development of this syndrome, to maintain a responsible degree of communication with family members, and to be certain no members are ignorant of the consequences of failing to undergo early screening.

Biochemical Screening of MTC

Measurement of the serum calcitonin concentration after administration of a substance which stimulates calcitonin release remains the "gold standard" for the diagnosis of hereditary MTC.

Provocative Stimulators of Calcitonin Release

The earliest histologic lesion observed in the thyroid gland of gene carriers for MEN 2A is C-cell hyperplasia. There is evidence that this histological lesion results from an expansion of the number of C-cells within the thyroid gland and is a precursor to multifocal MTC (Wolfe et al. 1973; Wolfe and DeLellis 1981). The increase in C-cell number over time results in greater basal or stimulated (pentagastrin, calcium, or pentagastrin and calcium) calcitonin concentrations in humans (Wolfe and DeLellis 1981) or in animal (DeLellis et al. 1979) models of this disease. At some point in this progression there is a clear separation between calcitonin values found in normal family members and those with histologic abnormalities of the C-cell. Studies initiated almost 20 years ago have demonstrated that identification of affected individuals by this approach followed by total thyroidectomy has resulted in apparent cure (normal calcitonin values after a follow-up period of more than 10 years; Gagel et al. 1988).

The provocative test which has achieved most widespread acceptance is the bolus injection of pentagastrin (0.5 μg/kg body weight) with measurement of the serum calcitonin at 2, 5, 10, and 15 min after the injection

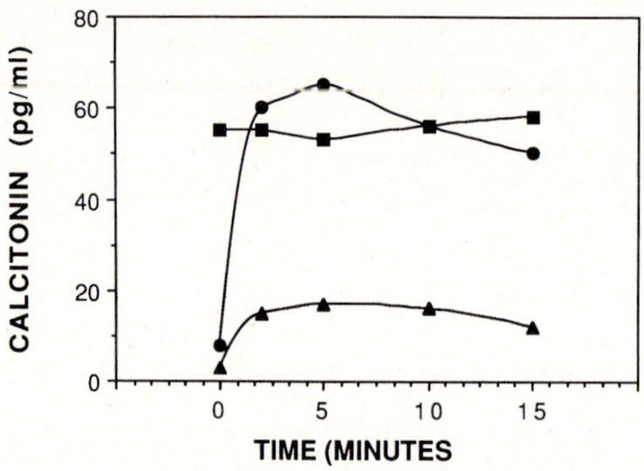

Fig. 2. Calcitonin response patterns after provocative stimulation with pentagastrin. Three types of calcitonin response patterns are depicted: a normal response (▲), a likely artifactual elevation of the serum calcitonin concentration with no further increase after provocative stimulation (■); and a response consistent with C-cell hyperplasia or early MTC (●). The *shaded region* shows the normal range of response

(Hennessey et al. 1973, 1974). Another variation of this test combines a 1-min calcium infusion with a pentagastrin injection (Wells et al. 1978). In general, the combination results in greater stimulation of calcitonin release. Finally, a short calcium infusion is an acceptable alternative in patients who cannot tolerate pentagastrin (Parthemore et al. 1974). Several types of response patterns may be observed. In both men and women there is normally an increase in the plasma calcitonin concentration after a provocative test (Fig. 2) with basal and stimulated calcitonin values being greater in men than in women (Deftos et al. 1980; Tiegs et al. 1986).

The decision as to which provocative test to use is less of an issue now than several years ago. The routine availability of sensitive and specific radioimmunoassays for calcitonin (Parthemore et al. 1974; Motte et al. 1987, 1988; Heath and Sizemore 1977) has standardized the measurement of normal plasma calcitonin concentrations, thereby eliminating some of the overlap between normal and abnormal seen when first generation assays were used (Deftos et al. 1971; Tashjian et al. 1974). In particular, artifactual elevations of serum calcitonin can be excluded by measurement in either two-site immunoradiometric (Motte et al. 1988) or extraction assays (Heath and Sizemore 1977). Nonetheless it is inevitable that some overlap between normal and early abnormal test results will exist.

Problems with Annual Pentagastrin Testing

There are limitations and drawbacks to screening by pentagastrin testing. Annual or more frequent screening from the age of 3 years is necessary to identify affected individuals, and the average child at risk for MEN 2 must be tested for 5–8 years (Gagel et al. 1982). Fortunately improved sensitivity of assays has lowered the mean age of diagnosis, but a minimum of 5 years of screening is likely. Some family members have difficulty complying with the necessity for annual testing.

Provocative tests are not dangerous and usually are well tolerated by children, but can be unpleasant. The authors are aware of a few patients who have developed pronounced symptoms, but this is unusual. It is *important* to provide the patient with a clear explanation of the symptoms (flushing, tingling of extremities, nausea, and tightness of the lower chest) likely to be experienced during a pentagastrin test, and reassurance that these symptoms will end less than 2 min after the injection.

Operative Decisions

In most cases the finding of two consecutive or nonconsecutive abnormal pentagastrin tests (as defined above) will lead to a decision to operate. In some children the differentiation between normal and abnormal may be less clear, making a longer period of follow-up and retesting necessary. The physician should not feel pressured into making a decision based on inadequate information. Continued testing or correlation with genetic information to be discussed below will, in most cases, clarify the diagnosis. The finding that C-cell hyperplasia may exist in apparently nonaffected members of some MEN 2 families has further complicated diagnostic efforts, but this phenomenon appears to be limited to a few families (Lips et al. 1987). Patients with phenotypic features of MEN 2B are an exception. Thyroidectomy should be performed at the earliest possible time after birth because of the high risk of early metastatic disease.

Screening for Pheochromocytoma

The primary goal of screening for pheochromocytoma in MEN 2 is to identify and treat patients prior to the development of the life-threatening manifestations of pheochromocytoma. It does not seem reasonable to perform bilateral adrenalectomy, with the incumbent risks of adrenal insufficiency, on all patients with MEN 2. Most clinicians, therefore, have adopted a compromise approach in which they screen for pheochromocytoma at regular intervals. An integrated measurement of catecholamine secretion such as a 12- or 24-h urine measurement of catecholamines or metanephrines, or repetitive measurement of plasma catecholamines (Vistelle et al. 1991) and a careful history has proven to be the most reliable approach to the diagnosis during routine screening.

Patients with increased catecholamine production will frequently complain of palpitations, tachycardia, nervousness or jitteriness and occasional headaches. Hypertension during the early phases of enhanced adrenal medullary growth is rare and may be attributable to the increased production of epinephrine relative to norepinephrine (Hamilton et al. 1978; Miyauchi et al. 1982; Gagel et al. 1988). The optimal frequency of screening is not completely clear although annual measurements appear to detect most pheochromocytomas prior to the development of significant symptoms (Fig. 3) (Gagel et al. 1975, 1988). Although abnormal accumulation of radioiodinated metaiodobenzylguanidine is an early characteristic of the adrenal lesion (Jones and Sisson 1983), there is concern that repetitive exposure to radiation might enhance the rate of growth or the malignant potential of the adrenal lesion. The diagnostic use of magnetic resonance imaging instead of radiation techniques such as computerized tomography may provide a safe alternative for more frequent imaging of the adrenal glands.

There is particular concern about the detection of pheochromocytoma in young women of childbearing years (20–40 years of age) because these are also the peak years for diagnosis of pheochromocytoma in MEN 2. Deaths have been reported as a result of catecholamine excess during labor and delivery (Chodankar et al. 1982; Moraca Kvapilova et al. 1985), and it is prudent to screen women at several points during the pregnancy to exclude this possibility. Because measurements of basal urine catecholamines may not detect small tumors which could become symptomatic during labor and delivery, the obstetrician and anesthesiologist should be alerted to the possibility of pheochromocytoma and take appropriate action to treat hypertension or tachycardia during labor and delivery.

Screening for Hyperparathyroidism

Each patient with MEN 2A should have an annual or biannual serum calcium measurement. The finding of elevated serum calcium and immunoreactive parathyroid hormone concentrations is usually indicative of primary hyperparathyroidism.

Use of Genetic Screening Tests for the Determination of Gene Carrier Status

The gene for MEN 2 has been mapped to the centromeric region of chromosome 10 (Mathew et al. 1987; Simpson et al. 1987). Subsequent studies have resulted in the mapping of MEN 2B and MTC – only syndromes to this same locus (Jackson et al. 1988; Lairmore et al. 1991). Subsequent efforts by several groups have resulted in a more detailed map of the disease gene region and the tentative assignment of the MEN 2 gene to the proximal long arm of chromosome 10.

Of particular significance for current management is the ability to utilize polymorphic DNA sequences closely linked to or flanking the MEN 2

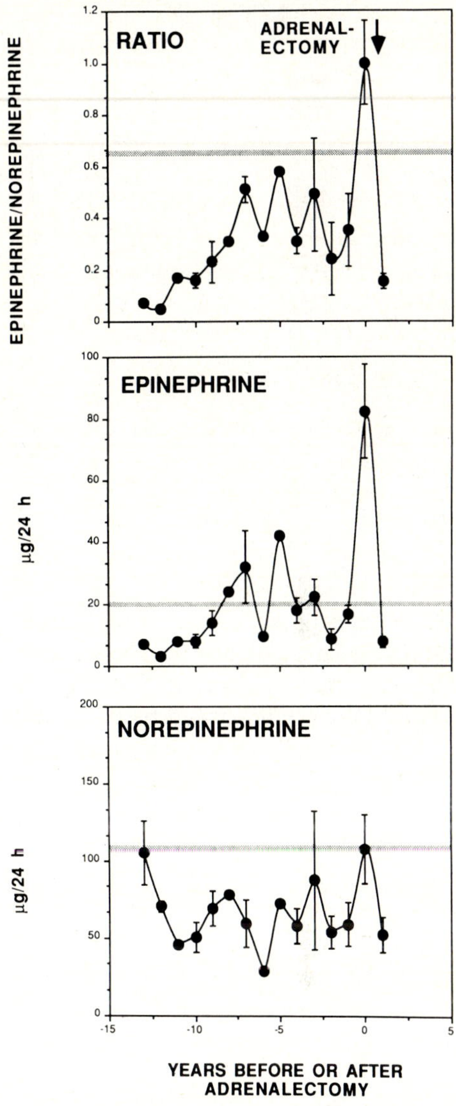

Fig. 3. Mean 24-h urine norepinephrine, epinephrine, and ratio of epinephrine to norepinephrine in 11 prospectively screened patients proved to have pheochromocytoma. Each *point* shows the mean values for each of these parameters from all available data on these 11 patients. The *gray line* shows the upper limit of normal. (Modified from Gagel et al. 1988)

locus to determine the gene carrier status for MEN 2. Polymorphic DNA sequences permit the separation of one parental allele from the other and permit tracking of the allele within a particular family. Several of the polymorphic DNA sequences for MEN 2 are so close to the disease gene that recombinant events (separation of the polymorphic DNA sequence and the disease gene for MEN 2) have not been observed (Fig. 4). This makes these alleles particularly useful for prediction of disease gene carrier status.

Several criteria must be met before a particular closely linked DNA sequence can become useful for diagnostic purposes. The first is that the

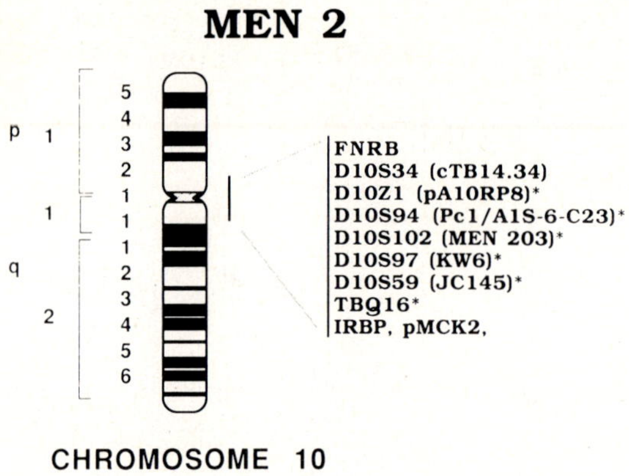

Fig. 4. Schematic diagram of chromosome 10 showing tentative ordering of polymorphic DNA sequences on chromosome 10. There has been no recombination with the MEN 2 locus observed for the DNA sequences indicated with an *asterisk*. This information was compiled from several sources as reviewed in Simpson (1991)

DNA sequences for a particular marker must be polymorphic in the MEN 2 family to be evaluated. By this is meant that it must be possible to separate the two alleles of a particular DNA sequence. Separation of the two alleles is generally accomplished by the finding of a restriction site in one copy of a particular gene (allele) that is not present in the other and which results in the two alleles being differently sized when separated by electrophoretic techniques. The technique is performed by restriction of DNA obtained from peripheral blood samples with a particular endonuclease, separation by an electrophoretic technique on the basis of size, transfer of the DNA to a nitrocellulose or nylon filter, and then hybridization with a radiolabeled DNA sequence which is closely linked to the disease gene. Exposure of the filter to X-ray film will show a pattern similar to that shown in Fig. 5.

In this example separation of parental alleles and those passed to each child is straightforward, making it possible to track the inheritance of a particular allele through several generations (Fig. 5). If a genetic disease is closely linked to a particular allele, it is possible to predict disease status by determining which allele is associated with the disease and then following the pattern of inheritance. Although the determination of risk is now routinely performed by computer analysis, interpretation in an informative family can frequently be performed by visual analysis. The first step in this process is to determine on which allele the disease gene is located (determine *phase*). The finding in Fig. 6 that allele B is inherited by an affected daughter from the affected mother (with it being obligatory that the other allele came from the unaffected father) establishes phase. It then becomes possible to determine which of the daughter's children carry the disease allele.

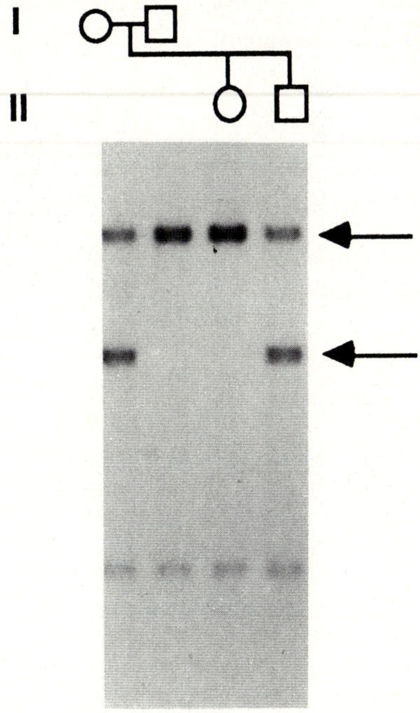

Fig. 5. Restriction fragment length polymorphism. DNA was isolated from all family members, restricted with *Bgl*II, separated by agarose electrophoresis, and then transferred to a nylon membrane. Hybridization with H4.IRBP was performed, followed by autoradiography. The restriction fragment length polymorphism in this family permits separation of parental alleles (*arrows*). The mother is heterozygous for the two alleles; the father is homozygous for the upper allele. One child is homozygous for the upper allele and the other heterozygous for the two alleles. There is a constant band shown at the bottom of the autoradiogram that is present in all family members and is likely to represent nonspecific binding of the radiolabeled DNA to genomic DNA. Reprinted by permission of the publisher from "The impact of gene mapping techniques on the management of multiple endocrine neoplasia type 2", by RF Gagel, Trends in Endocrinology and Metabolism 2:19–25. Copyright 1990 by Elsevier Science Publishing Co., Inc. (Gagel 1991)

There are several possible pitfalls associated with this type of analysis. There exists the possibility of a recombinant event between the closely linked marker and the disease gene resulting in incorrect assignation of clinical status (Fig. 7A). Another possibility is the inability to separate parental alleles, thereby making it impossible to establish phase (Fig. 7B). Finally, this technique may be informative in some family members but not others (Fig. 7C).

The validity of information obtained by utilization of closely linked markers is dependent upon the recombination rate of a particular polymorphic DNA sequence with the disease gene. Although it is believed that the currently available flanking DNA markers for MEN 2 may be several

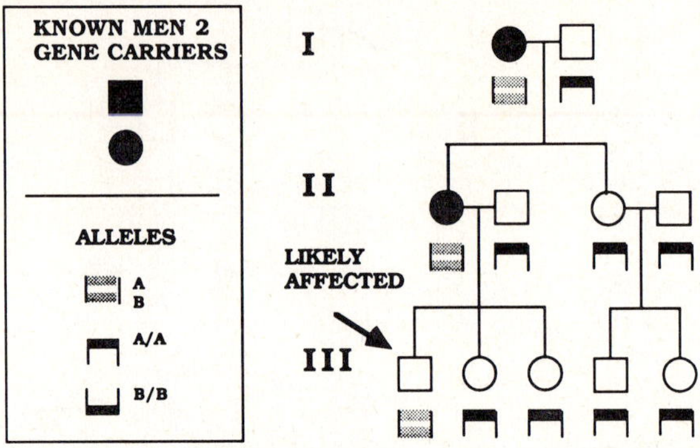

Fig. 6. Utilization of restriction fragment polymorphism with polymorphic DNA markers closely linked to the disease locus to predict disease in children of an affected parent. In this example, it is possible to predict (within the limitations described in the text) that patient III-1 is a likely gene carrier (he inherited allele A from his father and allele B – the allele on which the disease locus is located – from his mother), whereas III-2 and III-3 inherited allele A from the mother, making it likely they are not gene carriers. It is also possible to predict that the mother (II-3) and her children are not gene carriers. (From Gagel 1991) Reprinted by permission of the publisher from "The impact of gene mapping techniques on the management of multiple endocrine neoplasia type 2", by RF Gagel, Trends in Endocrinology and Metabolism 2:19–25. Copyright 1990 by Elsevier Science Publishing Co., Inc. (Gagel et al. 1991)

million bases from the disease gene, the finding of a low recombination rate in this region of chromosome 10 and the availability of at least six DNA sequences for which no recombination between the marker and the MEN 2 gene has been observed (Fig. 4) makes it possible to predict disease status for most family members when these probes or other sequences closer to the disease gene are used.

There are possible confounding issues. For example, there exists the remote possibility that a second nonchromosome-10 MEN 2 locus exists. Current information linking each of the forms of MEN 2 to the chromosome 10 locus make this unlikely; however, it is desirable to perform linkage analysis in a particular family to exclude this possibility if the family is large enough (>10 affected family members). A second confounding factor may be incorrect assignation of paternity leading to an incorrect diagnosis.

How Should Genetic Information Be Used?

Although gene carrier status can now be predicted with near certainty, there still exists the very small possibility of a recombinant event resulting in the incorrect prediction of disease status. The information obtained by genetic testing should be treated in a similar manner as information obtained re-

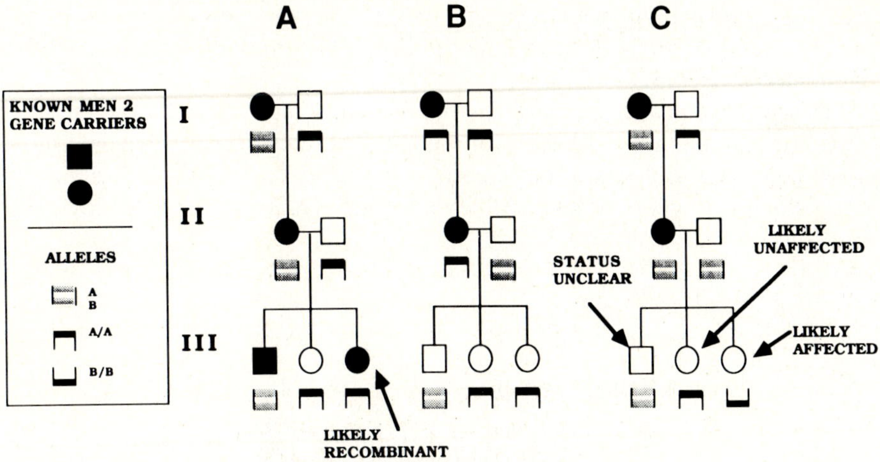

Fig. 7 A–C. Restriction fragment length polymorphism patterns that make it impossible to predict disease status with certainty. **A** Recombination. The clinical status of each member of this family is known with certainty. The pattern of inheritance observed in III-3 could only have been caused by a recombination event. **B** Inability to determine phase. It is not possible to predict the disease status of the individuals in the third generation. Although the disease is linked to allele A, it is not possible to determine *which* allele A is linked to the disease gene in the two affected individuals (I-1 and II-1). It, therefore, is not possible to predict the disease status of any of the individuals in the third generation. **C** Noninformative. In this example, it is possible to establish phase (the disease gene is linked to allele B), but it is possible to establish carrier status in only III-2 and III-3; for III-1, it is not possible to determine from which parent allele B was inherited. Reprinted by permission of the publisher from "The impact of gene mapping techniques on the management of multiple endocrine neoplasia type 2", by RF Gagel, Trends in Endocrinology and Metabolism 2:19–25. Copyright 1990 by Elsevier Science Publishing Co., Inc. (Gagel 1991)

garding the age-related probability of development of MTC (Gagel et al. 1982). Here, it was possible to predict that an individual older than 35 years of age had a subsequent probability of development of MTC of less than 5%. Because the probability of development of disease was low, it did not seem reasonable to continue testing at frequent intervals for likely unaffected family members. A recommendation was made that the frequency of testing be reduced and eventually discontinued. A similar type of approach could be applied to the family member for whom genetic tests predict noncarrier status. The likelihood of an incorrect prediction is low, but the implications of missing the diagnosis so great that pentagastrin testing should be performed, albeit at a reduced frequency.

How to manage the patient considered to be a gene carrier by genetic testing is not clear at present. There exists the small possibility (<0.1%) of incorrectly predicting gene carrier status, making it imprudent to make a recommendation for thyroidectomy without correlative calcitonin results.

An individual patient with positive genetic tests and normal calcitonin test results, however, may elect to undergo thyroidectomy rather than repetitive pentagastrin testing.

This particular decision will be complicated in most cases by the fact that a parent will make the decision for a child. These choices will become more clearly defined and somewhat easier to make when the MEN 2 gene has been cloned. It will then be possible to predict gene carrier status with 100% certainty.

References

Cance WG, Wells SA (1985) Multiple endocrine neoplasia type IIa. Curr Probl Surg 22:1–56

Carney JA, Sizemore GW, Sheps SG (1976a) Adrenal medullary disease in multiple endocrine neoplasia, type 2. Am J Clin Pathol 66:279–285

Carney JA, Go VLW, Sizemore GW, Hayles AB (1976b) Alimentary-tract ganglioneuromatosis, a major component of the syndrome of multiple endocrine neoplasia type 2b. N Engl J Med 295:1287–1291

Carney JA, Sizemore GW, Hayles AB (1978) Multiple endocrine neoplasia type 2b. Pathol Annu 8:105–153

Carney JA, Sizemore GW, Hayles AB (1979) C-cell disease of the thyroid gland in multiple endocrine neoplasia, type 2b. Cancer 44:2173–2183

Chodankar CM, Abhyankar SC, Deodhar KP, Shanbhag AM (1982) Sipple's syndrome (multiple endocrine neoplasia) in pregnancy – case report. Aust N Z J Obstet Gynaecol 22:243–244

Chong GC, Beahrs OH, Sizemore GW, Woolner LH (1975) Medullary carcinoma of the thyroid gland. Cancer 35:695–704

Deftos LJ, Bury AE, Habener JF, Singer FR, Potts JT Jr (1971) Immunoassay for human calcitonin. II. Clinical studies. Metabolism 20:1129–1137

Deftos LJ, Weisman MH, Williams GW, Karpf DB, Frumar AM, Davidson BJ, Parthemore JG, Judd HL (1980) Influence of age and sex on plasma calcitonin in human beings. N Engl J Med 302:1351–1353

DeLellis RA, Nunnemacher G, Bitman WR, Gagel RF, Tashjian AH Jr, Blount M, Wolfe HJ (1979) C-cell hyperplasia and medullary thyroid carcinoma in the rat. An immunohistochemical and ultrastructural analysis. Lab Invest 40:140–154

Dyck PJ, Carney JA, Sizemore GW, Okazaki H, Brimijoin WS, Lanbert EH (1979) Multiple endocrine neoplasia type 2b: phenotype recognition, neurological features and their pathological basis. Ann Neurol 6:302–314

Farndon JR, Leight GS, Dilley WG, Baylin SB, Smallridge RC, Harrison TS, Wells SA (1986) Familial medullary thyroid carcinoma without associated endocrinopathy: a distinct clinical entity. Br J Surg 73:278–281

Frank K, Raue F, Gottswinter J, Heinrich U, Meybier H, Ziegler R (1984) Importance of early diagnosis and follow-up in multiple endocrine neoplasia (MEN IIB). Eur J Pediatr 143:112–116

Gagel RF (1991) The impact of gene mapping techniques on the diagnosis of multiple endocrine neoplasia type 2. Trends Endocrinol Metab 2:19–25

Gagel RF, Melvin KE, Tashjian AH Jr, Miller HH, Feldman ZT, Wolfe HJ, DeLellis RA, Cerviskinner S, Reichlin S (1975) Natural history of the familial medullary thyroid carcinoma-pheochromocytoma syndrome and the identification of preneoplastic stages by screening studies: a five-year report. Trans Assoc Am Physicians 88:177–191

Gagel RF, Jackson CE, Block MA, Feldman ZT, Reichlin S, Hamilton BP, Tashjian AH Jr (1982) Age-related probability of development of hereditary medullary thyroid carcinoma. J Pediatr 101:941–946

Gagel RF, Tashjian AH Jr, Cummings T, Papathanasopoulos N, Kaplan MM, DeLellis RA, Wolfe HJ, Reichlin S (1988) The clinical outcome of prospective screening for multiple endocrine neoplasia type 2a. An 18-year experience. N Engl J Med 318:478–484

Gagel RF, Levy ML, Donovan DT, Alford BR, Wheeler T, Tschen JA (1989) Multiple endocrine neoplasia type IIa associated with cutaneous lichen amyloidosis. Ann Intern Med 3:802–806

Griffiths AM, Mack DR, Byard RW, Stinger DA, Shandling B (1990) Multiple endocrine neoplasia IIb, an unusual cause of chronic constipation. J Pediatr 116:285–288

Grün R, Eberle F (1981) Multiple endocrine neoplasia type II (MEN II). Ergeb Inn Med Kinderheilkol 46:151–201

Hamilton BP, Landsberg L, Levine RJ (1978) Measurement of urinary epinephrine in screening for pheochromocytoma in multiple endocrine neoplasia type II. Am J Med 65:1027–1032

Heath H III, Sizemore GW (1977) Plasma calcitonin in normal man: differences between men and women. J Clin Invest 60:1135–1140

Heath H III, Sizemore GW, Carney JA (1976) Preoperative diagnosis of occult parathyroid hyperplasia by calcium infusion in patients with multiple endocrine neoplasia type 2a. J Clin Endocrinol Metab 43:428–435

Hennessey JF, Gray TK, Cooper CW, Ontjes DA (1973) Stimulation of thyrocalcitonin secretion by pentagastrin and calcium in 2 patients with medullary thyroid carcinoma of the thyroid. J Clin Endocrinol Metab 36:200–203

Hennessey JF, Wells SA, Ontjes DA, Cooper CW (1974) A comparison of pentagastrin injections and calcium infusion as provocative agents for the detection of medullary carcinoma of the thyroid. J Clin Endocrinol Metab 39:487

Hill CS, Ibanez ML, Samaan NA, Ahearn MJ, Clark RL (1973) Medullary (solid) carcinoma of the thyroid gland, an analysis of the MD Anderson Hospital experience with patients with the tumor, its special features, and its histogenesis. Medicine (Baltimore) 52:141–171

Jackson CE, Norum CE, O'Neal LW, Nikolai TF, Delaney JP (1988) Linkage between MEN 2b and chromosome 10 markers linked to MEN 2a. Am J Hum Genet 43:A147

Jadoul M, Leo JR, Berends HH, Ooms ECM, Buurke EJ, Vasen HFA, Seelen PJ, Lips CJM (1989) Pheochromocytoma-induced hypertensive encephalopathy revealing MEN IIa syndrome in a 13 year-old boy. Horm Metab Res Suppl 21:46–49

Jones BA, Sisson JC (1983) Early diagnosis and thyroidectomy in multiple endocrine neoplasia, type 2b. J Pediatr 102:219–223

Kakuda K, Carney A, Sizemore GW (1985) Medullary carcinoma of thyroid, biologic behavior of sporadic and familial neoplasm. Cancer 55:2818–2821

Keiser JR, Beaven MA, Doppmann J, Wells B, Buja LM (1973) Medullary thyroid carcinoma, pheochromocytoma, and parathyroid disease. Ann Intern Med 78:561–579

Khairi MRA, Dexter RN, Burzynski NJ, Johnston CC (1975) Mucosal neuroma, pheochromocytoma and medullary thyroid carcinomas multiple endocrine neoplasia type 3. Medicine (Baltimore) 54:89–112

Khan AH, Desjardins JG, Youssef S, Gregoire, Seidman E (1987) Gastrointestinal manifestations of Sipple syndrome in children. J Pediatr Surg 22:719–723

Lairmore TC, Howe JR, Korte JA, Dilley WG, Aine L, Aine E, Wells SAJ, Donis Keller H (1991) Familial medullary thyroid carcinoma and multiple endocrine neoplasia type 2B map to the same region of chromosome 10 as multiple endocrine neoplasia type 2A. Genomics 9:181–192

Lips KJ, van der Sluys Veer J, Struyvenberg A, Alleman A, Leo JR, Wittebol P, Minder WH, Kooiker CJ, Geerdink RA, van Vaes PF, Hackeng WH (1981) Bilateral occurrence of pheochromocytoma in patients with the multiple endocrine neoplasia syndrome type 2A (Sipple's syndrome). Am J Med 70:1051–1060

Lips CJM, Leo JR, Berends MJH, Minder WH, Blok APR, Geerdink RA, Hackeng WHL, Roelofs JMM, Vasen HFA, Vette JK (1987) Thyroid C-cell hyperplasia and micronodules in close relatives of MEN 2A patients: pitfalls in early diagnosis and reevaluation of criteria for surgery. Henry Ford Hosp Med J 35:133–138

Mahaffey SM, Martin LW, McAdams AJ, Ryckman FC, Torres M (1990) Multiple endocrine neoplasia type IIb with symptoms suggesting Hirschsprung's disease: a case report. J Pediatr Surg 25:101–103

Markey WS, Rayn WG, Economou SG, Sizemore GW, Arnand CD (1973) Familial medullary carcinoma and parathyroid adenoma without pheochromocytoma. Ann Intern Med 78:898–1005

Mathew CG, Chin KS, Easton DF, Thorpe K, Carter C, Liou GI, Fong SL, Bridges CD, Haak H, Kruseman AC, Schifter S, Hansen HH, Telenius H, Telenius-Berg M, Ponder BAJ (1987) A linked genetic marker for multiple endocrine neoplasia type 2A on chromosome 10. Nature 328:527–528

Melvin KEW, Tashjian AH, Miller HH (1972) Studies in familial medullary thyroid carcinoma. Recent Prog Horm Res 28:399–470

Miyauchi A, Masuo K, Ogihara T, Takai S, Matsuzuka F, Kuma K, Maeda M, Kumahara Y, Kosaki G (1982) Urinary epinephrine and norepinephrine excretion in patients with medullary thyroid carcinoma and their relatives. Nippon Naibunpi Gakkai Zasshi 58:1505–1516

Moraca Kvapilova L, Op de Coul AA, Merkus JM (1985) Cerebral haemorrhage in a pregnant woman with a multiple endocrine neoplasia syndrome (type 2A or Sipple's syndrome). Eur J Obstet Gynecol Reprod Biol 20:257–263

Motte P, Ait-Abdellah M, Vauzelle P, Gardet P, Bohuon C, Bellet D (1987) A two-site immunoradiometric assay for serum calcitonin using monoclonal antipeptide antibodies. Henry Ford Hospital Med J 35:129–132

Motte P, Vauzelle P, Gardet P, Ghillani P, Caillou B, Parmentier C, Bohuon C, Bellet D (1988) Construction and clinical validation of a sensitive and specific assay for serum mature calcitonin using monoclonal anti-peptide antibodies. Clin Chim Acta 174:35–54

Nunziata V, Giannattasio R, di Giovanni, D Armiento MR, Mancini M (1989) Hereditary localized pruritus in affected members of a kindred with multiple endocrine neoplasia type 2A (Sipple's syndrome). Clin Endocrinol (Oxf) 30:57–63

Parthemore JG, Bronzert D, Roberts G, Deftos LJ (1974) A short calcium infusion in the diagnosis of medullary thyroid carcinoma. J Clin Endocrinol Metab 39:108–111

Ponder BA, Ponder MA, Coffey R, Pembrey ME, Gagel RF, Telenius-Berg M, Semple P, Easton DF (1988) Risk estimation and screening in families of patients with medullary thyroid carcinoma. Lancet 1:397–401

Raue F, Frank K, Meybier H, Ziegler R (1985) Pheochromocytoma in multiple endocrine neoplasia. Cardiology 72 Suppl 1:147–149

Raue F, Komposch G, Ziegler R (1986) Mucosal neuromas of the lips and tongue, early symptoms of multiple endocrine neoplasia type IIb. Dtsch Zahnärztl Z 41:1000–1001

Saad MF, Ordonez NG, Rashid RK, Guido JJ, Hill CS, Hichey RC, Sakmaan NA (1984) Medullary carcinoma of the thyroid: a study of the clinical features and prognostic factors in 161 patients. Medicine 63:319–342

Schimke RN, Hartmann WH (1965) Familial amyloid-producing medullary thyroid carcinoma and pheochromocytoma, a distinct genetic entity. Ann Intern Med 63:1027–1031
Simpson NE (1991) The exploration of the locus or loci for the syndromes associated with medullary thyroid cancer (MTC) on chromosome 10. In: Brandi ML, White E (eds) Hereditary tumors. New York, Raven, pp 55–67
Simpson NE, Kidd KK, Goodfellow PJ, McDermid H, Myers S, Kidd JR, Jackson CE, Duncan AM, Farrer LA, Brasch K (1987) Assignment of multiple endocrine neoplasia type 2A to chromosome 10 by linkage. Nature 328:528–530
Sipple JH (1961) The association of pheochromocytoma with carcinoma of the thyroid gland. Am J Med 31:163–166
Steiner AL, Goodmann AD, Powers SR (1968) Study of a kindred with pheochromocytoma, medullary thyroid carcinoma, hyperparathyroidism, and Cushing's disease: MEN, type II. Medicine (Baltimore) 47:371–409
Stjernholm MR, Freudenbourg JC, Mooney HS, Kinney FJ, Deftos LJ (1980) Medullary carcinoma of the thyroid before age 2 years. J Clin Endocrinol Metab 51:252–253
Tashjian AH Jr, Wolfe HJ, Voelkel EF (1974) Human calcitonin: immunologic assay, cytologic localization and studies on medullary thyroid carcinoma. Am J Med 56:840–849
Telander RJ, Zimmermann D, van Heerden JA, Sizemore GW (1986) Results of early thyroidectomy for medullary thyroid carcinoma in children with multiple endocrine neoplasia type 2. J Pediatr Surg 21:1190–1194
Telander RJ, Zimmermann D, Sizemore GW, van Heerden JA, Grant CS (1989) Medullary carcinoma in children, results of early detection and surgery. Arch Surg 128:841–843
Tiegs RD, Body JJ, Barta JM, Heath H III (1986) Secretion and metabolism of monomeric human calcitonin: effects of age, sex, and thyroid damage. J Bone Miner Res 1:339–349
Vasen HFA, Nieuwenhuyzen-Krusemann AC, Berkel H, Benkers EK, Delprat CC, von Doorn RG, Geerdink RA, Haak HR, Hackeng WH, Koppenschaar HPF, Krenning EP, Lamberts SWJ, Lekkerkerker FJF, Michels RPJ, Moers AMJ, Pieters GFFM, Wiersinga WM, Lips CJM (1987) Multiple endocrine neoplasia syndrome type 2: the value of screening and central registration, a study of 15 kindreds in the Netherlands. Am J Med 83:847–852
Vistell R, Grulef H, Fay R, Delisle MJ, Caron J (1991) High permanent plasma adrenaline levels: a marker of adreual medullary disease in medullary thyroid carcinoma. Clin Endocrinal 34:133–138
Wells SA Jr, Baylin SB, Linehan WM et al. (1978) Provocative agents and the diagnosis of medullary carcinoma of the thyroid gland. Ann Surg 188:139–141
Wells SA, Dilley WG, Farndon JA, Leight GS, Baylin SB (1985) Early diagnosis and treatment of medullary thyroid carcinoma. Arch Intern Med 145:1248–1252
Williams ED, Pollock DJ (1966) Multiple mucosal neuromata with endocrine tumours: a syndrome allied to von Recklinghausen's disease. J Pathol Bacteriol 91:71–80
Wolfe HJ, DeLellis RA (1981) Familial medullary thyroid carcinoma and C-cell hyperplasia. Clin Endocrinol Metab 10:351–365
Wolfe HJ, Melvin KEW, Cervi-Skinner SJ et al. (1973) C-cell hyperplasia preceding medullary thyroid carcinoma. N Engl J Med 289:437–441

Imaging Methods for Medullary Thyroid Cancer

C. Reiners

Klinik für Nuklearmedizin, Universitätsklinikum Essen, Hufelandstraße 55,
W-4300 Essen, FRG

Introduction

Imaging of multiple endocrine neoplasia (MEN) syndromes is a challenge not only for the radiologist but for every physician engaged in ultrasonography (US), conventional radiology, computerized tomography (CT), magnetic resonance imaging (MRI), and scintigraphy (SC). Doppman (1985) called the MEN syndromes "a nightmare" for the diagnostician because of the difficulty of detecting and localizing small tumors or even only hyperplasia of endocrine organs. Nevertheless, the primary aim of all efforts is detection of preclinical stages of organ involvement, as it is only in those early stages that curative therapy of medullary thyroid cancer (MTC) may be possible. On the other hand, sensitive imaging methods are needed for follow-up to localize suspected recurrences or metastases of MTC in patients with elevated serum tumor markers. In this context, the diagnostic efficacy of US, SC, CT, and MRI must be discussed. Additionally, the clinical value of fine needle aspiration (FNA) biopsy has to be considered.

Primary Diagnosis

The diagnostician may encounter a primary diagnosis of MTC with incidental pheochromocytoma in an index case of a family with hereditary MTC. More frequently, suspicion of MTC arises after a pathological result in a known MTC kindred is obtained from family screening using the pentagastrin stimulation test. Imaging procedures have to be used to localize the suspected thyroid tumors (Table 1). In addition, in patients with suspected MEN syndrome (MEN IIa or IIb), accompanying pheochromocytomas have to be diagnosed.

Table 1. Imaging techniques in patients with MEN 2: primary diagnosis

MTC:	– Sonography – Thyroid scintigraphy (^{99m}Tc) – Aspiration biopsy (complementary)
Pheochromocytoma	– Sonography – CT – MRI – Adrenal scintigraphy (^{123}I MIBG)

MTC, medullary thyroid carcinoma; CT, computed tomography; MRI, magnetic resonance imaging; MIBG, metaiodobenzyl guanidine.

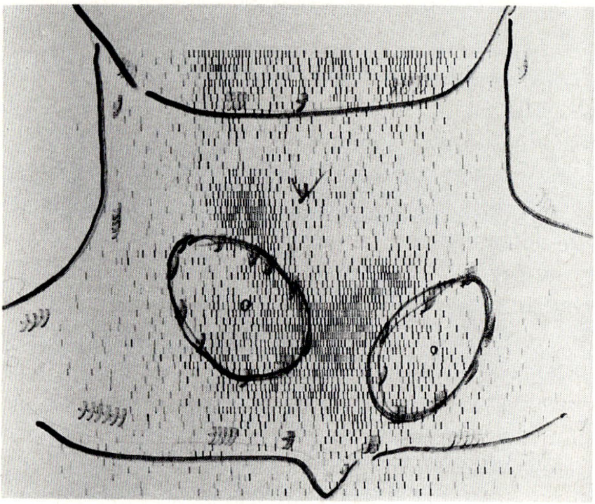

Fig. 1. ^{99m}Tc pertechnetate thyroid scan of a 50-year-old female with bilateral medullary thyroid carcinoma

Scintigraphy

Today, thyroid scanning is performed routinely using ^{99m}Tc pertechnetate. Figure 1 shows the incidental findings in a 50-year-old woman who was operated on for bilateral, large thyroid nodules. Typically, MTCs that were detectable scintigraphically as cold nodules were localized histologically in the lateral portions of both lobes.

Figure 2 shows the results of pentagastrin screening and pertechnetate SC in two sons of the patient mentioned above. The thyroid glands of both

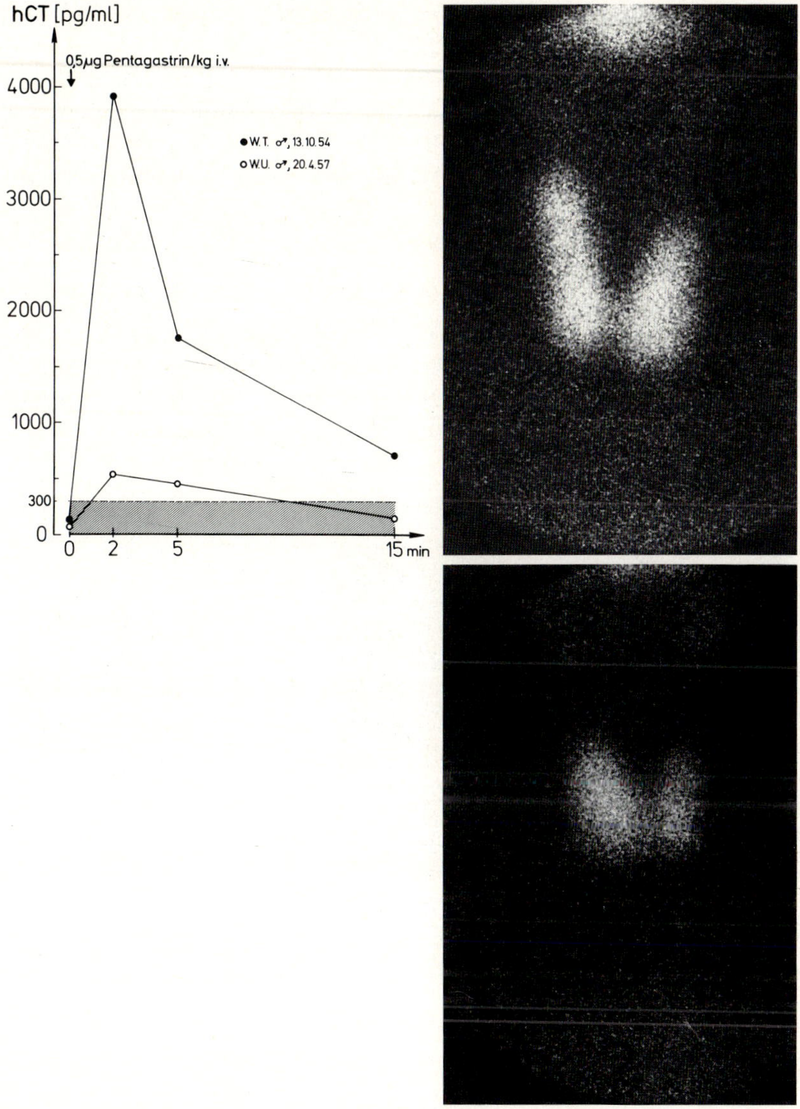

Fig. 2. Pathological increases of serum calcitonin after stimulation with 0.5 μg pentagastrin per kilogram of body weight iv in two brothers with hereditary medullary thyroid cancer. Thyroid scans were without abnormality

patients harbored small bilateral MTCs (diameters approx. 4 mm and 6 mm respectively). These early tumor stages could not be detected as cold nodules by pertechnetate SC (Fig. 2). The limited spatial resolution of SC with negative contrast does not allow localization of cold lesions smaller than approx. 1 cm.

Theoretically, SC with positive contrast using different radiopharmaceuticals with tumor affinity (see below), such as Tl-201 chloride, ^{99m}Tc(V) dimercaptosuccinic acid (DMSA) or radiolabeled anti-carcinoembryonic antigen (anti-CEA) antibodies should be better suited to tumor detection before surgery. Experiences with these techniques in primary diagnosis of MTC are limited; the main interest in tumor SC is focused on follow-up.

Sonography

In patients with suspected MTC, information about thyroidal and nodal involvement may be best derived using US. Figure 3 shows the thyroid sonogram of a patient with MEN IIa. Typically, the tumor in the right lobe is echointense whereas the left-sided tumor is hypointense.

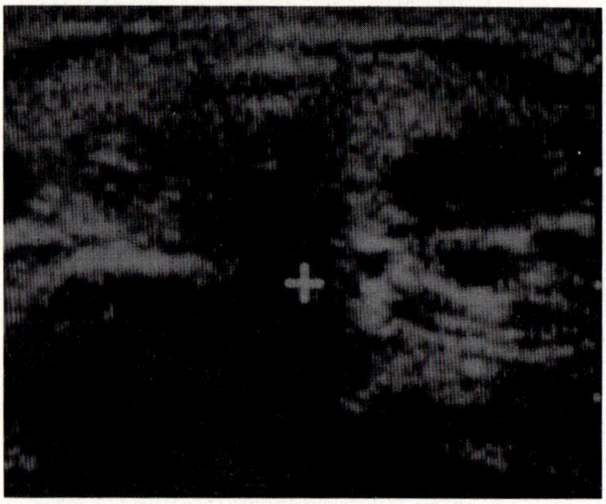

Fig. 3. Transversal sonogram of the neck (7.5 MHz transducer) from a patient with bilateral medullary thyroid cancer, left mass is hypoechogenic whereas right mass shows bright echos, possibly due to calcifications. (Example kindly provided by Priv.-Doz. Dr. Dr. Th. Olbricht, Department for Endocrinology, Essen University)

Table 2. Sonography of the thyroid: sensitivity in primary diagnosis of medullary thyroid carcinoma. (Schwerk et al. 1985)

Site	Size (mm)	hCT (pg/ml)		Sonogram
		Basal	Stimulated	
Hyperplasia	0	95	455	–
Unilateral	6	125	988	–
Bilateral	4/12	196	438	+
Unilateral	10	356	526	+
Bilateral	8/16	223	2924	+
Bilateral	30/14	637	966	+
Bilateral	14/12	664	1446	+
Bilateral	10/11	1338	9980	+
Bilateral	50/15	>10000	–	+
Unilateral	40	>10000	–	+

Schwerk et al. (1985) evaluated the diagnostic sensitivity of the US investigation in patients with hereditary MTC after laboratory screening. In this study (Table 2), tumors could be localized sonographically in 8 of 10 patients with pathological calcitonin (hCT) levels after pentagastrin stimulation. The lower limit of detectability with high frequency transducers

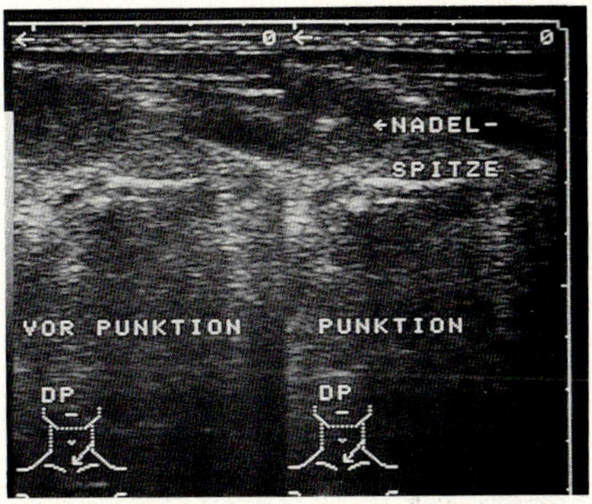

Fig. 4 Ultrasonographically guided fine needle aspiration biopsy of a thyroid lesion (*bright reflex*, needle tip)

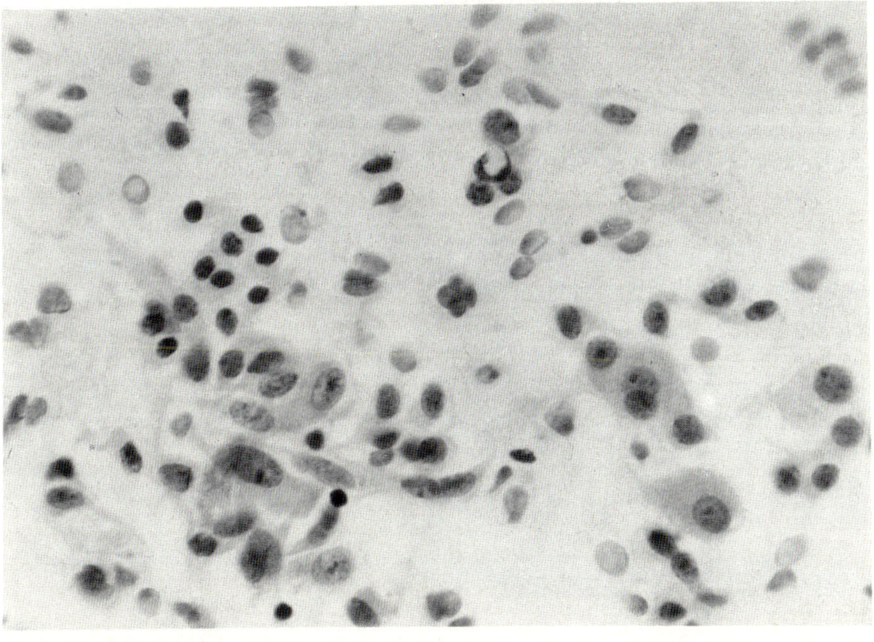

Fig. 5. Cytological appearance of medullary thyroid cancer. Roundish, prismatic to spindle-shaped, predominantly disseminated and often binucleated cells. Frequently eccentrically positioned nucleoli, moderate coarseness of chromatin pattern and rarely nuclear inclusions. (Slide kindly provided by Prof. Dr. R. Schäffer, Institute for Pathology, University of Giessen) H&E, ×40

(5–7.5 MHz) lies in the range of 3–4 mm. Compared to SC, CT, and MRI, US is a very simple and sensitive method for the detection of even small thyroidal lesions.

Fine Needle Aspiration Biopsy

In patients with suspected thyroidal lesions, diagnosis should be completed with (FNA) biopsy before surgery. Today, a sensitivity and specificity of aprox. 90% (Reiners et al. 1986a) can be achieved by ultrasonographically guided FNA (Fig. 4).

If FNA confirms the clinical suspicion for MTC (Fig. 5), the surgeon should follow a radical strategy and try to remove the thyroid and the lymph nodes totally. In addition, in patients in whom MTC is highly suspected according to FNA and/or serum level of hCT, diagnostic screening for pheochromocytoma by laboratory investigations and imaging procedures should be performed before surgery.

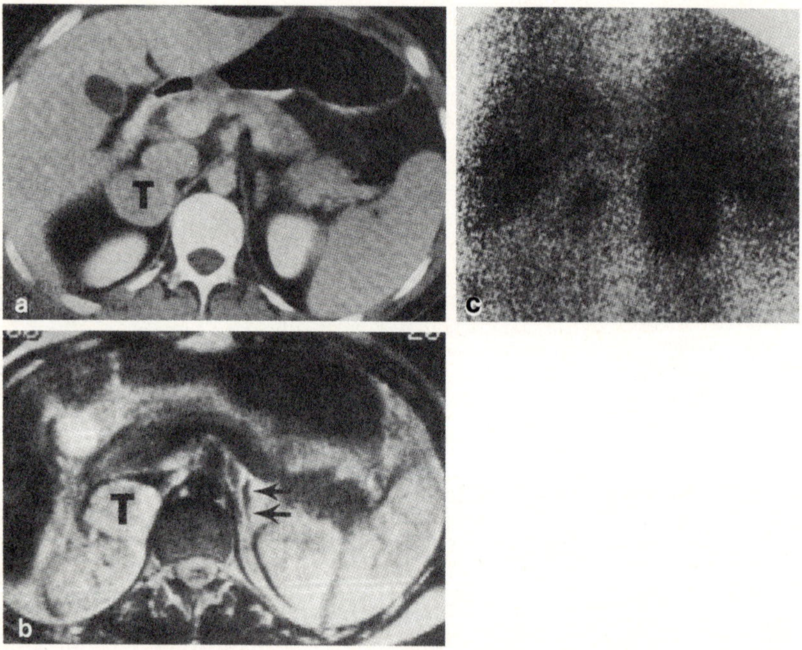

Fig. 6 a–c. Imaging in a patient with bilaterally proved pheochromocytoma in a patient with MEN 2B syndrome (Quint et al. 1987). **a** False-negative CT for left adrenal tumor. Scan shows only the large right adrenal tumor (*T*). **b** T2-weighted MR tomogram delineates large right adrenal mass better (*T*) but left adrenal appears normal as well (*arrows*). **c** ^{123}I MIBG scintigram (posterior view) shows large right and smaller left adrenal tumor clearly

Screening for Pheochromocytoma

Pheochromocytomas may also be localized by US, but the sensitivity of US (approx. 55%) for the detection of adrenal masses is not very high, as Georgi et al. (1984) pointed out. In their patients with various adrenal masses, Georgi et al. (1984) reached a sensitivity of approx. 90% with CT scanning.

Nearly identical results were presented by Francis et al. (1983) with CT (sensitivity 87%) in the primary diagnosis of a larger series of patients with pheochromocytomas. However, the group from Ann Arbor, where radiolabeling of metaiodobenzyl guanidine (MIBG) – a noradrenaline receptor ligand – had been developed (Wieland et al. 1980) got a better diagnostic sensitivity of 97% with ^{131}I MIBG scanning (Fig. 6) (Francis et al. 1983).

The sensitivity of MRI for primary diagnosis of pheochromocytoma has been evaluated by different groups. Quint et al. (1987) showed that T2-weighted images are much better suited for the delineation of pheochromocytomas than T1-weighted tomograms. Reinig et al. (1986) demonstrated earlier by semi-quantitative analysis that the adrenal mass/liver intensity ratio of T2 signals allows a clear cut separation of pheochromocytomas from adrenal adenomas (Fig. 7).

However, in some cases, pheochromocytomas may be undetectable by both MRI and CT; only the MIBG scan shows the metabolic activity of the adrenal tumor (Kafaghi et al. 1991; see Fig. 6). The comparison of studies published recently comparing the diagnostic performance of MRI, CT, and MIBG scanning yields the highest sensitivity for adrenal imaging by MIBG SC (Table 3). This view can be confirmed by the experiences of the Würzburg group (Spiegel et al. 1988). Patients with clinically occult pheo-

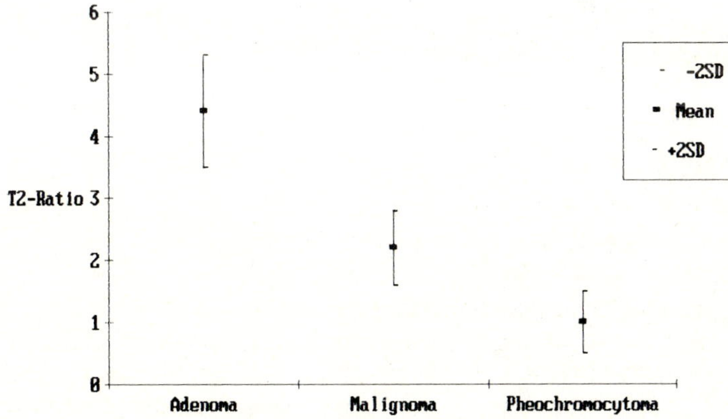

Fig. 7. Ratio of T2 signals from adrenal mass and liver, determined with MRI in patients with benign adrenal adenoma, adrenal malignoma and pheochromocytoma. (Reinig et al. 1986)

Table 3. MRI, CT, and MIBG scintigraphy: sensitivity in primary diagnosis of pheochromocytoma

	MRI	CT	MIBG scan
Mathieu et al. (1987)	10/10	9/10	8/10
Quint et al. (1987)	18/20	14/20	20/20
Velchik et al. (1989)	12/17	16/19	17/19
Total	40/47	39/49	45/49
Percentage	85%	80%	92%

MRI, magnetic resonance imaging; CT, computed tomography; MIBG, metaiodobenzyl guanidine.

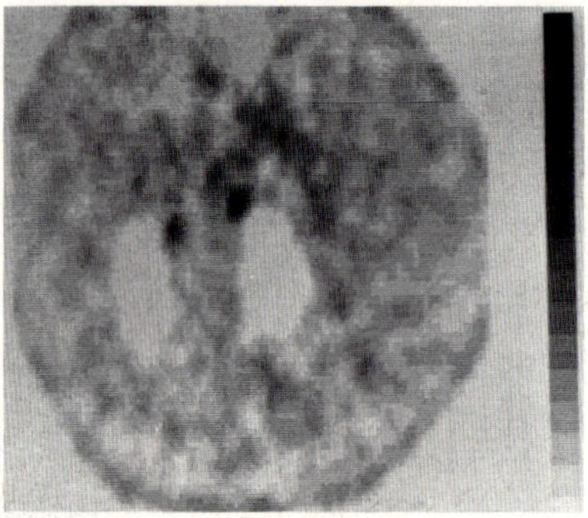

Fig. 8. ^{123}I MIBG scan in a patient with MEN IIa syndrome and small bilateral, clinically occult pheochromocytomas, showing pathological accumulation of the tracer in both adrenals

chromocytomas were investigated, including, for example, a patient where small tumors could only be delineated in the MIBG scan (Fig. 8). Spiegel et al. (1988) were able to show that MIBG SC is the most sensitive method for diagnosis of adrenal involvement in four out of six MEN IIa patients with clinically occult pheochromocytomas.

Staging and Follow-Up

In MTC, total resection of the tumor and possibly the lymph nodes is the only means of curing the patient of tumor disease. Prognosis is better if there is no nodal involvement primarily. Therefore, precise staging should be performed in patients with suspected MTC before surgery. Later on, the patient has to be followed up closely. Typically, the highly sensitive tumor markers hCT and CEA indicate a suspicion for recurrent or metastatic MTC. If recurrences or secondaries can be detected and localized early on, repeated surgical interventions may guarantee long periods of remission.

The whole spectrum of today's imaging procedures should be used for follow-up (Table 4); each method has its special uses. US is best suited to

Table 4. Imaging techniques in patients with MEN II: staging and follow-up

MTC	Sonography (neck, liver) X-Ray/CT/MRI (lung, mediastinum) Tumor scintigraphy (^{123}I MIBG, T1-201 chloride, ^{99m}Tc(V) DMSA, anti-CEA MAB)
Pheochromocytoma	Sonography (abdomen) CT/MRI (abdomen) Tumor scintigraphy with ^{123}I MIBG (whole body screening)

MTC, medullary thyroid carcinoma; CT, computed tomography; MRI, magnetic resonance imaging; MIBG, metaiodobenzyl guanidine; DMSA, dimercaptosuccinic acid; CEA, carcinoembryonic antigen; MAB, monoclonal antibody.

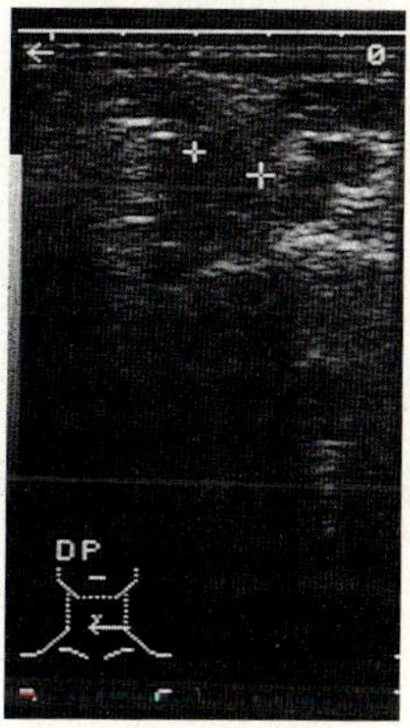

Fig. 9. Transversal sonogram of the neck (5 MHz transducer) in a patient with a small lymph node metastasis medial from the carotid artery and the jugular vein

routine examination of the neck, supplemented by conventional X-ray imaging, CT, or MRI in patients with suspected mediastinal or pulmonary involvement. With respect to SC, encouraging results have been published recently with different tracers.

Sonography

US allows the detection of nodal involvement and local recurrences in MTC rather precisely (Fig. 9). The Heidelberg group (Frank et al. 1987; Raue et al. 1989) evaluated the validity of US compared to palpation and CT in a larger series of MTC patients. Sonography which is quite easy to perform and may be repeated without limitations is superior even to CT in the follow-up of MTC (Table 5).

Sonography can also be used for the detection of liver metastases. As Fig. 10 shows, MTC metastases often show intense calcifications (Becker et al.

Table 5. Palpation, sonography and CT: sensitivity for the detection of local recurrences in medullary thyroid carcinoma. (Raue et al. 1989)

Examination	No. of patients	Positive findings *n*	%
Palpation	48	25	52
Sonography	27	21	78
Computed tomography	23	16	69

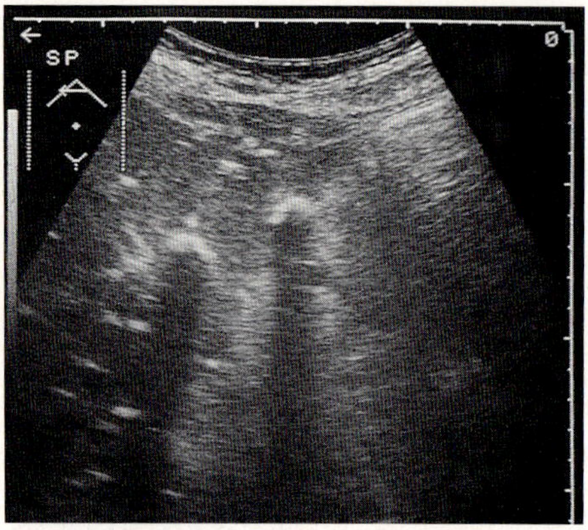

Fig. 10. Transversal sonogram of the abdomen (3.5 MHz sector scanner) in a patient with MEN IIa and calcifying liver metastases of medullary thyroid cancer

1986; Gorman et al. 1987), as is also the case with pulmonary metastases – as can be seen from the X-ray film (Fig. 11).

Scintigraphy

Metaiodobenzyl Guanidine

MIBG scanning should be used for primary diagnosis and follow-up of pheochromocytoma (Sisson et al. 1984; Spiegel et al. 1988; Valk et al. 1981). In addition, whole body scanning with this compound may also show tracer accumulation in recurrences or metastases of MTC (Endo et al. 1984). The most comprehensive study published up to now with MIBG for follow-up of MTC is the French cooperative study (Baulieu et al. 1987). The comparison of positive findings on MIBG scans in patients with elevated calcitonin levels (Table 6) yielded the highest sensitivity for hereditary MTC compared to sporadic MTC cases. However, the maximal sensitivity was not higher than 50%, which is unsatisfying in routine follow-up. This is in agreement with recent reports which yield an overall diagnostic sensitivity of MIBG SC for detection of MTC of only 31% (Table 7).

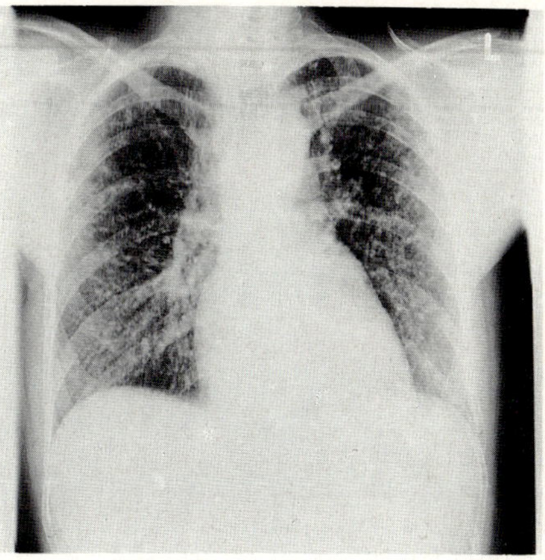

Fig. 11. Thorax X-ray of a patient with MEN IIa and calcifying lung metastases of medullary thyroid cancer (same patient as in Fig. 10)

Table 6. MIBG scintigraphy: sensitivity for the detection of recurrences and metastases in medullary thyroid carcinoma (French Cooperative Study). (Baulieu et al. 1987)

	Group	MIBG scan	
		n	%
I	hCT normal	0/11	0
II	hCT elevated (sporadic MTC)	3/24	13
III	hCT elevated (hereditary MTC)	7/15	42

Table 7. Sensitivity of $^{131}I/^{123}I$ MIBG scan in follow-up of medullary thyroid cancer

Reference	*n*
Hilditch et al. (1986)	1/5
Coutris et al. (1986)	2/2
Clarke et al. (1987)	4/16
Baulieu et al. (1987)	10/35
Hoefnagel et al. (1988)	3/11
Perdrisot et al. (1988)	2/6
Becker et al. (1989)	0/5
Cabezas et al. (1989)	2/8
Sandrock et al. (1989)	2/7
Guerra et al. (1989)	10/24
Troncone et al. (1989)	9/19
Verga et al. (1989)	1/12
	46/150 (31%)

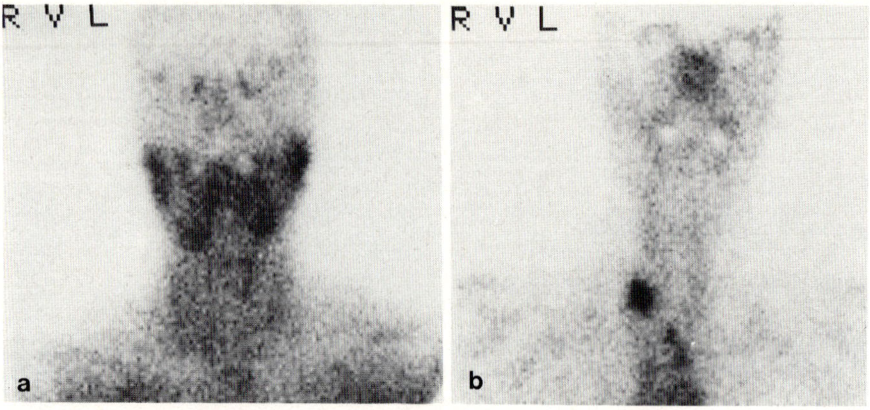

Fig. 12 a,b. Scintigrams of the neck in a patient with a right-sided recurrence of medullary thyroid cancer. **a** False-negative ^{201}Tl chloride scan. **b** Pathological accumulation of ^{99m}Tc(V)DMSA in the lesion

Table 8. Sensitivity of T1-201 scintigraphy in follow-up of medullary thyroid cancer

Reference	*n*
Talpos et al. (1985)	5/10
Arnstein et al. (1986)	2/2
Holub et al. (1987)	20/34
Hoefnagel et al. (1988)	11/12
Rufini et al. (1989)	4/5
Sandrock et al. (1989)	2/7
	44/70 (63%)

Tl-201 Chloride

For several years, Tl-201 has been used for scintigraphic imaging of recurrences and metastases in different histological types of thyroid cancer. According to our own experiences in more than 200 patients, Tl-201 SC is best suited for follow-up of follicular or papillary cancers which especially in cases of oncocytic variants do not take up radioiodine (Müller et al. 1990). The first patient with Tl-201 accumulation in MTC tumor tissue was reported in 1980 (Parthasarathy et al. 1980). Hoefnagel et al. (1988) evaluated systematically Tl-201 scanning in MTC patients; they found a tumor accumulation in 11 out of 12 patients with elevated serum calcitonin levels. Our own experiences with Tl-201 in MTC are not so satisfying; Fig. 12 a shows an example of a negative Tl-201 scan in a patient with a MTC recurrence in the right neck. On the whole, the diagnostic sensitivity of Tl-201 SC for follow-up of MTC falls in the range of 62% (Table 8).

Table 9. Preparation of $^{99m}Tc(V)$ DMSA

1.	Put 925 MBq of $^{99m}Tc\ O_4^-$ (in 2.5 ml of 0.9% NaCl) into an empty elution vial
2.	Add 0.1 ml aqua pro injectione +0.2 ml $NaHCO_3$
3.	Mix and check pH value (set point pH 8)
4.	Put this solution into a commercial lyophilized DMSA kit (1.2 mg DMSA, 0.31 mg Sn(II) Cl); mix gently for 15 min
5.	Quality control: Paper chromatography with *N*-butanol + acetic acid + H_2O

Pentavalent $^{99m}Tc(V)$ DMSA

Pentavalent $^{99m}Tc(V)$ DMSA was first used by the Japanese group of Ohta et al. (1984) for follow-up of MTC. After 5 years of our own experiences in more than 100 investigations, we now prefer this compound for tumor scanning in MTC. Figure 12b compares a high accumulation of $^{99m}Tc(V)$ DMSA – which is diagnostic without any doubt in a patient with recurrent MTC – with a negative T-201 scan (Fig. 12a).

It was recognized by Ikeda et al. (1977) that various ^{99m}Tc DMSA complexes – in the trivalent, tetravalent, and pentavalent state – behave biochemically quite differently. The trivalent $^{99m}Tc(III)$ DMSA complex with its high cortical accumulation is used routinely for renal scanning; it has to be prepared by reconstitution of ^{99m}Tc pertechnetate with DMSA at pH 5. The preparation at pH 8 yields the pentavalent $^{99m}Tc(V)$ DMSA anion (Dahir et al. 1989; Ikeda et al. 1977; Ramamoorthy et al. 1987), which has a structure comparable to the orthophosphate ion. Pentavalent DMSA therefore has an affinity to bony structures, as well as to certain tumors like MTC (Ohta et al. 1984; Ramamoorthy et al. 1987; Reiners 1988; Wulfrank et al. 1989). It is known from the literature that bone-seeking radiopharmaceuticals like ^{99m}Tc–labeled phosphonates sometimes accumulate in MTC tumor tissue (Becker et al. 1989; Johnson et al. 1984; Reuter et al. 1983; Shigeno et al. 1984).

The preparation of pentavalent $^{99m}Tc(V)$ DMSA by modification of commercial DMSA kits is quite simple (Kujath and Panitz 1989; Ramamoorthy et al. 1987; Westera et al. 1985). The only manipulation consists in alkalization of the ^{99m}Tc pertechnetate solution before adding it to the preparation vial with "cold" DMSA (Table 9).

In 1987, we began an open prospective study in patients with recurrent or metastatic MTC, comparing $^{99m}Tc(V)$ DMSA SC with clinical findings, tumor markers, US, CT, and with other scintigraphic procedures like Tl-201 scans or immunoscintigraphy using anti-CEA antibodies (Reiners 1988). Up to now, 62 MTC patients have been investigated. Including repeated scans, we performed more than 100 scans with $^{99m}Tc(V)$ DMSA in MTC patients; 600 MBq of the pentavalent complex prepared with a commercial DMSA kit were injected (Table 9). Routinely, we acquired multiple planar camera

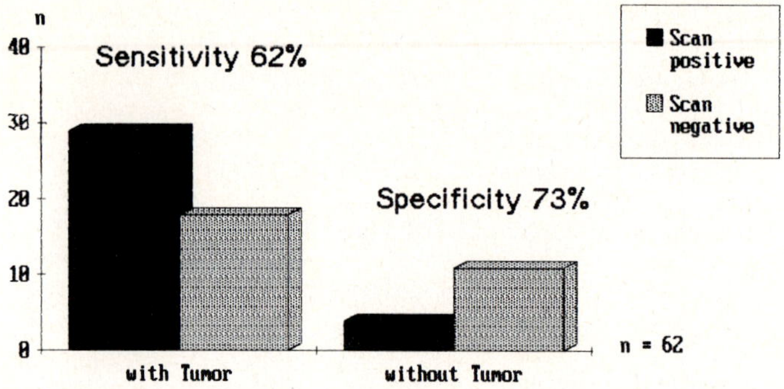

Fig. 13. Diagnostic efficacy of $^{99m}Tc(V)DMSA$ scanning in 62 patients with medullary thyroid cancer. Overall sensitivity amounts to 62% and specificity to 73%

images of the whole body 6h after intravenous injection. In most cases, single photon emission computed tomography (SPECT) scans of neck and thorax were added.

Figure 13 summarizes our results of $^{99m}Tc(V)$ DMSA scanning in follow-up of MTC: tumor localization was possible in 29 out of 47 patients with elevated serum levels of hCT (sensitivity 62%); four patients without elevation of the tumor marker showed unspecific uptake of pentavalent DMSA in skeletal lesions such as fractures (specificity 73%).

On the whole, a sensitivity of 62% and a specificity of 73% seems to be little less than excellent. But it has to be stressed that in 23 out of the 47 patients with "active" tumor, DMSA scanning was the only imaging procedure which was able to detect and localize the tumor. Those patients were referred to the surgeon again; in only one patient with a suspected metastasis to the spine was it not possible to confirm the tumor lesion by surgery. To conclude, DMSA scanning yields clinically very relevant information in approx. 50% of patients with recurrent or metastatic MTC.

Up to now, the most extensive experiences with SC in the follow-up of 253 MTC patients were gathered with $^{99m}Tc(V)$ DMSA (Table 10). The overall sensitivity of 68% corresponds quite well to the sensitivity of 62% in our own relatively large series.

Immunoscintigraphy with Anti-CEA Antibodies

As early as 1982 (Berché et al. 1982; Sullivan et al. 1982), radiolabeled antibodies against CEA were used for tumor localization in MTC. For comparison, Fig. 14 shows the accumulation of a ^{99m}Tc-labeled anti-CEA antibody (Fig. 14a) and the uptake of $^{99m}Tc(V)$ DMSA (Fig. 14b) in a liver metastasis of MTC. According to our experiences, tumor uptake of pentavalent $^{99m}Tc(V)$ DMSA is higher than the accumulation of radiolabeled CEA antibodies in most patients with MTC (Reiners et al. 1986b).

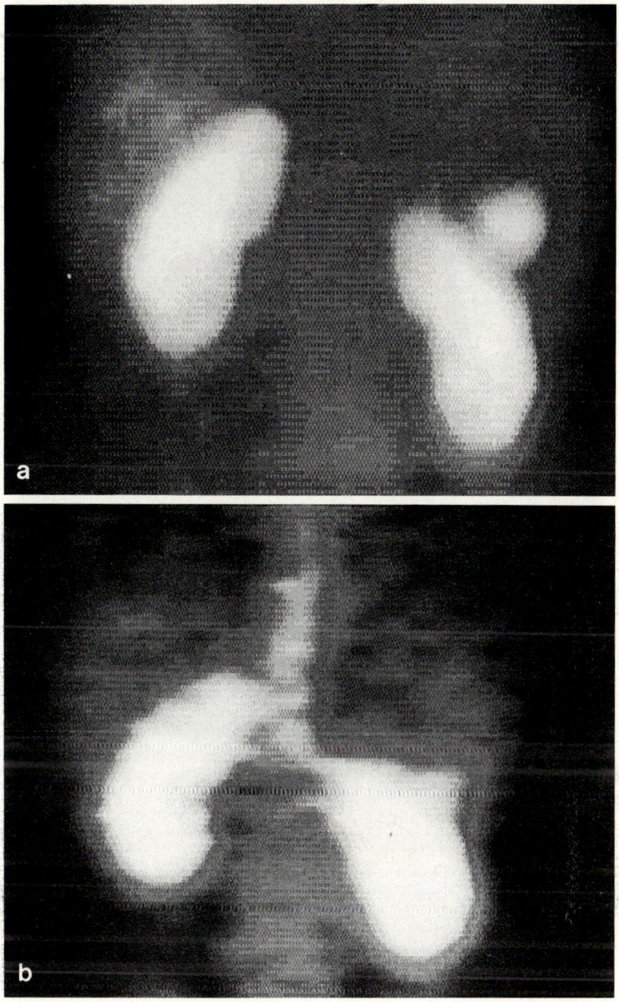

Fig. 14 a,b. Scintigrams (posterior view) of the lumbar region of a patient with a liver metastasis from medullary thyroid cancer. **a** Intense uptake of $^{99m}Tc(V)DMSA$ **b** Only slight uptake of ^{99m}Tc-labeled anti-CEA antibody

However, several studies published very recently give a more promising judgement about the diagnostic performance of CEA immunoscintigraphy for follow-up of MTC. Table 10 shows that the sensitivity of anti-CEA SC lies in the same order of magnitude as the sensitivity of $^{99m}Tc(V)$ DMSA SC (Table 11). Because of the different approaches of both imaging procedures, diagnostic sensitivity possibly may increase if they are combined.

Another field of interest lies in the development of radiolabeled monoclonal antibodies against calcitonin, which is more specific and sensitive

Table 10. Sensitivity of $^{99m}Tc(V)$ DMSA scintigraphy in follow-up of medullary thyroid cancer

Reference	*n*
Hilditch et al. (1986)	0/16
Endo et al. (1987)	14/19
Holub et al. (1987)	4/8
Hoefnagel et al. (1988)	2/3
Patel et al. (1988)	12/15
Becker et al. (1989)	2/5
Clarke et al. (1989)	28/32
Guerra et al. (1989)	16/19
Rodrigues et al. (1989)	14/10
Troncone et al. (1989)	11/14
Urcancioglu et al. (1989)	12/15
Verga et al. (1989)	3/12
Wulfrank et al. (1989)	1/5
Castellani et al. (1991)	7/15
Mojiminiyi et al. (1991)	9/10
Reiners (1991)	29/47
	174/257 (68%)

Table 11. Sensitivity of CEA immunoscintigraphy in follow-up of medullary thyroid cancer

Reference	*n*
Sullivan et al. (1982)	0/5
Parmentier et al. (1984)	4/10
Reiners et al. (1986)	3/6
Hoefnagel et al. (1986)	6/7
Edington et al. (1988)	1/1
Cabezas et al. (1989)	7/10
Becker et al. (1989)	0/5
Troncone et al. (1989)	2/3
Sandrock et al. (1989)	6/7
Scheidhauer et al. (1990)	7/12
Zanin et al. (1990)	1/1
	49/82 (60%)

for MTC than CEA (Gautvik et al. 1982; Guilletau et al. 1985; Samaan et al. 1987). However, such antibodies for human application are not yet available. Concerning routine follow-up of MTC, a general drawback of immunoscintigraphy has to be kept in mind: human anti-mouse antibodies (HAMA) induced by monoclonal anti-CEA or anti-hCT antibodies, may restrict repeated applications of radiolabeled murine immunoglobulins. The problem with HAMA is not an increased risk for allergic reactions but a lack of tumor uptake of the radiolabeled antibody.

Conclusions

The main indication for imaging procedures in primary diagnosis of MEN II is the early localization of preclinical tumor stages in patients with suspected disease after laboratory screening. For MTC, sonography of the neck is the method of first choice because it has a high sensitivity for the localization of primary tumors and regional lymph nodes. Before surgery, mediastinal involvement can be best excluded by CT.

According to recent studies, ^{123}I MIBG SC seems to be mandatory in every patient with suspected MTC before surgery of the thyroid. Clinical occult pheochromocytomas may be detected first by metabolic scanning with MIBG. Today, T2-weighted MRI scans seem to be best suited to the exact delineation of adrenal tumors before surgery.

In staging and follow-up, imaging procedures should localize resectable residues, recurrences, or metastases of MTC. Again, US is best suited to the detection of recurrences or metastases in the neck. Routine screening for lung secondaries can be performed by conventional X-ray imaging. If there are supicious lesions in the lung or mediastinum, CT is the best method for exact delineation.

Today, ^{99m}Tc(V) DMSA scanning seems to be the scintigraphic procedure of first choice for follow-up of MTC and should be applied especially in patients with negative or equivocal findings of routine imaging procedures like sonography, X-ray imaging, CT, or MRI. Because of the different methodological approaches, immunoscintigraphy with anti-CEA antibodies has to be considered as a complementary scintigraphic procedure, especially in patients with negative results of ^{99m}Tc(V) DMSA SC and high tumor marker levels.

References

Arnstein NB, Juni JE, Sisson JC, Lloyd RV, Thompson NW (1986) Recurrent medullary thyroid carcinoma of the thyroid demonstrated by thallium-201 scintigraphy. J Nucl Med 27:1564–1568

Baulieu JL, Guilleteau D, Delisle MJ, Perdrisot R, Gardet P, Delepine N, Baulieu F, Dupont JL, Talbot JN, Coutris G (1987) Radioiodinated meta-iodobenzylguanidine uptake in medullary thyroid cancer. Cancer 60:2189–2194

Becker W, Spiegel W, Reiners C, Börner W (1986) Besonderheiten bei der Nachsorge des C-Zellkarzinoms. Nuklearmediziner 9:167–181

Becker W, Börner W, Reiners C (1989) Tc-99m-(V)-DMSA: the new sensitive and specific radiopharmaceutical for imaging metastases of medullary thyroid carcinomas? Horm Metab Res Suppl 21:38–42

Berché C, Mach J-P, Lumbroso J-D, Langlais C, Aubrey F, Buchegger F, Carrel S, Rougier P, Parmentier C, Tubiana M (1982) Tomoscintigraphy for detecting gastrointestinal and medullary thyroid cancers: first clinical results using radiolabelled monoclonal antibodies against carcinoembryonic antigen. Br Med J 285:1447–1451

Cabezas RC, Berna L, Estorch M, Carrio I, Garcia-Ameijeiras A (1989) Localization of metastases from medullary thyroid carcinoma using different methods. Henry Ford Hosp Med J 37:169–172

Castellani MR, Crippa F, del Bo L, Gasparini M, Grassi M, Maffioli L, Cusumano F, Bombardieri E, Buraggi GL (1991) Tc-99m(V) DMSA scintigraphy in diagnosis of occult recurrences of medullary thyroid carcinoma: preliminary results. In: Schmidt HAE, van der Schoot JB (eds) Nuclear medicine. State of the art in Europe. Schattauer, Stuttgart, pp 334–336

Clarke SEM, Lazarus CR, Maisey MN (1987) Radionuclide imaging in medullary thyroid carcinoma: evaluation of two new radiopharmaceuticals. Henry Ford Hosp Med J 35:124–126

Clarke SEM, Lazarus CR, Maisey MN (1989) Experience in imaging medullary thyroid carcinoma using 99mTc(V)dimercaptosuccinic acid (DMSA). Henry Ford Hosp Med J 37:167–168

Coutris G, Talbot JN, Kabla G, Calmettes C, Milhaud G (1986) Uptake of I-131-MIBG by medullary carcinoma of thyroid in familial cases. Eur J Nucl Med 12:77–79

Dahir ND, Hesslewood SR, Jack DB (1989) Preparation and protein binding of pentavalent Tc DMSA. In: Schmidt HAE, Buraggi GL (eds) Nuclear medicine. Trends and possibilities in nuclear medicine. Schattauer, Stuttgart, p 131

Doppman JL (1985) Multiple endocrine syndromes – a nightmare for the endocrinologic radiologist. Semin Roentgenol 20:7–16

Edington HD, Watson CG, Levine G, Tauxe WN, Yousem SA, Unger M, Kowal CD (1988) Radioimmunimaging of metastatic medullary carcinoma of the thyroid using an In-111-labeled monoclonal antibody to CEA. Surgery 104:1004–1010

Endo K, Shiomi K, Kasagi K, Konish J, Torizuka K, Nakao K, Tanimura H (1984) Imaging of medullary thyroid cancer with I-131-MIBG. Lancet 233

Endo K, Ohta H, Torizuka K, Horiucht K, Yomoda I, Yokoyama A (1987) Technetium-99m(V)-DMSA in the imaging of medullary thyroid carcinoma. J Nucl Med 28:252–253

Francis IR, Glazer GM, Shapiro B, Sisson JC, Gross BH (1983) Complementary roles of CT and I-131-MIBG scintigraphy in diagnosing pheochromocytoma. AJR 141:719–725

Frank K, Raue F, Lorenz D, Herfart C, Ziegler R (1987) Importance of ultrasound examination for the follow-up of medullary thyroid carcinoma: comparison with other localization methods. Henry Ford Hosp Med J 35:122–123

Gautvik KM, Svindahl K, Skretting A, Stenberg B, Myhre L, Ekeland A, Johannesen JV (1982) Uptake and localization of I-131-labeled anti-calcitonin immunoglobulins in rat medullary thyroid carcinoma tissue. Cancer 50:1107–1114

Georgi M, Hofbauer J, Weiss H, Keller EW, Wunschik F, von Mittelstadt G, Linder M (1984) Wertigkeit von Sonographie, Computertomographie und Angiographie in der Nebennierendiagnostik. RÖFO 140:373–379

Gorman B, Charboneau JW, James EM, Reading CC, Wold LE, Grant CS, Gharib H, Hay ID (1987) Medullary thyroid carcinoma: Role of high-resolution ultrasound. Radiology 162:147–150

Guerra UP, Pizzocaro C, Terzi A, Giubbini R, Maira G, Pagliani RP, Bestagno M (1989) New tracers for the imaging of medullary thyroid carcinoma. Nucl Med Commun 10:285–295

Guilletau D, Baulieu J-L, Besnard J-C (1985) Medullary thyroid carcinoma imaging in an animal model: use of radiolabeled anticalcitonin F(ab')2 and meta-iodobenzyl guanidine. Eur J Nucl Med 11:198–200

Hilditch TE, Conell JMC, Murray T, Reed NS (1986) Poor results with technetium-99m-(V)-DMSA and I-131-MIBG in the imaging of medullary thyroid carcinoma. J Nucl Med 27:1150–1153

Hoefnagel CA, Voute PA, de Kraker J, Marcuse HR (1986) Detection and treatment of neural crest tumors using I-131-meta-iodobenzylguanidine. In: Schmidt HAE, Ell PJ, Britton KE (eds) Nuclear medicine in research and practice. Schattauer, Stuttgart, pp 474–476

Hoefnagel CA, Delprat CC, Zanin D, van der Schoot JB (1988) New radionuclide tracers for the diagnosis and therapy of medullary thyroid carcinoma. Clin Nucl Med 13:159–165

Holub V, Nemec J, Neradilova M, Benova M, Blazek T, Dusek M (1987) Positive scintigraphy of medullary thyroid cancer using 201-Tl and alkalized 99m-Tc-DMSA. Radiobiol Radiother 28:640–645

Horiuchi K, Yomoda I, Okta H, Endo K, Yokoyama A (1991) Search for polynuclear pentavalent technetium complex of dimercaptosuccinic acid Tc(V)-DMS tumour localization mechanism. Eur J Nucl Med 18:796–800

Ikeda I, Inoue O, Kurata K (1977) Preparation of various Tc-99m-dimercaptosuccinate complexes and their evaluation as radiotracers. J Nucl Med 18:1222–1229

Johnson DG, Coleman RE, McCook TA, Dale JK, Wells SA (1984) Bone and liver images in medullary carcinoma of the thyroid gland: concise communication. J Nucl Med 25:419–422

Kafaghi FA, Shapiro B, Fischer M, Sisson JC, Hutchinson R, Beierwalter WH (1991) Phaechromocytoma and functioning paraganglioma in childhood and adolescence: role of iodine 131 metaiodobenzylguanidine. Eur J Nucl Med 18:191–198

Kujath C, Panitz N (1989) Vereinfachte Präparation von 99m-Tc(V)-DMSA. Nuklearmediziner 12:291–293

Mathieu E, Despres E, Delepine N, Taieb A (1987) MR imaging of the adrenal gland in Sipple's disease. J Comput Assist Tomogr 11:790–794

Mojiminiyi OA, Udelsman R, Soper NDW, Shepstone BJ, Dudley NE (1991) Clinical application of Tc-99m(V)DMSA scintigraphy in patients with medullary carcinoma of the thyroid (MTC). In: Schmidt HAE, van der Schoot JB (eds) Nuclear medicine. The state of the art in Europe. Schattauer, Stuttgart, pp 344–346

Müller SP, Guth-Tougelidis B, Piotrowski B, Farahati J, Reiners C (1990) Tl-201 scintigraphy in the follow-up of eosinophilic thyroid carcinoma. J Nucl Med 31:767

Ohta H, Yamamoto K, Endo K, Mori T, Hamanaka D, Shimazu A, Ikekubo K, Makimoto K, Iida Y, Konishi J, Morita R, Hata N (1984) A new imaging agent for medullary carcinoma of the thyroid. J Nucl Med 25:323–325

Parmentier C, Lumbroso J, Schlumberger M, Gardet P, Mach J-P, Berché C, Rougier P, Caillou B, Tubiana M (1984) Immunoscintigraphie avec tomographie d'émission dans les cancers de la thyroide. Ann Med Interne (Paris) 135:345–350

Parthasarathy KL, Shimaoka K, Bakshi SP, Razack MS (1980) Radiotracer uptake in medullary carcinoma of the thyroid. Clin Nucl Med 5:45–48

Patel MC, Petel RB, Ramamoorthy N, Krishna BA, Sharma SM (1988) Clinical evaluation of 99mTc(V)-dimercaptosuccinic acid (DMSA) for imaging medullary carcinoma of thyroid and its metastasis. Eur J Nucl Med 13:507–510

Perdrisot R, Rohmer V, Lejeune JJ, Bigorgne JC, Jallet P (1988) Thyroid uptake of MIBG in Sipple's syndrome. Eur J Nucl Med 14:37–38

Quint LE, Glazer GM, Francis IR, Shapiro B, Chenevert TL (1987) Pheochromocytoma and paraganglioma: comparison of MR imaging with CT and I-131 MIBG scintigraphy. Radiology 165:89–93

Ramamoorthy N, Shetye SV, Pandey PM, Mani RS, Patel MC, Patel RB, Ramanathan P, Krishna BA, Sharma SM (1987) Preparation and evaluation of

99mTc(V)DMSA complex: studies in medullary carcinoma of the thyroid. Eur J Nucl Med 12:623–628

Raue F, Winter J, Frank-Raue K, Lorenz D, Herfarth C, Ziegler R (1989) Diagnostic procedure before reoperation in patients with medullary thyroid carcinoma. Horm Metab Res Suppl 21:31–34

Reiners C (1988) Tumorszintigraphie mit Tc-99m-V-DMSA: Lokalisation von Rezidiven und Metastasen des C-Zell-Karzinoms der Schilddrüse. Nuklearmediziner 11:123–131

Reiners C (1991) Nuklearmedizinische Diagnostik des medullären Schilddrüsenkarzinoms und des Sipple-Syndroms. Med Welt 42:1001–1006

Reiners C, Becker W, Spiegel W, Börner W, Müller H-A (1986a) Schildrüsendiagnostik: Nutzen von Sonographie, Szintigraphie und Punktionszytologie für die Praxis. Intern Welt 10:294–304

Reiners C, Eilles C, Spiegel W, Becker W, Börner W (1986b) Immunoscintigraphy in medullary thyroid cancer using an I-123- or In-111-labelled monoclonal anti-CEA antibody fragment. Nuklearmedizin 25:227–231

Reinig JW, Doppman JL, Dwyer AJ, Johnson AR, Knop RH (1986) Adrenal masses differentiated by MR. Radiology 158:81–84

Reuter E, Bethge N, Matthes M, Koppenhagen K (1983) Tc99m-phosphonates for imaging of amyloid in C-cell carcinoma. Eur J Nucl Med 8:398–400

Rodrigues M, Vieira MR, Santos R, Limbert E (1989) Clinical evaluation of 99mTc(V)-dimercaptosuccinic acid (DMSA) for follow-up of patients with medullary thyroid carcinoma. Eur J Nucl Med 15:522

Rufini V, Troncone L, Giordano A, Daidone MS (1989) Evaluation of diagnostic effectiveness of new scintigraphic techniques in medullary thyroid carcinoma (MTC). Eur J Nucl Med 15:473

Samaan NA, Yang K-P (1987) Localization of radiolabeled monoclonal antibody to calcitonin in rat medullary thyroid carcinoma allografts. Henry Ford Hosp Med J 35:153–156

Sandrock D, Blossey H-C, Steinroeder M, Munz DL (1989) Contribution of different scintigraphic techniques to the management of medullary thyroid carcinoma. Henry Ford Hosp Med J 37:173–174

Scheidhauer K, Puskas C, Sciuk J, Brandau W, Bartenstein P, Schober O (1990) CEA-Immunszintigraphie in der Nachsorge des medullären Schilddrüsen-Ca. Nuklearmedizin 29:A50

Schwerk WB, Grün R, Wahl R (1985) Ultrasound diagnosis of C-cell carcinoma of the thyroid. Cancer 55:624–630

Shigeno C, Fukunaga M, Yamamoto I, Dokoh S, Morita R, Hino M, Torizuka K (1984) Accumulation of Tc-99m phosphorus compounds in medullary carcinoma of the thyroid. Report of two cases. Clin Nucl Med 7:297–298

Sisson JC, Shapiro B, Beierwaltes WH (1984) Scintigraphy with I-131 MIBG as an aid to the treatment of pheochromocytomas in patients with the multiple endocrine neoplasia type 2 syndromes. Henry Ford Hosp Med J 32:254–261

Spiegel W, Eilles C, Becker W (1988) Die Szintigraphie chromaffiner Tumoren mit Metajodobenzylguanidin (MIBG). Nuklearmediziner 11:109–121

Sullivan DC, Silva JS, Cox CE, Haagensen DE, Harris CC, Birner WH, Wells SA (1982) Localization of I-131-labeled goat and primate anti-carcinoembryonic antigen (CEA) antibodies in patients with cancer. Invest Radiol 17:350–355

Talpos GB, Jackson CE, Froelich JW, Kambouris AA, Block MA, Tashijan AH (1985) Localization of residual medullary thyroid cancer by thallium/technetium scintigraphy. Surgery 98:1189–1196

Troncone L, Rufini V, DeRosa G, Testa A (1989) Diagnostic and therapeutic potential of new radiopharmaceutical agents in medullary thyroid carcinoma. Henry Ford Hosp Med J 37:178–184

Urgancioglu I, Üzüm F, Özker K (1989) 99mTc(V)-DMSA scanning of the follow-up patients with medullary thyroid carcinoma. Eur J Nucl Med 15:540

Valk TW, Frager MS, Gross MD, Sisson JC, Wieland DM, Swanson DP, Mangner TJ, Beierwaltes WH (1981) Spectrum of pheochromocytoma in multiple endocrine neoplasia. A scintigraphic portrayal using I-131-I-metaiodobenzylguanidine. Ann Intern Med 94:762–767

Velchik MG, Alavi A, Kressel HY, Engelmann K (1989) Localization of pheochromocytoma: MIBG, CT, and MRI correlation. J Nucl Med 30:328–336

Verga U, Muratori F, DiSacco G, Banfi F, Libroia A (1989) The role of radiopharmaceuticals MIBG and (V)DMSA in the diagnosis of medullary thyroid carcinoma. Henry Ford Hosp Med J 37:175–177

Westera G, Gadze A, Horst W (1985) A convenient method for the preparation of 99mTc(V)dimercaptosuccinic acid (99mTc(V)DMSA). Int J Appl Radiat Isot 36:311–312

Wieland DM, Wu J-L, Brown LE, Mangner TJ, Swanson DP, Beierwaltes WH (1980) Radiolabeled adrenergic neuron-blocking agents: adrenomedullary imaging with I-131 iodobenzylguanidine. J Nucl Med 21:349–353

Wulfrank DA, Schelstrate KH, Small F, Fallais CJ (1989) Analogy between tumor uptake of technetium(V)-99m dimercaptosuccinic acid (DMSA) and technetium-99m-MDP. Clin Nucl Med 14:588–593

Zanin DEA, van Dongen A, Hoefnagel CA, Bruning PF (1990) Radioimmunscintigraphy using iodine-131-anti-CEA monoclonal antibodies and thallium-201 scintigraphy in medullary thyroid carcinoma: a case report. J Nucl Med 31:1854–1855

Therapeutic Procedure in Medullary Thyroid Carcinoma

Surgical Strategies and Methods for the Treatment of Metastasizing Medullary Thyroid Carcinoma

H.J. Buhr, F. Kallinowski, and C. Herfarth

Abteilung 2.1, Chirurgische Universitätsklinik, Klinikum der Universität, Im Neuenheimer Feld 110, W-6900 Heidelberg, FRG

Introduction

The medullary thyroid carcinoma (MTC) exhibits several biological peculiarities. The early formation of metastases in the local lymph nodes of the neck region and of the proximal mediastinum is of particular importance for the development of therapeutic regimens (Bergholm et al. 1989; Buhr et al. 1991; Duh et al. 1989; Graze et al. 1978). Considering patients with elevated basal calcitonin values which were detected during family screening programs Wells et al. (1978b) demonstrated in 50% a lymph node involvement. Patients with clinically manifest tumors suffered in 71% from local metastases. Similarly, metastases in the neck lymph nodes were found in 9% and mediastinal secondaries in 8% of patients with clinically occult familial C-cell carcinomas characterized by normal basal calcitonin levels but pathological elevations upon pentagastrin stimulation. The prognostic relevance of lymph node metastases is demonstrated by the classic work of Woolner et al. (1969). The 10-year survival rate of patients without lymph node involvement reached 85% and was not significantly different to a reference population. In patients with lymph node involvement it was significantly reduced to 42%. These reports were further substantiated by other authors (Bergholm et al. 1989; Roka et al. 1982; Saad et al. 1984; Schröder et al. 1988; Wahl et al. 1987). Since distant metastases occur only late in the natural history of the disease, surgical eradication of lymph node metastases can prolong the patient's life and even achieve higher cure rates (Tisell et al. 1986). Since the tumor cells are relatively radio- and chemoresistant, surgical intervention is highly indicated (Pertursson 1988; Samaan et al. 1988; Scherübl et al. 1990).

Recent Results in Cancer Research, Vol. 125

Lymphatic Drainage System of the Thyroid

Knowledge of the lymphatic tree and the drainage system of the thyroid gland is of paramount importance for the surgical therapy of medullary thyroid cancer. The book *Die Lymphbahnen der menschlichen Schilddrüse* by Eickhoff and Herberhold (1968) can serve as a reference text. According to these authors, the intrathyroidal lymphatic vessels are separated in three sections. Firstly, the lymphatic tree arises in the perifollicular space. Secondly, these lymphatic capillaries combine at the borders of the individual thyroid lobules to form the perilobular lymphatic net. Thirdly, the lobular vessels run into large trabecular lymphatic ducts which connect to the extrathyroidal lymphatic drainage system. The border between the intra- and extrathyroidal lymphatic system has to be drawn at the transition from the trabecular connecting ducts and the lymphatic vessels of the fibrous capsule of the thyroid. In the capsule, the first lymphatic vessels characterized by an invariate presence of intravascular valves can be found. The dense reticular lymphatic network of the capsule is the collecting point of all intrathyroidal lymphatic vessels. However, at the dorsal aspect of the thyroid gland, a regular arrangement of lymphatic vessels could not be detected by these authors. Since the thyroid gland is in this area connected to the trachea by dense fibrous tissue, the presence of a rich network of lymphatic vessels cannot be expected. The majority of lymphatic vessels of the capsule run in conjuntion with the vasculature and only a few follow individual pathways. The lymphatic vessels of the capsule lead to particular areas on the surface of the thyroid gland from which the further drainage system arises. The distribution of these feeding points varies only little and can be found in different individuals at constant places. Analogous to the penetrating points of the thyroidal vasculature, lymphatic vessels arise from the upper pole of both lobes concomitant with the superior thyroid artery and vein, at the middle of both lateral aspects accompanying the inferior thyroid artery, and at the lower pole with the inferior thyroid veins. Further lymphatic vessels arise separately from the vasculature at the inner, upper, and lower aspects of the thyroid gland. These vessels run independently and unaccompanied by any blood vessels to their regional lymph nodes. The collecting lymph vessels of the upper poles are the largest draining ducts of the entire organ. These vessels are fed from both ventral and dorsolateral areas of the thyroid. There are connections between the proximal and caudal drainage systems contributing to the possibility of metastases in areas remote from the primary tumor. The draining lymphatic vessels of the thyroid are connected to various groups of regional lymph nodes. Vessels from the upper inner poles reach praelaryngeal lymph nodes whereas the ones from the lower inner poles run to praetracheal lymph nodes. Laterally arising vessels of the upper outer pole, of the thyroid edge, and of the lower outer pole can be attributed to the deep lateral lymph nodes.

The jugular truncus and its larger contributaries constitute the collecting ducts for the lymphatic fluid of the head and neck. The internal jugular vein serves as a guideline for the neck lymphatics. The lymphatic fluid from the thyroid gland flows via the superficial and deep neck lymph nodes to the jugular truncus. However, judging from clinical experience, connections must exist to lymph nodes situated far lateral of the internal jugular vein in the lateral triangle of the neck. On careful dissection of all lymph nodes of the neck for metastazing C-cell carcinoma, tumor-involved lymph nodes are frequently found far lateral between the fascicles of cervical nerves. In order for this to occur, tumor cells must jump nodes between the thyroid gland and these lateral lymphatics since intermediate nodes are histologically tumor free.

Diagnostic Modalities

Plasma Calcitonin Assay

Calcitonin constitutes a tumor marker with excellent specificity and sensitivity both for primary diagnosis and postoperative follow-up. Calcitonin levels in the serum should be measured twice a year as a postoperative follow-up after curative total thyroidectomy. In the case of normal basal calcitonin levels, stimulation tests with pentagastrin should be performed once a year. For these stimulation tests, 0.5 μg pentagastrin/kg body weight are injected i.v. rapidly within 15 s after drawing a blood sample for basal calcitonin values, followed by the collection of blood samples after 2, 5, 7, and 10 min. If occult medullary thyroid cancer tissue persists severalfold elevations of blood calcitonin can be detected as rapidly as 2 min after pentagastrin stimulation. This confirms the diagnosis of a C-cell carcinoma recurrence or a metastasis. In most patients with strict follow-up, this pathological elevation of pentagastrin-stimulated calcitonin levels is the first indicator for a recurrence or the presence of micrometastases depending on the length of the "tumorfree" postoperative interval (DeLellis et al. 1978; Goltzmann et al. 1974; Raue et al. 1983; Raue 1985; Wells et al. 1978a, 1982). In some cases, pathological elevations of pentagastrin-stimulated calcitonin values can be detected long before any imaging techniques yield positive results. In these instances, selective venous catheterization with repeated blood sampling as described below can be recommended for site localization of the pathological calcitonin production (Block et al. 1980; Mrad et al. 1989; Norton et al. 1980).

Imaging

As a first approach, ultrasonography of the neck should be performed. Enlarged cervical lymph nodes sometimes with infiltration of surrounding

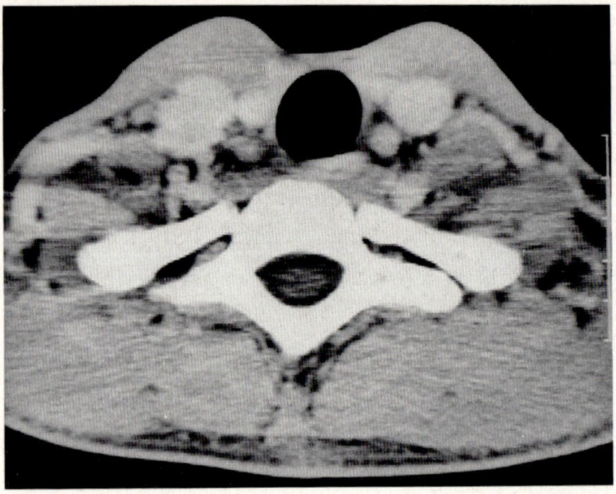

Fig. 1. Transverse contrast computer-tomographic scan of the cervical region. The tumor extends posterior of the right internal jugular vein with compression of its posterior wall

structures can be detected under favorable circumstances (Schwerk et al. 1985; Simeone et al. 1982). The preoperative search for metastases should also include posterior–anterior and lateral chest X-ray films and ultrasonographic scans of the liver. Distant metastases to the bones need to be excluded by skeletal scintigraphy.

A computer tomographic investigation of the neck is not mandatory since micrometastases cannot be visualized. In case of the ultrasonographic detection of enlarged neck nodes, computer tomography can further clarify the extent of the tumor and a possible involvement of surrounding structures. Figure 1 illustrates lymph node metastases of a 31-year-old male with a metastasizing MTC of the multiple endocrine neoplasia (MEN) type. Three years ago, a total thyroidectomy was performed in a small hospital in his home country, Cyprus. Postoperatively, basal serum calcitonin levels were persistently elevated. He has since presented at our department with palpable lymph nodes at the right side of the neck. Selective venous catheterization confirmed these nodes as a likely site for calcitonin production. A modified radical neck dissection and a transcervical mediastinal dissection were recently performed. Following this procedure, basal calcitonin and carcinoembryonic antigen (CEA) values were reduced but still in the pathological range. Therefore, a modified radical neck dissection of the left-hand side is planned after completion of the appropriate diagnostic procedures.

A computer-tomographic investigation must be performed if mediastinal metastases are suspected either on clinical grounds or on plain X-ray films (Fig. 2). After diagnosis of a pT2N1b MTC, the patient shown in Fig. 2 underwent a total thyroidectomy and a bilateral neck dissection in an

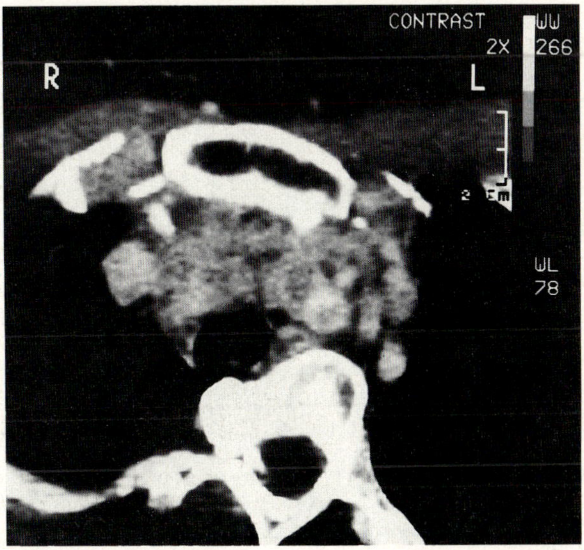

Fig. 2. Transverse contrast computer-tomographic scan of the upper mediastinum. Retrosternal tumor recurrence of a C-cell carcinoma which in caudal scans encased the arterial vessels and occluded the left brachiocephalic vein. (Scoliosis of the spine due to poliomyelitis)

outside hospital. Despite radical treatment at a comparatively early stage of the primary tumor, the patient was later diagnosed to have mediastinal metastases. His poor prognosis may partially be explained by the presence of positive lymph nodes at the time of primary treatment (Fig. 2).

Selective Venous Catheterization

In all cases, selective venous catheterization with repeated collection of blood samples is the most appropriate preoperative investigation for occult persistent MTC. Blood samples are collected repeatedly without pentagastrin stimulation after the superselective catheterization of veins in the neck, the mediastinum, and the abdomen and are consecutively analyzed for calcitonin concentrations. Any elevation above basal calcitonin values is indicative of a tumor localization in the tributary tissue region. With such a detailed mapping, the exact tumor site can be attributed to a particular neck region and the surgeon can commit himself to a unilateral neck dissection. Furthermore, lymph node tumors in the mediastinum can be detected and the suspicion of distant metastases (e.g., in the liver) can be raised (Gautwick et al. 1989). A selective venous catheterization is necessary before any reoperation is considered. Figure 3 depicts the calcitonin concentrations

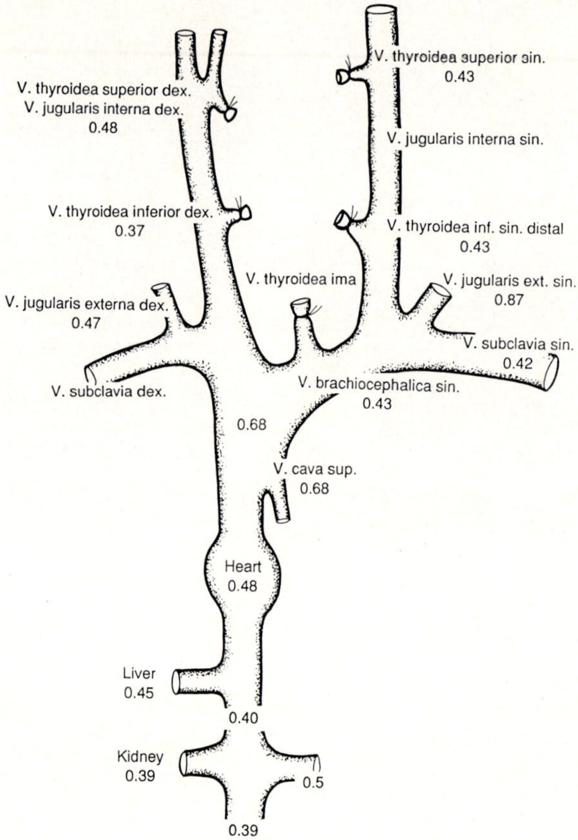

Fig. 3. Calcitonin concentrations (μg/l) in blood samples collected at the respective sites during selective venous catheterization in a 62-year-old white male 7 years after total thyroidectomy for MEN 2A

determined from selective venous catheterization in a 57-year-old white male suffering from MEN type 2A. Eleven years previously, a right-sided pheochromocytoma was removed. Four years later, a total thyroidectomy had to be performed for a medullary thyroid carcinoma. Postoperatively, elevated calcitonin levels persisted. Within the last months before proceeding to a selective venous catheterization a progressive increase of the calcitonin and CEA concentrations was observed. Ultrasound investigations demonstrated an enlarged node on the left-hand side of the neck with reduced echogenicity. The histological examination following a modified radical neck dissection confirmed tumor tissue in the venous and arterial sheath, the paralaryngeal, the center of the lateral triangle of the neck, and in the former thyroid bed adjacent to the recurrent nerve.

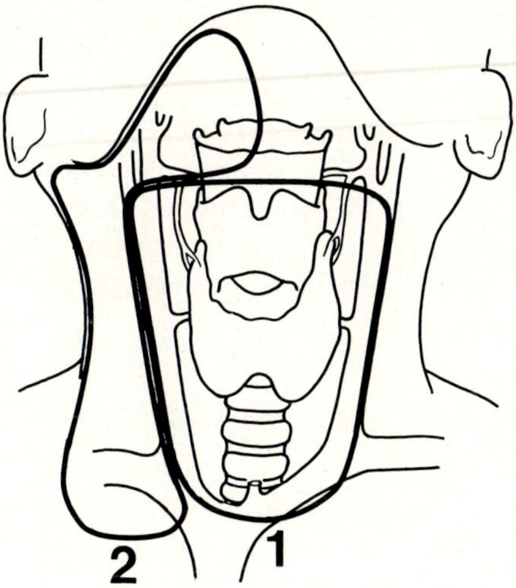

Fig. 4. Schematic drawing of surgical land marks in the neck region. Compartment 1 is the area which needs to be included into the total thyroidectomy as initial treatment. Compartment 2 is the area removed during a modified radical neck dissection as described in the text

Surgical Strategy

Oncological Considerations

Any operative strategy must consider the biological properties of C-cell carcinoma which have been recognized within the last 20 years. The most important observation for the surgeon is the fact that this tumor entity metastasizes early into the regional lymph nodes of the neck and the upper mediastinum, whereas distant metastases occur only late during tumor growth (Woolner et al. 1969). Besides defining the operative strategy, the involvement of neck lymph nodes is also of prognostic relevance (Böckdahl et al. 1985; Saad et al. 1984; van Heerden et al. 1990; Woolner et al. 1969), leading to an extensive dissection of neck nodes already at the time of the primary surgical intervention. This is of particular importance since malignant C-cells are resistant to radioiodine treatment due to a lack of uptake; only minimally sensitive to conventional chemotherapy; and virtually nonresponsive to percutaneous radiotherapy. Thus, any loss of momentum with the only potentially curative treatment, namely surgery, destines the patient to a gloomy future and reduces his chances of survival.

Primary Treatment

A surgical intervention can be recommended in cases of inadequate primary surgery (Block et al. 1978; Russell et al. 1983; Telander et al. 1986; Wells et al. 1978b). Possible indications include residual thyroid tissue or incomplete removal of the central lymphatic compartment. According to Fig. 4, the primary operation must include total thyroidectomy with complete removal of the dorsal capsule and an extensive dissection of the central lymph node compartment. Here, the selective removal of obviously enlarged lymph nodes (so-called berry picking) is insufficient. Rather, the fatty and lymphatic tissue has to be excised completely and en bloc including small, but visually unidentifiable lymph nodes. The operative field (Fig. 4) has to be extended laterally to the vascular sheath, proximally to the carotid bifurcation, and caudally to the left brachiocephalic vein (compartment 1).

Microsurgical Technique for Treatment of Recurrences and Micrometastases

The surgical approach to occultly persisting micrometastases which are obvious only by minimally elevated calcitonin levels cannot be standardized at this point in time due to limited clinical experiences on the natural course of this condition. In 1986, Tisell et al. presented for the first time their method and experience with the treatment of asymptomatic metastasizing medullary thyroid cancers. With the aid of magnifying glasses, this group performs a microsurgical technique aiming at the complete dissection of the neck. Following the pioneering work of Tisell et al. (1986), we have been performing a similar microsurgical lymph node dissection in our department since 1988 (Buhr et al. 1990). During this procedure, the lateral, central, and proximal mediastinal lymph node compartments are surgically removed independently of the extent of primary surgery. Evaluating the reoperations performed at our department ($n = 40$), an insufficient extirpation even of the central lymph node compartment became evident in all cases. This meant that solely a thyroidectomy had been performed previously. In particular, paratracheal lymph nodes were tumor infiltrated. Before attempting a second surgical intervention, the report of the previous, usually externally performed surgery and the details of the histological examination have to be carefully evaluated in order to assess the extent of the central lymph node dissection at the time of primary surgery. Further preoperative investigations include a direct laryngoscopy and a fluoroscopic evaluation in order to assure full function of the laryngeal and phrenic nerves.

Our operative strategy for recurrent surgery of palpable or – with imaging techniques – visualizable tumor or of occult micrometastases includes the following.

In any one session, a neck dissection is, in our department, performed only on one side since the required time frequently extends beyond 5 and up to 8 h. Over the years the operation time has been progressively shortened due to increased experience and the employment of magnifying lenses, recently leading to operation times of just under 3.5 h. One should start with the side localized by highest calcitonin concentrations after selective venous catheterization.

Chirurgische Universitätsklinik Heidelberg
Direktor: Prof. Dr. Ch. Herfarth

Patient

Dokumentation

Name

Medulläres Schilddrüsencarcinom:
Systematik der cervico- und mediastinalen
Lymphadenektomie

Datum

Links ◯ Rechts ◯

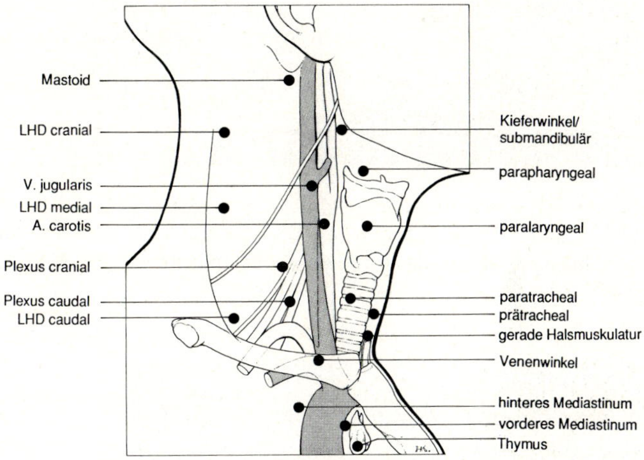

Fig. 5. Documentation sheet for the standardized documentation of excised lymphatic tissue

The operation is performed strictly according to a set schema. All excised tissue is carefully recorded in the newly designed documentation sheet (Fig. 5). Only in this fashion can routes of metastases be exactly evaluated. For the surgeon, it is very important to gain a multitude of samples with precisely detailed particulars regarding localization and extent in order to reach an adequately detailed histological evaluation.

Problems can be encountered during preparation if the neck region was percutaneously irradiated following previous surgery. In this case, extensive scar formation can occur involving vessels and various nerves. The scar tissue can be so dense that anatomical structures can no longer be distinguishable thus limiting the extent of surgery. A carotis angiography is recommended if a previous irradiation can be substantiated from the patient's history. This investigation can yield information on a possible dislocation of the arteries or infiltration of the vessel wall. In our department, four patients were operated on after receiving irradiation treatment between 4 and 12 years earlier. In two patients, extensive scar tissue was encountered in the center of the irradiation field which excluded a preservation of anatomical structures, thus limiting the extent of surgery. Figures

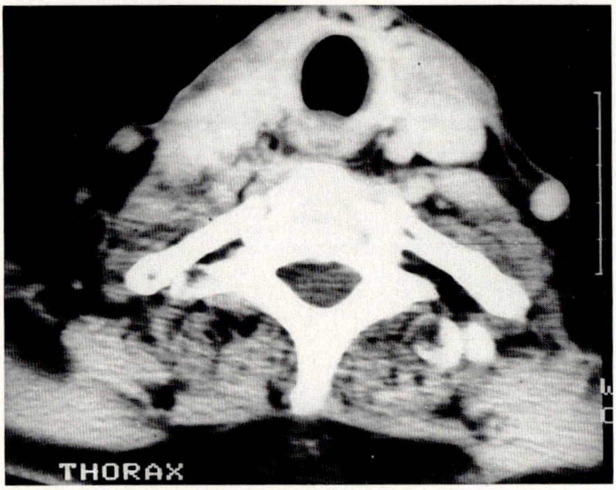

Fig. 6. Tumor recurrence after radiation therapy. Transverse contrast computer-tomographic scan at the level of the thyroid cartilage. The position of the right internal jugular vein is replaced by tumor; the right carotid artery cannot be delineated

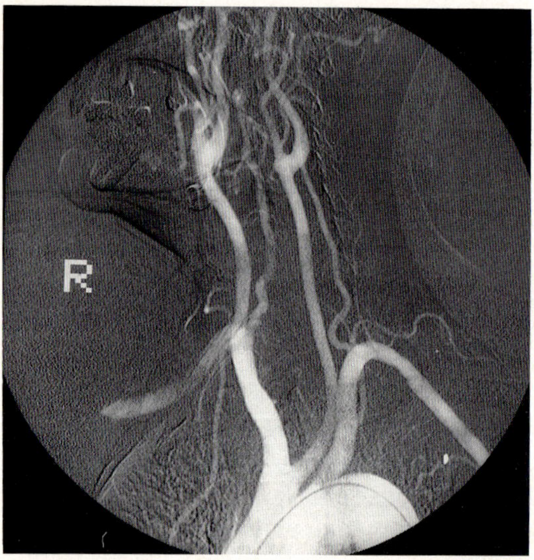

Fig. 7. Tumor recurrence after radiation therapy. Angiography, arterial phase: Posterior displacement of the right common carotid artery; no compression or tumor invasion

6–8 show a 64-year-old patient 2 years after a thyroidectomy for an MTC. Postoperatively, a percutaneous radiation therapy had been commenced (60 Gy). Clinically, dense and marginally mobile scar tissue was palpable in the right side of the neck. Sonographically, a large and slightly inhomo-

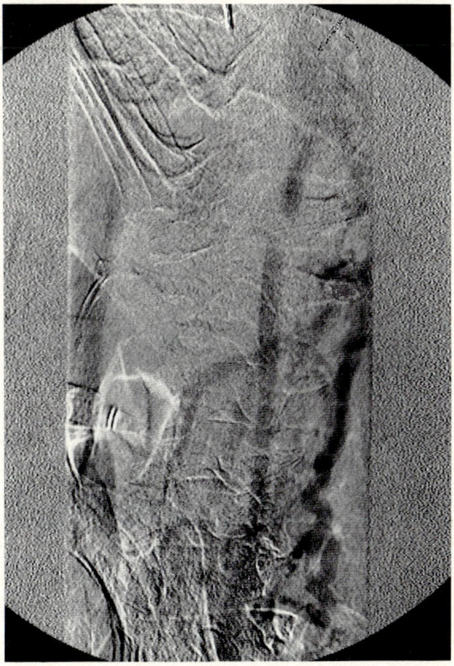

Fig. 8. Tumor recurrence after radiation therapy. Angiography, venous phase: Occlusion of lower portion of internal jugular vein with abundant collaterals. Intraoperatively, the vein was patent but severely compressed

geneous mass was demonstrated in the middle of the right neck. Figure 6 depicts relevant results of a computer-tomographic investigation. It shows two lymph node metastases, one in the region of the thyroid cartilage ventral of the carotid artery and a second one more caudally located between the carotid artery and the internal jugular vein. Serum calcitonin levels were elevated to 7.3 ng/ml (normal levels are <0.3 ng/ml). A transaortic angiography with selective imaging of the right carotid artery indicated a dislocation of this vessel medially but failed to demonstrate any sign of intravascular tumor infiltration (Fig. 7). On venography, the right internal jugular vein was occluded or subtotally compressed in its lowest third for a distance of about 1 cm (Fig. 8). In another department, a neck dissection was unsuccessfully attempted, failing at a tumor-surrounded carotid artery; in our department, the neck dissection was performed using sharp dissection in the plane of the adventitia of the carotid artery (Fig. 9). Intraoperatively, the computer tomographically visualized lymph nodes were found to be tumor infiltrated. Due to the previous radiation therapy, the vessel wall was severely scarred. Nevertheless, sharp dissection of the carotid artery and en bloc resection of the tumor tissue was possible. In the other two patients, scar formation was much less pronounced leaving the major anatomical landmarks subject to easy preparation.

During surgery, the patient is placed on a heating pad in order to avoid a potentially dangerous reduction in body temperature. A transurethral

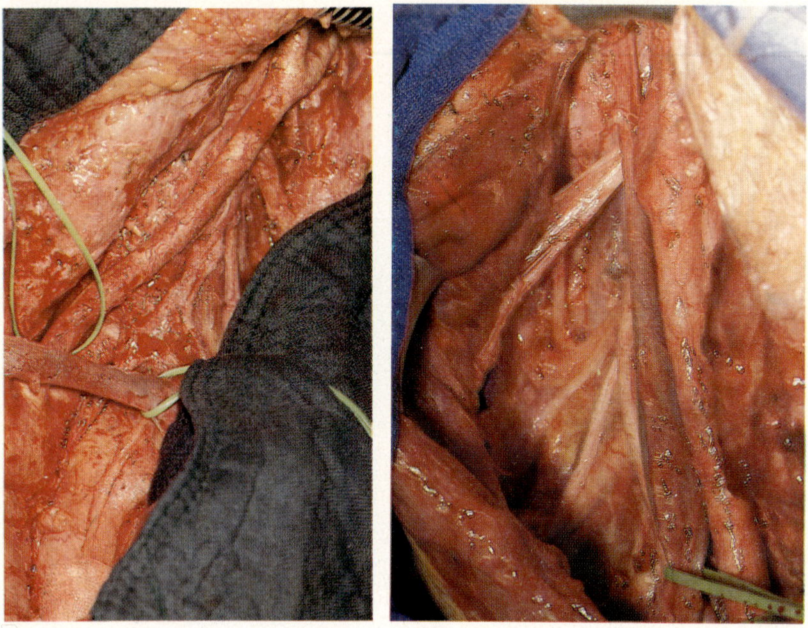

Fig. 9. View of the operative site of the central (*left*) and lateral (*right*) compartment

catheter is inserted for a more adequate anesthesiological monitoring during the operative procedure.

Palliative Approach

Palpable or imaged tumor nodes should be surgically removed without delay (Chong et al. 1975; Rossi et al. 1980). Surgical therapy should only be restricted in cases in which grossly advanced disease reduces the likelihood of both palliation and increased survival. In the analysis by Rossi et al. (1980) a purely palliative intervention carried a poor prognosis in patients with sporadic C-cell carcinoma: 90% of the palliatively operated patients died after a mean survival time of 15 months. In contrast, 54% of the curatively operated patients were still alive after a mean survival time of 48 months. However, palliative interventions have to be recommended if the quality of life is drastically reduced by surgically removable but not curable tumor masses, e.g., in the case of compression of large vessels. For example, we performed an extensive palliative dissection of a large mediastinal metastases in a 57-year-old patient. After modified radical microdissection of both sides of the neck a continuous basal calcitonin elevation was observed up to values of 3.3 ng/ml. The patient complained of a swelling of the left arm due to an outflow obstruction consistent with a pronounced venous filling of the subcutaneous veins of the upper left arm. Computer tomography demonstrated extensive lymph node metastases in the anterior and posterior mediastinum. In this patient, a pronounced kyphoscoliosis preexisted due to a polio infection during adolescence. The phlebography confirmed the occlusion of the left brachiocephalic vein and the formation of adequate collateral blood-conducting channels. Based on clinical experiences, it was decided that a palliative reduction of the tumor mass might delay the death of the patient due to suffocation. Using a transsternal approach, the tumor could be grossly reduced. Intraoperatively, a complete tumor related occlusion of the brachiocephalic vein on the left side was obvious which explained the venous inflow obstruction on the left side. Furthermore, a moderate compression of the superior vena cava was evident with a pending complete occlusion within a short time interval. Further, a progressive mechanical obstruction of the trachea was demonstrated. So far, the slowly growing tumor has not yet again reached a size which could endanger the patient's life.

Postoperative Evaluation

After the unilateral neck dissection further diagnostic procedures are performed: determination of basal and pentagastrin-stimulated calcitonin concentrations; sonography; and, if indicated, another selective catheterization of the neck veins. Only with these additional investigations can a decision for a possible neck dissection of the contralateral side be reached.

Microsurgical Technique

Access

The region of the neck is draped, leaving the ear lobe, the angle of the jaw, and the tip of the chin exposed. Laterally, the posterior neck region and caudally, the proximal 10 cm of the chest are included in the surgical field. After excision of the scar from previous surgery, the incision is extended along the anterior edge of the sternocleidomastoid muscle up to the angle of the jaw. Then, the sternocleidomastoid muscle is completely mobilized in order to be able to transect it at a later stage between two clamps if needed. This procedure can increase exposure and completeness of dissection in the lateral region of the neck.

Central Compartment

The internal jugular vein is separated in the roximal and the distal direction from the surrounding tissue. Using the plane of the adventitia this is possible even after extensive scarring due to previous surgery or radiation therapy. All ventrally running veins (Kocher's vein, facial vein, etc.) are ligated and transected. Proximally, the internal jugular vein is followed up to the base of the skull. The same procedure is performed with the carotid artery. Similarly, the adventitial plane is recommended for dissection as it is best suited for preparation after previous surgery. Keeping this in mind, scarring after thyroidectomy is rarely a problem.

The carotid bifurcation is first dissected free. Then, the internal carotid artery is prepared to the base of the skull, similar to the internal jugular vein. After isolating the artery and the vein, the vagal nerve is also dissected free from its surrounding tissues, whereby careful attention must be paid to the preservation of the perineural tissues. Under these conditions, all nerves can be dissected for most of their course without increasing the risk of postoperative dysfunction extensively. The ansa cervicalis is proximally ligated and resected. Next, all lymphatic tissue extending from the lower jaw to the cervical spine is removed in several portions. The digastric muscle is separated. Below this muscle, the hypoglossal nerve is identified and dissected for a longer distance. The submandibular gland is encountered during this procedure and preserved. In order to achieve this, several small veins draining the face have to be ligated in this area. Caudally, the preparation is continued along the pharynx, identifying the hyoid bone. Along the pharynx the superior laryngeal nerve with its accompanying vessels is encountered. The diameter of this nerve is highly variable and great care has to be exerted not to accidentally damage the nerve. The nerve is followed up to its junction with the larynx. Here, it penetrates the laryngeal membrane at the upper edge of the larynx at 11 or 1 o'clock. The external carotid artery with its branches is also dissected free and the superior thyroid artery is ligated and resected at its origin. The tissue is then dissected from the cervical spine, carefully paying attention to the sympathetic nerves in order to avoid a possible postoperative Horner's syndrome (miosis, ptosis, enophthalmus).

The recurrent nerve is identified before any further preparation of the laryngeal region is attempted. This is best achieved in virgin tissue where no scarring can be expected. Once this is successfully done the nerve is again followed caudally and identified in its course. During this preparative step, the common carotid artery is dissected free. Cranially, the recurrent nerve runs along the esophagus in the tracheoesophageal groove obliquely to the larynx, entering the lower laryngeal edge at 5 and 7 o'clock. In this way, the recurrent nerve is first identified in its caudal portion at the esophagus and then followed for its complete length. Thus, the nerve can be dissected from scar tissue in the thyroid bed without damage. Again, the perineural tissue has to be preserved. After identification of the complete course of the recurrent nerve the next portion of lymphatic tissue is removed down to the spine; the parathyroid glands, however, have to be preserved. If the vascular supply of the parathyroid glands has to be sacrificed due to technical or tactical reasons the parathyroid tissue is stored in order to permit a replantation into the sternocleidomastoid muscle at a later time. The inferior thyroid artery is dissected in a similar manner to the superior thyroid artery and resected at its origin.

After finally removing the last portion of lymphatic tissue down to the cervical spine, carefully paying attention to the sympathetic nerves, the pretracheal tissue can be approached. Sternothyroid, sternohyoid and omohyoid muscles are transected if necessary. The scar tissue in the former thyroid bed is now completely removed taking any residual thyroid tissue including the thyroid capsule and any additional lymph nodes with it. Continuing along the trachea caudally, the lymphatic and fatty tissue from the anterior mediastinum is removed to the level of the brachiocephalic vein. Additionally, the thymus is removed by blunt dissection using the cervical approach. This is possible without extensive bleeding. On the operation table, the thymus is serially cut and macroscopically examined for additional parathyroid tissue which is also preserved for later reimplantation. In lean patients the transcervical removal of pretracheal tissue is possible up to 1–2 cm below the brachiocephalic vein. After preparation of the anterior mediastinum the posterior mediastinum is dissected. Here again, the recurrent nerve has to be preserved. Then, the lymphatic and fatty tissue between trachea, esophagus, superior vena cava, and subclavian vein is carefully resected.

Lateral Compartment

After complete removal of the medial compartment to the internal jugular vein one proceeds to the dissection of the lateral compartment (Fig. 9). Here, it is intended to remove the tissue between the internal jugular vein and the trapezoid muscle. In order to gain better access the sternocleidomastoid muscle is transected. The preparation starts proximally at the mastoid bone. In this cranial and lateral neck region the tissue is interspersed with very dense connective tissue. Therefore, it can be difficult to isolate and preserve the parotid gland. However, we have never postoperatively encountered problems due to a resection of the caudal pole of the parotid gland. Proceeding caudally, the accessory nerve is dissected and isolated. Next, the minor occipital nerve and branches of the cervical plexus (segments II–IV, N. auricularis magnus, N. transversus colli, Rr. musculares, Nn. supraclaviculares) are isolated removing the lymphatic tissue completely but preserving the musculature (M. splenius capitis, M. levator scapulae, M. trapezius). All branches of the plexus are freed for several centimeters. Small retractors are used to carefully keep the nerves away from the dissection area without causing traction injuries. Even further caudally, the brachial plexus is encountered. Medially in the direction of the jugular vein, the phrenic nerve runs on the anterior scalenus muscle originating from C3-C5. This nerve must be preserved.

The preparation proceeds caudally to the clavicle, identifying the subclavian vein. In this supraclavicular area the fatty and lymphatic tissue is very loose and easily dissectable. On the left-hand side, the thoracic duct has to be carefully preserved on its course out of the thorax aperture arching into the left subclavian vein. A variety of other lymphatic vessels empty into the thoracic duct necessitating careful ligation of any lymphatics encountered. Otherwise, long-standing lymph fistulas can occur. In one patient, we observed a lymphatic fistula producing 2–3 l/day which persisted for several weeks postoperatively. The leakage eventually closed itself under conservative therapy. A ligation of the truncus is possible without any problems but transfixing sutures should be avoided since such sutures can by themselves lead to microinjuries, again giving rise to lymph fistulas.

In one patient, we combined the left-sided neck dissection with a median sternotomy to perform a lymphadenectomy of the anterior and posterior mediastinum. This was a 49-year-old male patient who was diagnosed 1 year previously as suffering from MTC after the excision of an enlarged cervical lymph node. Subsequently, a total thyroidectomy was performed in an outside hospital. Postoperative calcitonin and CEA levels were persistently elevated. A selective venous catherization revealed two possible sites of calcitonin production in the left lower neck and in the area of the brachiocephalic vein, thus further pointing towards persistent metastases in these regions. We performed a modified radical dissection of the left side of the neck and of the mediastinum after a transsternal mediastinotomy in one session. The histological examination demonstrated tumor tissue in the following regions: distally in the lateral triangle of the neck, in the supraclavicular fossa, at the brachiocephalic venous trunk and in the hilar region of the left lung. Postoperatively, calcitonin and CEA values were markedly reduced but still elevated. Therefore, the dissection of the contralateral side of the neck is planned.

After careful hemostasis the procedure is finished. Redon drains are placed into the posterior mediastinum and the lateral neck region (both no. 14) and paratracheally (no. 10). Before closing the skin, any divided muscle is rejoined and parathyroideal tissue reimplanted into the sternocleidomastoid muscle marking the site with clips. Next, the subcutaneous tissue is readapted and the skin is closed with interrupted sutures. The redon drains are partially drawn after 2 days and completely removed on the fifth day if a lymphatic fistula does not occur.

In conclusion, the surgical procedure is characterized by a complete removal of the lymphatic and fatty tissue of the neck from the cervical spine to the mastoid and from the trachea to the upper mediastinum, preserving all important anatomical structures.

Clinical Experiences

In our department, we performed 51 neck dissections on 40 patients between May 1988 and May 1991. The mean age was 46 years. So far, 20 patients with 31 neck dissections have been evaluated. In four patients, calcitonin levels were suppressed even after pentagastrin stimulation. Basally suppressed calcitonin values were also found in ten patients who exhibited pathological elevations upon pentagastrin stimulation. In a further four patients, the calcitonin concentrations in the serum were markedly reduced by the extensive lymphadenectomy but still persisted in the pathological range. The rate of permanent complications was bearable in these patients. Most complications were minor and of transient nature. Persistent nerve lesions were observed in 10% of patients. It can be concluded that the microsurgical lymph node dissection can still achieve serological cures or pronounced tumor reductions even after years of suffering from metastasizing C-cell carcinoma. Tisell et al. (1986) reported elevated survival rates after extensive neck dissection. Due to a limited observation period, we can not yet comment on this claim.

References

Bergholm U, Adami HO, Bergström R, Johansson H, Lundell G, Telenius-Berg M, Akerström G (1989) Clinical characteristics in sporadic and familial medullary thyroid carcinoma. Cancer 63:1196–1204

Block MA, Jackson CHE, Tashjian AH (1978) Management of occult medullary thyroid carcinoma. Arch Surg 113:368–372

Block MA, Jackson CE, Greenwald KA, Yott JB, Tashjian AH (1980) Clinical characteristics distinguishing hereditary from sporadic medullary thyroid carcinoma. Treatment complications. Arch Surg 115:142–148

Böckdahl M, Tallroth E, Auer G, Forsslund G, Grawberg PO, Lundell G, Löwhagen G (1985) Prognostic value of nuclear DNA content in medullary thyroid carcinoma. World J Surg 9:980–987

Buhr HJ, Lehnert T, Raue F (1990) New operative strategy in the treatment of metastasizing medullary carcinoma of the thyroid. Eur J Surg Oncol 16:366–369

Buhr HJ, Raue F, Herfarth C (1991) Spezielle Tumorbiologie und Chirurgie des C-Cell-Carcinoms. Chirurg 62:529–535

Chong GC, Beahrs OH, Sizemore GW, Woolner LH (1975) Medullary thyroid carcinoma of the thyroid gland. Cancer 35:695–704

DeLellis RA, Rule AH, Spiler I, Nathason I, Tashjian AH, Wolfe I (1978) Calcitonin and carcinoembryonic antigen as tumor markers in medullary thyroid carcinoma. Am J Clin Pathol 70:587–591

Duh QY, Sancho JJ, Greenspan FS, Hunt TK, Galante M, de Lorimier AA, Conte FA, Clark OH (1989) Medullary thyroid carcinoma. The need for early diagnosis and total thyroidectomy. Arch Surg 124:1206–1210

Eickhoff W, Herberhold C (1968) Die Lymphbahnen der menschlichen Schilddrüse. Springer, Berlin Heidelberg New York

Gautwick KM, Talle K, Hager B, Jorgensen OG, Aas M (1989) Early liver metastases in patients with medullary carcinoma of the thyroid gland. Cancer 63:175–180

Goltzmann D, Potts JT, Ridgeway EC, Maloof F (1974) Calcitonin as a tumor marker. N Engl J Med 290:1035–1039

Graze K, Spiler IJ, Tashjian AH, Melvin KEW, Cervi-Skinner S, Gagel RF, Miller HH, Wolfe HJ, DeLellis RA, Leape L, Feldman ZT, Reichlin S (1978) Natural history of familial medullary thyroid carcinoma. N Engl J Med 299:980–985

Mrad MDB, Gardet P, Roche A, Rougier PL, Calmettes C, Motte PL, Parmetier C (1989) Value of venous catheterization and calcitonin studies in the treatment and management of clinically inapparent medullary thyroid carcinoma. Cancer 63: 133–138

Norton JA, Doppman JL, Brennan MF (1980) Localization and resection of clinically inapparent medullary carcinoma of the thyroid. Surgery 87:616–622

Pertursson SR (1988) Metastatic medullary thyroid carcinoma. Complete response to combination chemotherapy with dacarbazine and 5-fluorouracil. Cancer 62: 1899–1903

Raue F (1985) Diagnostik des medullären Schilddrüsencarcinoms. Dtsch Med Wochenschr 110:1334–1337

Raue F, Schmidt-Gayk H, Ziegler R (1983) Tumormarker beim C-Zell-Karzinom. Dtsch Med Wochenschr 108:283–287

Roka R, Niederle B, Fritsch A, Krisch K, Schemper M (1982) Chirurgische Therapie des medullären Schilddrüsenkarzinoms. Dtsch Med Wochenschr 107:132–138

Rossi RL, Cady B, Meissner WA, Wool MS, Sedgwich CE, Werber J (1980) Nonfamilial medullary thyroid carcinoma. Am J Surg 139:554–560

Russell CF, van Heerden JA, Sizemore GW, Edis JA, Taylor WF, Remine WH, Carney JA (1983) The surgical management of medullary thyroid carcinoma. Ann Surg 197:42–48

Saad MF, Ordonez NG, Rashid RK (1984) Medullary carcinoma of the thyroid: a study of the clinical features and prognostic factors in 161 patients. Medicine (Baltimore) 63:319–342

Samaan NA, Schultz PN, Hickey RC (1988) Medullary thyroid carcinoma: prognosis of familial versus sporadic disease and the role of radiotherapy. J Clin Endocrinol Metab 67:801–805

Scherübl H, Raue F, Ziegler R (1990) Kombinationstherapie von Adriamycin, Cisplatin und Vindesin beim C-Zell-Karzinom der Schilddrüse. Onkologie 13: 198–202

Schröder S, Böcker W, Baisch H, Bürk CG, Arps H, Meiners I, Kastendieck H, Heitz PU, Klöppel G (1988) Prognostic factors in medullary thyroid carcinomas. Cancer 61:806–816

Schwerk WB, Grün R, Wahl R (1985) Ultrasound diagnosis of C-cell carcinoma of the thyroid. Cancer 55:624–630

Simeone J, Daniels G, Müller P (1982) High resolution real time ultrasonography of the thyroid. Radiology 145:431–435

Telander RL, Zimmerman D, van Heerden JA, Sizemere GW (1986) Results of early thyroidectomy for medullary thyroid carcinoma in children with multiple endocrine neoplasia type 2. J Pediatr Surg 21:1190–1194

Tisell LE, Hansson G, Jansson S, Salander H (1986) Reoperation in the treatment of asymptomatic metastasizing medullary thyroid carcinoma. Surgery 99:60–66

Van Heerden JA, Grant CS, Gharib H, Hay JD, Ilstrup DM (1990) Longterm course of patients with persistent hypercalcitoninemia after apparent curative primary surgery for medullary thyroid carcinoma. Ann Surg 212:395–401

Wahl RA, Branscheid D, Goretzki PE, Röher HD (1987) Chirurgische Therapie des C-Zell-Karzinoms. In: Wörner W, Reimers C (eds) Schilddrüsenmalignome, Diagnostik, Therapie und Nachsorge. Schattauer, Stuttgart, pp 267–280

Wells SA, Haagensen DE, Lineham WH, Farrell RE, Dilley WG (1978a) The detection of elevated plasma levels of carcinoembryonic antigen in patients with suspected or established medullary thyroid carcinoma. Cancer 42:1498–1503

Wells SA, Bauglin SB, Gamm DS, Farrell RE, Dilley WG, Preissig SH, Lineham WM, Cooper CW (1978b) Medullary thyroid carcinoma: relationship of method of diagnosis to pathologic staging. Ann Surg 188:377–383
Wells SA, Baylin SB, Leight GS, Dale J, Dilley WG, Farndon JR (1982) The importance of early diagnosis in patients with hereditary medullary thyroid carcinoma. Ann Surg 195:595–599
Woolner LB, Beahrs OH, Black MB, McCanahey WM, Keating FR (1969) Long-term survival rates. UICC Monogr Ser 12:326–330

Surgical Management of MEN 2

H. Dralle, G.F.W. Scheumann, J. Kotzerke, and E.G. Brabant*

Klinik für Abdominal- und Transplantationschirurgie, Medizinische Hochschule Hannover, Konstanty-Gutschow-Straße 8, W-3000 Hannover 61, FRG

Introduction

The multiple endocrine neoplasia (MEN) syndromes are genetically transmitted endocrinopathies. In both types of MEN syndrome, usually one organ predominantly is affected; however, the individual manifestation of the disease with regard to time and extent of organ involvement varies considerably. Unlike in MEN 1, in MEN 2 surgical treatment represents the therapy of choice for each part of the disease.

Surgical management of MEN 2 patients includes (a) preoperative diagnostic procedures identifying the organ(s) involved and the extent of accompanying morphological and functional disturbances, (b) preoperative medical treatment of patients with pheochromocytoma (PCC) before adrenalectomy, and perioperative alphareceptor blockade at the time of cervical intervention in patients with precursor forms of PCC (adrenomedullary hyperplasia) not yet considered for adrenalectomy, (c) surgical strategy in patients with synchronous multiorgan manifestation, and finally (d) the surgical technique of thyroid, parathyroid, and adrenal gland resection.

Although surgery generally is regarded as the treatment of choice in MEN 2, the extent of surgical resection of the involved endocrine organs is still debatable. In adrenomedullary disease, some centers recommend bilateral total adrenalectomy in all MEN 2 patients with adrenomedullary diseases (van Heerden et al. 1984); others reported conclusive results with a more conservative surgical procedure removing both adrenal glands only in the case of proven bilateral PCC (Tibblin et al. 1983; Jansson et al. 1984; Hamberger et al. 1987; Gagel et al. 1988; Dralle et al. 1989; Decker and Wells 1989). With regard to medullary thyroid carcinoma (MTC), prognosis

* We are grateful to Mrs. G. Martin for typing the manuscript and drawing the graphs.

has been proven to be significantly worsened by the development of lymph node metastases (Woolner et al. 1968; Saad et al. 1984; Schröder et al. 1988). However, the extent of lymph node surgery in the initial operation is still controversial (Samaan et al. 1989; Block 1990) and requires further studies including quantitative assessment of the relation of primary tumor size to lymphogenous spread of regional lymph nodes (Dralle et al. 1992).

The purpose of this study is to present our current surgical strategy for MEN 2 patients, with particular reference to the surgical approach in adrenomedullary and multiglandular disease and a new surgical technique of compartment-oriented microdissection of cervical lymph nodes in metastatic MTC.

Clinical Manifestations of the MEN 2 Syndrome: Surgical Considerations

The MEN 2 syndrome appears in two variants. MEN 2A is defined as "the MEN 2 syndrome without the mucosal neuroma phenotype," MEN 2 as "the MEN 2 syndrome with the mucosal neuroma phenotype" (Gagel et al. 1989). Recently, a third form of hereditary non-MEN 2 MTC (MTC without PCC) has been separated from the MEN 2A-associated MTC (Farndon et al. 1986). Whether these two forms of hereditary MTC represent discrete clinical entities or should be considered as part of a spectrum of tumor liability is not yet known (Sobol et al. 1989). The majority of hereditary cases belong to the MEN 2A (70%) or familial non-MEN 2A variant (17%–24%); only 6%–13% are of the mucosal neuroma phenotype (MEN 2B) (Saad et al. 1984; Brunt and Wells 1987; Raue et al. 1990).

Although tissue involvement varies within families, there are some major differences between MEN 2A and MEN 2B patients regarding the occurrence, mean age at diagnosis, and biological behavior of the associated endocrine neoplasms, which are of importance for the surgical management of MEN 2 patients.

Medullary Thyroid Carcinoma

According to recent genetic studies, MTC in MEN 2A and MEN 2B as well as hereditary MTC in patients without PCC is suggested to be due to the same gene locus (Sobol et al. 1989). Age of onset, and clinical severity of the disease may differ significantly between these types. In contrast to MEN 2B MTC, which is diagnosed more and more already during childhood (Russel et al. 1983; Brunt and Wells 1987; Telander et al. 1989), mean age at diagnosis of MEN 2A MTC is the third (Brunt and Wells 1987) and fourth decade (Raue et al. 1990). Regarding clinical course, MTC tends to be less aggressive in families without PCC, and less in MEN 2A than in

MEN 2B (Kakudo et al. 1985; Brunt and Wells 1987; Duh et al. 1989; Block 1990). Age- and tumor stage-correlating studies comparing hereditary, non-MEN 2A MTC, MEN 2A, and MEN 2B cases are lacking and there is, in particular, no study to illustrate the different clinical results in MEN 2A versus MEN 2B MTC patients despite the same age of manifestation, primary tumor size, and lymph node status, of which the latter has been confirmed to be the most important prognostic factor for all types of hereditary and the sporadic variant of MTC (Woolner et al. 1968; Saad et al. 1984; Schröder et al. 1988; Dralle et al. 1992). Thus, for the present, surgical management should be exclusively aligned to tumor stage, i.e., tumor size and lymph node involvement, and not to the clinical variant of hereditary MTC involved.

Parathyroid Disease

The incidence and type of morphological and functional changes of the parathyroid glands in MEN 2A varies considerably in different series (20%–100%) (Chong et al. 1975; Heath et al. 1976; Saad et al. 1984; Wells et al. 1985). This phenomenon was presumed to be due to the variability in MEN 2A gene expression in different families. MEN 2B patients show only in a few cases (2.4%, Khairi et al. 1975) abnormalities of the parathyroid glands; the majority of them present no clinical, biochemical, or morphological evidence of parathyroid disease (Heath et al. 1976; Norton et al. 1979; Carney et al. 1980). Thus, the association of parathyroid disease with MEN 2 is regarded as being genetically determined and not a response to elevated calcitonin or catecholamine levels; this is confirmed by the lack of increased frequency of parathyroid diseases in sporadic MTC and PCC.

In contrast to histopathological changes observed in many MEN 2A parathyroid glands that have been surgically removed, clinical evidence of hyperparathyroidism (HPT) is much less frequent and, when present, usually mild. Wells et al. (1975) found in about 50% of their patients all four glands involved while in the remaining group one, two, or three glands were enlarged. Parathyroid pathology varies considerably in the excised glands, and the whole spectrum from focal hyperplasia up to true adenomas has been reported; however, there is no correlation to serum calcium and/or parathyroid hormone (PTH) concentrations (Steiner et al. 1968; Block et al. 1975; Saad et al. 1984). In view of the clinical expression of MEN 2A parathyroid disease, which is consistently dissimilar to primary HPT (pHPT) in MEN 1, surgical management is emphasized to preserve parathyroid function, i.e., to identify all parathyroid glands during cervical exploration, but to remove only the grossly enlarged glands. In case of four-gland involvement, subtotal parathyroidectomy (Block 1990) or total parathyroidectomy with parathyroid autotransplantation (Brunt and Wells 1987) is indicated.

Adrenomedullary Disease

Development of adrenomedullary neoplasms in MEN 2 is proceeded by several stages starting with focal or diffuse hyperplasia, followed by nodule formation. PCC represents the end stage of this MEN 2-associated disease. Characteristically, different stages of the hyperplastic and neoplastic changes of the adrenal medulla coexist within both adrenal glands, thus comparable to pathomorphological findings in MEN 2 MTC, and fit Knudson's two-mutational model for the initiation of cancer (Knudson 1971; Block et al. 1980).

Surgical management of patients with adrenomedullary disease in MEN 2 is continuously controversial in regard to time and the extent of adrenal resection (total bilateral versus unilateral or subtotal adrenalectomy), due to the inconsistent frequency of adrenal involvement between MEN 2 families, the frequency of asynchronous adrenomedullary changes in both glands, and the rare occurrence of metastatic and extraadrenal manifestation.

PCC is observed in about 50% of MEN 2 patients (Saad et al. 1984; Wells et al. 1985; Gagel et al. 1988); 50%–80% of MEN 2 PCCs are bilateral, although about 40%–50% of these appear metachronously with an interval of several years. In 36 MEN 2 patients studied by Gagel et al. (1988) and Tibblin et al. (1983), 15 patients initially developed bilateral PCC, and 8 out of 21 patients with unilateral PCC at first manifestation required the removal of the contralateral adrenal gland subsequently because of PCC. Due to the need for adrenocortical replacement therapy with the risk of addisonian state or at least discomfort with the mode of hormone supplementation (Telenius-Berg et al. 1989), some centers now prefer a more conservative approach to hereditary adrenomedullary disease (Jansson et al. 1984; Hamberger et al. 1987; Gagel et al. 1988; Dralle et al. 1989; Decker and Wells 1989). The patient is followed regularly after unilateral or subtotal adrenalectomy to detect PCC in the contralateral or rest of the ipsilateral gland, as after bilateral total adrenalectomy to control adrenocortical substitution therapy. Under these conditions the prophylactic removal of a macroscopically normal gland seems to be inappropriate.

Although the possibility of developing a malignant PCC is raised in favor of total bilateral adrenalectomy in MEN 2, it is rare in MEN 2 patients (4/75, 5.3%, malignant PCCs in a collected series of six institutions from Westfried et al. (1978), Tibblin et al. (1983), van Heerden et al. (1984), Saad et al. (1984), Jansson et al. (1984), Dralle et al. (1989) and proved to be no more frequent in families with one patient bearing a malignant PCC (Carney et al. 1976a; Westfried et al. 1978). Moreover, the metastatic process has been uninfluenced by total bilateral adrenalectomy in the affected patients. MEN 2B patients seems to have the same risk of malignant PCC as has been observed in the MEN 2A families (Carney et al. 1976b).

Extraadrenal PCC/paraganglioma, which is associated in sporadic cases more frequently with metastatic course (30%–40%) than adrenomedullary neoplasms (2%–12%) (Melicow 1977; van Heerden et al. 1982), has rarely been observed in MEN 2 patients (Marks and Channick 1974); the association to MEN 2 therefore has to be further investigated.

Mucosal Neuromata Syndrome (MEN 2B)

Patients with MEN 2B syndrome are characterized by mucosal ganglioneuromatosis and/or marfanoid habitus without vascular disease. Unlike parathyroid abnormalities that occur rarely in MEN 2B, the pathomorphology of C-cell and adrenomedullary diseases is indistinguishable from that of MEN 2A. However, MEN 2B MTC occurs at a younger age, metastasizes earlier and has shorter tumor doubling times (Jackson et al. 1984); it is therefore associated with a significantly higher mortality.

MEN 2B syndrome is observed in about 50% of patients without family history of the disease (Khairi et al. 1975; Saad et al. 1984). Due to the characteristic phenotype, the syndrome can often be diagnosed in the first decade of life. Regarding the biological aggressiveness of MEN 2B MTC, it has been suggested that thyroidectomy should be performed in MEN 2B patients as soon as the phenotype is recognized and before stimulated calcitonin levels are increased (Thompson 1984).

Gastrointestinal tract abnormalities are common in MEN 2B patients (Khairi et al. 1975). As in the oral cavity, a disseminated ganglioneuromatosis is found throughout the alimentary tract. Carney et al. (1976c) reported 5 cases out of 16 MEN 2B patients with megacolon, leading to surgical intervention in 4. Thus, alimentary tract abnormalities in MEN 2B patients require greater attention at least during the postoperative course after cervical or adrenal gland surgery.

Results of Surgical Treatment

Between 1975 and 1990, 25 patients belonging to 11 families with MEN 2 were surgically treated at the Medizinische Hochschule Hannover (MHH). Twenty-three patients showed the MEN 2A, two patients the MEN 2B variant, the latter with no family history. There were 15 women and 10 men; the associated diseases are presented in Table 1. Regarding the age at first surgical treatment, no differences were observed between patients with MTC only (35 ± 15 years) and patients with two or more MEN 2A-related endocrinopathies (36 ± 14 years). MTC was present in all patients. In 5 out of 16 patients with MTC and PCC, MTC preceded the manifestation of adrenomedullary disease; in 9 of these patients MTC and PCC were detected synchronously, and in 2 patients PCC preceded MTC. Biochemical and clinical evidence of pHPT was established in four patients developing

Table 1. Clinical manifestation of medullary thyroid carcinoma, primary hyperparathyroidism, and pheochromocytoma in 25 patients belonging to 11 families with MEN 2A or MEN 2B syndrome

	MEN 2A (n = 23)	MEN 2B (n = 2)
MTC only	8	1
MTC ± pHPT + PCC	15	1
MTC + pHPT + PCC	4	–
MTC + PCC		
Synchronous	8	1
Metachronous	7	–
PCC		
Unilateral	9	1
Bilateral synchronous	4	–
Bilateral metachronous	2	–
Parathyroid disease	6	–
Hyperplasia, normocalcemia	2	
Primary hyperparathyroidism	4	

Data from the Medizinische Hochschule Hannover 1975–1990.
MTC, medullary thyroid carcinoma; pHPT, primary hyperparathyroidism; PCC, pheochromocytoma.

the full expression of MEN 2A. In addition, three patients operated on because of MEN 2A MTC showed parathyroid hyperplasia in the excised glands, but without hypercalcemia or clinical signs of pHPT. One young patient out of the whole series died because of metastasizing MTC 2 years after thyroidectomy; all other patients are currently alive.

Medullary Thyroid Carcinoma

The results of surgical treatment of 25 patients with MEN 2 MTC, treated from 1975 to 1990 at the MHH, are summarized in Table 2. From 1975 to 1985 the standard procedure in cases of sporadic or familial MTC was total thyroidectomy with lymphadenectomy of macroscopically enlarged or presumably tumor-infiltrated cervical lymph nodes (symptomatic lymphadenectomy). Since 1986, total thyroidectomy is combined with systematic lymphadenectomy of the central lymph node compartment in all patients. If central or lateral lymph nodes are suspicious or proven to be metastatic, ipsilateral systematic lymphadenectomy of the lateral compartment is added. Transsternal systematic lymphadenectomy of the upper mediastinum is performed in the case of lower cervicocentral, cervicolateral-suprajugular, and upper mediastinal lymph node metastases. (Dralle et al. 1992).

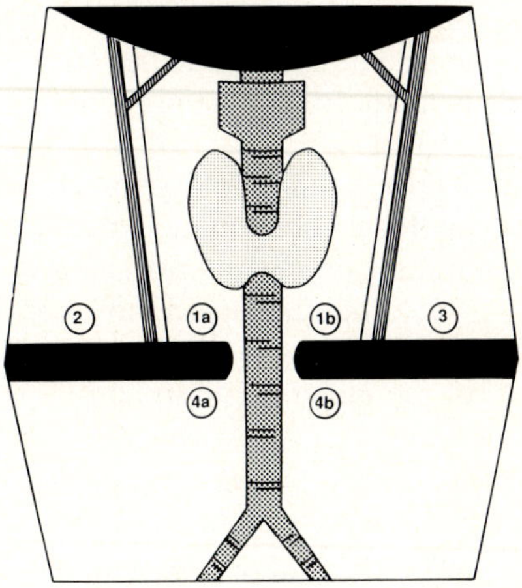

Fig. 1. Compartment classification of regional lymph nodes in the neck and upper mediastinum

Technique of Systematic Lymphadenectomy in the Neck and Upper Mediastinum. In contrast to different forms of symptomatic lymphadenectomy comprising the removal of one or more macroscopically tumor involved lymph nodes with or without interstitial adipose tissue, the principle of systematic, compartment-oriented lymphadenectomy is the en-bloc microdissection of anatomically defined whole compartments with the enclosed adipose, lymph node, and connective tissue. If the tumor is confined to these parts of tissues, all other anatomical structures, e.g., nerves, vessels, and muscles, as well as the trachea and esophagus are identified and preserved, serving as surgical landmarks during compartmentectomy.

Compartment Classification of Regional Lymph Nodes in the Neck and Upper Mediastinum (Fig. 1). Four regional lymph node compartments have been defined:

1. Central compartment (C1), right (C1a) and left (C1b) from the trachea (paratracheal lymph nodes), between trachea and the jugular vein, and from the hyoid bone down to the brachiocephalic veins. Most lymph nodes belonging to this compartment are arranged between inferior thyroid pole, recurrent laryngeal nerve and trachea, presumably representing the first region of lymph node metastases in thyroid cancer (Russel et al. 1963). Submandibular as well as paratracheal lymph nodes anatomically belong to the central compartment; however, concerning lymphangic spread of tumor cells, submandibular lymph nodes such as the parajugular lymph nodes function as a second region of lymphogenous spread.
2. Lateral compartments (C2, right; C3, left) are arranged between jugular vein (medial), subclavian vein (lower margin), trapezoid muscle and accessory nerve (lateral) and the hypoglossal nerve (cranial). To remove

this compartment completely, transsection of the sternocleidomastoid and omohyoid muscle and careful preparation of the adipose and lymphoid tissue anterior, between and posterior to the brachial plexus is necessary.
3. Upper mediastinal compartment (C4) is removed by a transsternal approach. Systematic lymphadenectomy of this area comprises the preparation of the inferior paratracheal lymph nodes down to the tracheal bifurcation and the removal of the infraclavicular praetracheal, paracaval, and paraesophageal lymph nodes within the anterior and posterior area of the upper mediastinum.

Results of Systematic, Compartment-Oriented Lymphadenectomy in MEN 2 MTC (Table 2). Regarding thyroid resection all patients were treated with no less than total thyroidectomy. The value of systematic versus symptomatic lymphadenectomy was analyzed by comparing patients with systematic lymphadenectomy (n = 14) with those who had only symptomatic or no kind of lymph node resection (n = 9). The results can be summarized as follows:

1. Results of calcitonin testing after pentagastrin stimulation were negative in 13 out of 14 MEN 2A MTC patients undergoing systematic lymphadenectomy (93%) compared with only 3 out of 9 MEN 2A MTC patients without systematic lymphadenectomy (33%).
2. Concerning the patients with pT1 ($<$10 mm) primary tumors (n = 12), all seven patients with systematic lymphadenectomy, but only two out of five patients without systematic lymphadenectomy had negative results of calcitonin testing after pentagastrin stimulation. As shown in Table 2, two patients (Nos. 302, and 305) with primary tumors of 5 and 8 mm diameter had proven lymph node metastases within the central compartment. Thus, from these results systematic lymphadenectomy at least of the central compartment seems to be clearly indicated in all MEN 2A MTC patients regardless of the primary tumor size.
3. Regarding ipsilateral systematic lymphadenectomy, the present data support its application in primary tumors exceeding 10 mm in diameter, at least in the case of tumor-involved central lymph nodes.
4. In contrast to cervical systematic lymphadenectomy, the value of transsternal systematic lymphadenectomy of the upper mediastinum remains to be elucidated. We observed only 1 out of 25 MEN 2A MTC patients with mediastinal lymph node metastases. This patient did not benefit substantially from this procedure.
5. Permanent recurrent laryngeal nerve paralysis and hypocalcemia was documented in four patients; recurrent laryngeal nerve paralysis resulted in the only patient with a pT4 tumor and extensive cervical lymph node metastases (No. 501). Permanent hypocalcemia was assessed after total thyroidectomy without lymphadenectomy in two women (Nos. 204, and

206) and after total thyroidectomy with central lymphadenectomy in a third woman (No. 601). After initiating the microdissection method, which is performed with the aid of magnifying glasses, complications of the surgical procedure concerning parathyroid glands and/or cervical nerve dysfunction no longer occurred. Thus, systematic microdissection of cervical lymph nodes was not associated with a higher surgery-related morbidity than that found after limited dissection procedures.

Parathyroid Disease

Four out of 25 MEN 2A patients developed clinical and/or biochemical signs of pHPT (Table 3). Both MEN 2B patients showed no evidence of parathyroid dysfunction. Irrespective of the surgical procedure performed in patients with pHPT (excision of macroscopically enlarged glands, subtotal or total parathyroidectomy with autotransplantation) all patients were normocalcemic postoperatively, although showing some abnormalities of the PTH metabolism.

In addition to these four patients with pHPT, in eight normocalcemic patients one or two parathyroid glands were surgically excised and examined by light microscopy. Three out of these eight patients (Nos. 102, 302, and 305) revealed hyperplastic parathyroid glands; the remaining patients did not show any evidence of parathyroid hyperplasia. As observed in the four patients with pHPT, these normocalcemic MEN 2A patients also demonstrated abnormalities of PTH metabolism (increased intact PTH with normal 44–68 midregional PTH, and vice versa). The postoperative results in this group of MEN 2A patients suggest a more conservative surgical procedure with excision of only macroscopically enlarged parathyroids rather than routine subtotal or total parathyroidectomy with autotransplantation. However, persistent PTH abnormalities in serum may be found in surgically treated as well as in nontreated patients indicating persisting, but subclinical disturbances of PTH metabolism in MEN 2A patients.

Adrenomedullary Disease

Clinical findings and results of surgical treatment in MEN 2 patients with adrenomedullary disease are summarized in Table 4. Sixteen out of 25 MEN 2 patients (64%) developed significant adrenomedullary lesions, treated in six patients by bilateral, and in ten patients by unilateral adrenalectomy. From the former group, four patients were operated on synchronously, and two metachronously with a time interval of 5 and 9 years, respectively. That means that, from a total of 12 initially unilateral adrenalectomized patients, to date only two have needed a second intervention at the contralateral adrenal gland.

Table 2. Results of surgical treatment of 25 patients with MEN 2 MTC (MHH, 1975–1990)

Patient no.	MEN 2-variant, clinical manifestation, year of MTC operation	Patient's age at MTC operation (years)	Tumor stage (UICC 1987)	Largest tumor diameter (mm)		Surgical treatment of MTC	Histological findings			Follow-up[b]
							Thyroid		Lymph nodes[a]	
				r	l		r	l		
101	MEN 2A (MTC, pHPT, PCC), 1991	69	pT2bNOMO	16	6	TT, syst. LA C1	MTC	MTC	C1a: 0/7 C1b: 0/6	Ct: neg.
102	MEN 2A (MTC, pHPT, PCC), 1990	37	pT2bNOMO	4	15	TT, syst. LA C1 + 3	MTC	MTC	C1a: 0/29 C1b: 0/21 C3: 0/10	Ct: neg.
201	MEN 2A (MTC, PCC), 1973	45	PT2bNOMO	>30	>10	TT	MTC	MTC	–	CT: 1.82 μg/l/multiple small liver metastases of MTC, n.e. of l.r.
202	MEN 2A (MTC, pHPT, PCC), 1976	37	pT2bNOMO	20	40	TT	MTC	MTC	–	CT: 8.98 μg/l/sympt. cervical LA 5/79 and 4/84; multiple small liver metast. of MTC, n.e. of l.r.
203	MEN 2A (MTC, PCC), 1985	30	pT2bN1MO	35	25	TT, syst. LA C1, sympt. LA C2 + 3	MTC	MTC	C1a: 7/11 C1b: 2/5 C2: 4/7 C3: 0/X	Ct: 2.02 μg/l
204	MEN 2A (MTC), 1985	24	pT2bNOMO	10	20	TT, syst. LA C1, sympt. LA C2 + 3	MTC	MTC	C1a: 0/8 C1b: 0/4 C2: X/X C3: 0/5	Ct: neg.
205	NEN 2A (MTC), 1985	19	pT1bNOMO	5	6	TT	MTC	MTC	–	Ct: neg.

206	MEN 2A (MTC, PCC), 1985	21	pT1bNOMO	6	9	TT	MTC	MTC	–	Ct: neg.
301	MEN 2A (MTC, PCC) 1986	21	pT1bNOMO	6	3	TT	MTC	MTC	–	Ct: 1.53 µg/l
302	MEN 2A (MTC, PCC), 1988	22	pT1bN1AMO	4	8	TT, syst. LA C1	MTC	MTC PTC	C1a: 0/2 C1b: 1/5	Ct: neg.
303	MEN 2A (MTC), 1988	61	pT1bNOMO	10	10	TT, syst. LA C1	MTC	MTC	C1: 0/4	Ct: neg.
304	MEN 2A (MTC, pHPT, PCC), 1989	40	pT1bNOMO	10	3	TT, syst. LA C1	MTC	MTC	C1: 0/4	Ct: neg.
305	MEN 2A (MTC, PCC), 1989	19	pT1aN1aMO	5	–	TT, syst. LA C1	MTC	CCH	C1: 2/9	Ct: neg.
401	MEN 2A (MTC, PCC), 1979	23	pT2bNOMO	8	35	TT	MTC	MTC	–	Ct: 10.0 µg/l
501	MEN 2A (MTC), 1986	23	pT3bN1bMO	n.k.	>40	TT, sympt. LA C1	MTC	MTC	C1: ≥ 1/X	Systematic cervical (7/86) and mediastinal LA (8/86), death due to metastasizing MTC (3/88)
502	MEN 2A (MTC, PCC), 1986	48	pT1bNOMO	10	7	TT	MTC	MTC	–	Ct: 0.81 µg/l

Table 2 (*continued*)

Patient no.	MEN 2-variant, clinical manifestation, year of MTC operation	Patient's age at MTC operation (years)	Tumor stage (UICC 1987)	Largest tumor diameter (mm)		Surgical treatment of MTC	Histological findings			Follow-up[b]
							Thyroid		Lymph nodes[a]	
				r	l		r	l		
503	MEN 2A (MTC, pHPT, PCC), 1987	50	pT2bN1aMO	25	20	TT, syst. LA C1a + 2	MTC	MTC	C1 + 2: ⩾1/X	Ct: neg.
504	MEN 2A (MTC, PCC), 1988	63	pT1bNOMO	5	8	TT	MTC	MTC	–	Ct: neg.
601	MEN 2A (MTC, PCC), 1985	54	pT2bN1bMO	15	35	TT, syst. LA C1, sympt. LA C2 + 3	MTC	MTC	C1b: ⩾1/X C1a: ⩾1/X C2 + 3: 0/X	Ct: neg.
701	MEN 2A (MTC), 1986	23	pT2bN1aMO	15	3	TT, syst. LA C1 – 3	MTC	MTC	C1a: ⩾1/X C1b: 0/X C2 + 3: 0/X	Ct: neg.
801	MEN 2A (MTC), 1989	40	pT1aNOMO	–	8	TT, syst. LA C1	–	MTC	C1a: 0/X C1b: 0/2	Ct: neg.
802	MEN 2A (MTC), 1989	36	pT1aNOMO	1,5	–	TT, syst. LA C1	MTC	–	C1: 0/3	Ct: neg.
901	MEN 2A (MTC), 1990	62	–	–	–	TT, syst. LA C1	CCH	CCH	C1: 0/X	Ct: neg.

1001	MEN 28 (MTC), 1989	6	pT1bN1bMO	4	5	TT, syst. LA C1	MTC	MTC	C1a: 1/12 C1b: 5/7	Ct: post-op. neg.; now 0.37 μg/l
1101	MEN 2B (MTC, PCC), 1990	15	pT2bN1bMX	15	19	TT, syst. LA C1 – 3	MTC	MTC	C1a: ≥1/X C1b: ≥1/X C2: 27/27 C3: 6/14	Ct: 0.59 μg/l

r, right thyroid lobe; l, left thyroid lobe; TT, total thyroidectomy; syst. LA, systematic lymphadenectomy; sympt. LA, symptomatic lymphadenectomy; C1 – 4, cervicomediastinal lymph node compartment classification; MTC, medullary thyroid carcinoma; PTC, papillary thyroid carcinoma; n.k., not known; n.e. of l.r., no evidence of local recurrence.

[a] Lymph nodes C1 – 4, cervicomediastral lymph node compartment classification with description of the number of tumor involved, and the number of surgically excised lymph nodes (X, unknown number of surgically excised lymph nodes).

[b] Follow-up 5 ± 2.2 years, all patients were traced until March 1991; Ct, calcitonin testing after pentagastrin stimulation (0.5 μg Gastrodiagnost/kg body weight, given as an intravenous bolus injection, peripheral blood was drawn at 0, 2, and 5 min. after injection for Ct measurements); negative Ct testing are Ct serum concentrations <0.3 μg/l; positive Ct testing Ct >0.3 μg/l.

Table 3. Results of surgical treatment of pHPT in 4 out of 25 MEN 2 patients

Patient no.	Clinical evidence of pHPT	Parathyroidectomy		Histology	Follow-up[a]
		Year	Procedure		
101	Hypercalcemia	1963	Parathyroidectomy (one gland)	Nodular hyperplasia	Mild hypercalcemia
		1991	Parathyroidectomy[b] (left lower)	Nodular hyperplasia	Normocalcemic without medication; normal mid-regional (44–68) PTH (165 pg/ml), slightly increased intact PTH (61 pg/ml) in serum[c]
202	Bilateral renal calculi since 1956; hypercalcemia (3.15 mmol/l)	1976	Parathyroidectomy (left lower)	Adenoma	Normocalcemic without medication; normal mid-regional (44–68) PTH (78 pg/ml)
304	Hypercalcemia (3.18 mmol/l)	1989	Subtotal parathyroidectomy (left upper and lower, right lower)	Nodular hyperplasia of all three glands	Normocalcemic without medication; mid-regional (44–68) PTH 260 pg/ml, increased intact PTH (97 pg/ml) in serum
503	Hypercalcemia (2.68 mmol/l)	1987	Total parathyroidectomy with autotransplantation right sternocleidomastoid muscle	One adenoma (right upper gland); three normal parathyroid glands	Normocalcemic without medication; increased mid-regional (44–68) PTH (311 pg/ml) and intact PTH (181 pg/ml) in serum

Data from the Medizinische Hochschule Hannover, 1975–1990.
pHPT, primary hyperparathyroidism; PTH, parathyroid hormone.
[a] All patients were traced until March 1991.
[b] Parathyroidectomy was performed en bloc with total thyroidectomy and central systematic lymphadenectomy because of MTC.
[c] Normal values for mid-regional (44–68) PTH <300 pg/ml, and intact (1–84) PTH 12–55 pg/ml.

Table 4. Results of surgical treatment of adrenomedullary disease in 16 out of 25 MEN 2 patients

Patient no.	Clinical presentation	Preoperative localization	Adrenalectomy		Histology[a]	Follow-up[b]
			Year	Procedure		
101	Asymptomatic (screening)	Right adrenal PCC, positive US, CT scan, and 123-I BG scan; left adrenal gland with normal findings	1990	Right translumbal total adrenalectomy	Unifocal PCC, 5 cm, 16.5 g	Normotensive, normocatecholaminemic without antihypertensive drugs, uneventful course of thyroidectomy 3 months post adrenalectomy
102	Asymptomatic, check-up because of phlebothrombosis	Bilateral adrenal PCC, positive US, CT sc an, and 132-I BG scan	1990	Transperitoneal bilateral total adrenalectomy	Bilateral multifocal PCC, right 4 cm, 86 g; left 3.5 cm, 29 g	Normotensive, normocatecholaminemic with adrenocortical substitution, without antihypertensive drugs
201	Sustained hypertension	Right adrenal PCC, positive US. CT scan, and 131-I BG scan; left adrenal gland with normal findings	1988	Transperitoneal right total adrenalectomy	Unifocal PCC, 3.5 cm, 14.5 g	Normotensive, normocatecholaminemic with antihypertensive drugs
202	Sustained hypertension	Right adrenal PCC, positive US. CT scan, and 131-I BG scan; left adrenal gland with normal findings	1987	Transperitoneal right total adrenalectomy	Multifocal PCC, 3.0 cm, 57 g	Normotensive, slightly increased concentrations of epinephrine, norepinephrine, and dopamine in serum and urine, with antihypertensie drugs

Table 4 (*continued*)

Patient no.	Clinical presentation	Preoperative localization	Adrenalectomy		Histology[a]	Follow-up[b]
			Year	Procedure		
203	Asymptomatic (screening)	Right adrenal PCC, positive US, CT scan, 131-I BG scan, and MR tomography; left adrenal gland with normal findings	1988	Right translumbal total adrenalectomy	Unifocal PCC, 2.5 cm, 12.5 g	Normotensive, normocatecholaminemic without antihypertensive drugs
206	Palpitations	Left adrenal PCC, positive US, CT scan, 123-I BG scan, and MR tomography; right adrenal gland with normal findings	1990	Left translumbal subtotal adrenalectomy	Unifocal PCC, 4.5 cm, 27 g	Normotensive, normocatecholaminemic without antihypertensive drugs
301	Paroxysmal hypertension	n.k.	1973	Transperitoneal left total adrenalectomy	Unifocal PCC, 209 g	
	Recurrent paroxysmal hypertension	Right adrenal PCC, positive angiographic findings	1978	Paravertebral right adrenalectomy	Unifocal PCC, 8.0 cm, 90 g	
	Recurrent hypertension since 1985	Recurrent right adrenal PCC, positive US, 123-I BG scan, and CT scan	1990	Transperitoneal resection of PCC in right adrenal remnant	Unifocal PCC, 1.2 cm	Normotensive, normocatecholaminemic without antihypertensive drugs, adrenocortical substitution therapy

302	Asymptomatic (screening)	Bilateral adrenal PCC, positive US, CT scan, and 123-I BG scan	1988	Transperitoneal left total and right subtotal adrenalectomy	Unifocal right PCC (3.5 cm), multifocal left PCC (3.0 cm)	Normotensive, normocatecholaminemic, without antihypertensive or adrenocortical substitution therapy
304	Hypertension	n.k.	1967	Transperitoneal right total adrenalectomy	Unifocal PCC	Hypertensive till 1971
	Recurrent paroxysmal hypertension	Left adrenal PCC, positive angiography	1976	Paravertebral left total adrenalectomy	Unifocal PCC, 9 cm, 156 g	Normotensive without antihypertensive drugs, normocatecholaminemic, adrenocortical substitution therapy
305	Asymptomatic (screening)	Bilateral adrenal PCC, positive US, CT scan, and 123-I BG scan	1989	Transperitoneal left total and right subtotal adrenalectomy	Bilateral multifocal PCC, right 3 cm, 25 g; left 5 cm, 56 g	Normotensive without antihypertensive drugs, normocatecholaminemic, adrenocortical substitution therapy
401	Sweating	Right adrenal PCC, positive US, and CT scan	1985	Transperitoneal right total adrenalectomy	Unifocal PCC, 5 cm, 59 g	Normotensive, normocatecholaminemic without antihypertensive drugs
502	Sweating, palpitations	Right adrenal PCC, positive US, and CT scan	1987	Translumbal right total adrenalectomy	Multifocal PCC, 2.2 cm	Normotensive, normocatecholaminemic without antihypertensive drugs

Table 4 (*continued*)

Patient no.	Clinical presentation	Preoperative localization	Adrenalectomy		Histology[a]	Follow-up[b]
			Year	Procedure		
503	Sustained hypertension	Bilateral adrenal PCC, positive US, CT scan, 131-I BG scan, and MR tomography	1988	Transperitoneal bilateral total adrenalectomy with adrenocortical autotrans-plantation left forearm	Bilateral multifocal PCC, right 1.0 cm; left 1.8 cm	Normotensive, normocatecholaminemic without antihypertensive drugs, adrenocortical substitution therapy
504	Asymptomatic (screening)	Right adrenal PCC, positive US, CT scan, and 131-I BG scan	1987	Transperitoneal right total adrenalectomy	Multifocal PCC, 7.5 cm, 71 g	Normotensive, normocatecholaminemic without antihypertensive drugs
601	Paroxysmal hypertension	Left adrenal PCC, positive US, and CT scan	1985	Transperitoneal left total adrenalectomy	Unifocal PCC, 5.0 cm, 34 g	Normotensive, normocatecholaminemic without antihypertensive drugs
1101	Asymptomatic	Left adrenal PCC, positive US, CT scan, and 123-I BG scan	1990	Transperitoneal left total adrenalectomy	Unifocal PCC, 3.0 cm, 21.5 g	Normotensive, normocatecholaminemic without antihypertensive drugs

Data from the Medizinische Hochschule Hannover, 1975–1990.
PCC, pheochromocytoma; US, ultrasound; CT scan, computed tomography; BG, benzylguanidine; MR, magnetic resonance; n.k., not known.
[a] Histological diagnosis of main adrenal lesion, largest tumor diameter (cm), and total weight of the resected specimen (adrenal gland plus tumor).
[b] All patients were traced till March, 1991.

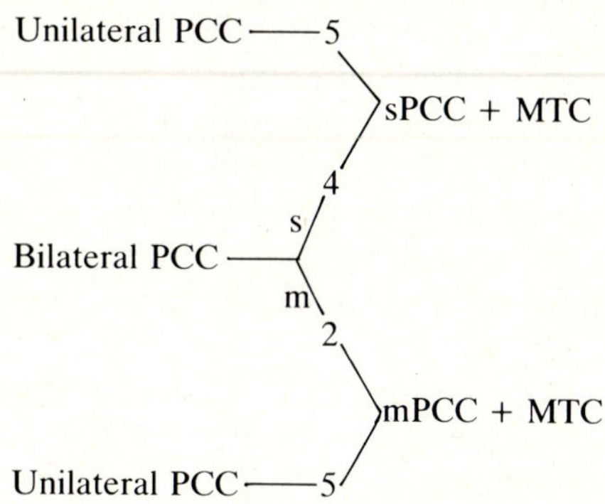

Fig. 2. Adreuomedullary disease in 25 MEN 2 patients. Data from the Medizinische Hochschule Hannover 1975–1990. *PCC*, pheochromocytoma; *MTC*, medullary thyroid carcinoma; *m*, metachronous occurrence; *s*, synchronous occurrence

Regarding the concurrent occurrence of MTC and PCC, in 9 out of 16 patients both these endocrinopathies were detected synchronously, 4 of them having bilateral synchronous PCC. In 7 out of 16 patients, PCC developed metachronously, 2 of them having bilateral metachronous PCC. Histological analysis revealed that seven out of ten unilateral PCC were unifocal neoplasms within the excised glands; on the other hand, only one out of the four synchronously occurring bilateral PCCs but both metachronously occurring bilateral PCCs were shown to be unifocal adrenal tumors.

In conclusion, about half of our MEN 2 patients with adrenomedullary disease developed PCC synchronously, or metachronously (Fig. 2). In no case could malignant tumor growth be established. Bilateral PCC occurred more frequently in patients with synchronous PCC and MTC than in those with metachronous PCC and MTC.

The last group of patients showed more often unilateral PCC and, in the two cases of synchronous MTC with bilateral PCC, PCC developed metachronously in both glands. Thus, only a few MEN 2 patients present with synchronous bilateral neoplastic adrenomedullary disease (4/25, 16%, in our series) supporting a more reserved approach to this part of the disease regarding the indication for surgery and the extent of adrenal gland resection.

Synchronously Occurring Bi-or Triendocrinopathies in MEN 2

Eleven out of 25 MEN 2 patients (44%) presented with bi-or triendocrinopathies synchronously. Two of them presented with MTC and pHPT (Nos. 202, and 304), two with MTC, pHPT, and PCC (Nos. 101, and 503), and seven with MTC and PCC (Table 5). In four patients with concurrent MTC and pHPT (Nos. 101, 202, 304, and 503; see Tables 2, 3) total thyroidectomy and parathyroidectomy were performed in a one-stage procedure. The indication for operation, extent of resection, and operative stress for the patient did not differ from that for one-gland disease. Depending on the extent of the disease and the physical condition of the patient, in nine patients with concurrent MTC and PCC cervical and adrenal operations were performed either in a one-stage (five patients), or in a two-stage procedure (four patients).

The postoperative course of all these patients with one- or two-stage procedures in synchronous MEN 2 endocrinopathies passed without major complications.

As for patients with PCC only, all patients with *concurrent MTC and PCC* were preoperatively treated with a high dosage of alpha-receptor blockage (mean dosage preoperatively 270 mg phenoxybenzamine) during a 13- to 25-day period (Grosse et al. 1990) to normalize the catecholamine-induced hemodynamic changes in PCC. Those patients from the two-stage procedure group, who underwent thyroidectomy first because of symptomatic MTC (Nos. 502, and 503), were treated perioperatively with high-dosage alpha-receptor blockage without any intraoperative or postoperative hemodynamic complications. The duration of postoperative hospital stay depended more on the type of adrenalectomy (unilateral versus bilateral) because of implementation of adrenocortical substitution therapy, rather than on the timing of surgical procedure (one-stage versus two-stage) (Table 5).

Thus, regarding postoperative hospital stay and surgical complications, timing of surgical intervention, i.e., one-stage, or two-stage-procedure with adrenalectomy first as routine procedure, or primary thyroidectomy in the case of dominating malignant cervical disease, may be performed individually according to the patient's physical and MEN 2-related condition, and if adequate alpha-receptor blocking pretreatment is performed.

Conclusions

MEN 2 represents a hereditary multiendocrinopathy with two predominant manifestations – MTC as an obligatory part and the prognostic pacemaker of the syndrome, and PCC, an optional part, but, like pHPT, sometimes the primary event of the syndrome with characteristic functional disturbances of the involved hormone metabolism. As a consequence of these different qualities of diseases in MEN 2, surgical strategy has to be adjusted accordingly to the individual biological significance of the oncological and/or functional disorder. In most cases, problems of surgical treatment turn out to be a result of inadequate resection of MTC but not of adrenomedullary disease. Family screening of MEN 2 kindreds is now becoming increasingly established in most countries; the patients involved die in most cases because of metastasizing MTC and not as a consequence of PCC compli-

Table 5. Surgical procedure in nine patients with synchronous MEN 2 MTC and PCC

Patient no.	One-stage procedure	Postoperative day of discharge from hospital	Compli-cations	Patient no.	Two-stage procedure		Postoperative day of discharge from hospital	Compli-cations
					Date	Procedure		
102	TT, syst. La C1 + 3, parathyroidectomy, transperitonal bilateral total adrenalectomy	17	–	101	Dec. 1990	Right translumbal total adrenalectomy	8	Intermittent brady-arrythmia
					March 1991	TT, syst. LA C1	4	–
302	TT, syst. LA C1, parathyroidectomy, transperitoneal left total and right subtotal adrenalectomy	19	–	502	Dec. 1986	TT	2	–
					July 1987	Translumbal right total adrenalectomy	7	–
305	TT, syst. LA C1, parathyroidectomy transperitoneal left total and right subtotal adrenalectomy	24	–	503	March 1987	TT, syst. LA C1 + 2	8	–
					May 1988	Transperitoneal bilateral total adrenalectomy with adrenocortical autotransplantation left forearm	15	–
601	TT, syst. LA C1, sympt. LA C2 + 3, transperitoneal left total adrenalectomy	9	–	504	Dec. 1987	Transperitoneal right total adrenalectomy	22	Pneumonia
					April 1988	TT	4	–
1101	TT, syst. LA C1 – 3, transperitoneal left total adrenalectomy	13	–					

Data from the Medizinische Hochschule Hannover, 1975–1990. For abbreviations, see Table 2.

cations. Considering the biological and socioeconomical conditions of MEN 2, the following surgical principles for MEN 2 treatment can be summarized (Fig. 3).

Medullary Thyroid Carcinoma

Although the occurrence of regional lymph node metastases is generally accepted as the most important unfavorable prognostic factor in both sporadic and hereditary MTC (Woolner et al. 1968; Schröder et al. 1988), there are only a few studies dealing with the tumor stage-related surgical procedure in MTC (Bigner et al. 1981; Dralle et al. 1992). Some authors experienced that cervical lymphadenectomy in patients with lymph node involvement at initial operation was unsuccessful in the eradication of metastatic disease (Jackson et al. 1983).

From our experience, classification of regional lymph node compartments, standardized compartment-oriented microdissection of cervical lymph nodes, and systematic evaluation of the exact number of lymph nodes surgically removed and metastatic nodes involved, are the inevitable conditions for a standardized therapy concept and success control. The following conclusions can be drawn from the present data (Fig. 3):

- Central systematic lymphadenectomy is essential for all stages of MTC. In patients with primary tumors not exceeding 10 mm in diameter and without central lymph node metastases (as proven intraoperatively by routine morphological methods) only 40% of patients without systematic central lymphadenectomy, but all patients with systematic central lymphadenectomy revealed normal calcitonin levels after pentagastrin stimulation postoperatively.
- Ipsilateral/cervicolateral systematic lymphadenectomy is recommended for all patients with primary tumors exceeding 10 mm in diameter, in the case of tumor-involved lymph nodes in the ipsilateral central compartment, or lymph node metastases within the ipsilateral/cervicolateral compartment.
- Bilateral systematic lymphadenectomy of central and lateral compartments is essential in primary tumors with bilateral lymph node metastases, as is observed in most MEN 2B patients.
- Transsternal mediastinal systematic lymphadenectomy is indicated in those patients showing enlarged or tumor-involved lymph nodes intraoperatively or preoperatively by imaging methods within the upper mediastinum. However, benefit on survival, "downstaging" of primary tumor stages, or significant effects on lowering calcitonin levels is observed only in few patients with such an advanced tumor stage.
- Reexploration of patients with symptomatic or asymptomatic MTC seems to be indicated to complete cervical compartmentectomy (see Buhr et al., this volume). However, success rates with regard to postoperatively

CCH/MTC

Exclusion
of
pHPT, PCC

CCH TT

MTC *<10 mm (T1N0M0)*
TT, central LA (C1a+b)

>10 mm, or LNM
(T2–4 N1 M0/1)
TT, central LA,
ipsilateral LA
(C1a+b, C2/3)

pHPT

Exclusion
of
CCH/MTC, PCC

1- to 3-gland disease
Removal of
enlarged glands

4- gland disease
Subtotal, or total
parathyroidectomy
with
autotransplantation

PCC

Exclusion
of
CCH/MTC, pHPT

Unilateral PCC
Unilateral adrenalectomy
(subtotal in unifocal, total
with multifocal PCC)

Bilateral PCC
Bilateral adrenalectomy
(bilateral total, or unilateral
total and contralateral sub-
total adrenalectomy)

Synchronous CCH/MTC and/or pHPT, and PCC

- Adequate pre-operative alpha-receptor blockade in all patients with adreno-medullary disease.
- Decision on one-or two-stage procedure with sequence of gland resection according to patients physical and MEN 2-related conditions.

Fig. 3. Surgical strategy for MEN 2 endocrinopathies. *CCH*, C-cell hyperplasia; *C1–4*, compartment classification (for details, see text); *LA*, systematic lymphadenectomy; *MTC*, medullary thyroid carcinoma; *pHPT*, primary hyperparathyroidism; *PCC*, pheochromocytoma; *TT*, total thyroidectomy; *LNM*, lymph node metastases

stimulated calcitonin levels (van Heerden et al. 1990) and patient survival are certainly reduced compared with primary interventions. Only in a few cases with subtle surgical procedures may patients be cured biochemically (Tisell et al. 1986; Dralle et al. 1992). Thus, adequate initial surgery remains the main objective in MTC treatment.

Parathyroid Disease

MEN 2 involvement of parathyroid glands is generally accepted as a minor complication of the disease. In some cases (9% in our series), pHPT may be the initial symptom of MEN 2A; in these and other affected patients, clinical course is usually mild compared with MEN 1 pHPT. Recurrent hypercalcemia after surgical treatment is rare, irrespective of the surgical method employed. For this reason most authors, including ourselves, favor a symptomatic approach to MEN 2 pHPT, consisting of resection of enlarged glands with preservation of the normal-sized ones. Only in the case of four-gland disease has subtotal or total parathyroidectomy with autotransplantation been recommended (Block 1990).

Adrenomedullary Disease

Adrenomedullary disease is a frequent but not always symptomatic part of MEN 2 syndrome. Surgical treatment is indicated in all patients with PCC proven by clinical or biochemical, and modern imaging methods independent of its individual symptomatology. The extent of initial surgery in MEN 2 adrenomedullary disease is still debatable. Based on the actual literature and our own results, a conservative approach to adrenal gland resection in MEN 2 patients is substantiated by the following arguments:

1. When present, adrenomedullary disease in MEN 2 always involves both adrenal glands; however manifestation is asynchronous in most patients. At least one-third of MEN 2 patients with adrenomedullary involvement (in our study 63%) remain symptom free after unilateral adrenalectomy (Tibblin et al. 1983).
2. Micronodule formation and adrenomedullary hyperplasia in the contralateral gland (Cho et al. 1980; Lips et al. 1981; van Heerden et al. 1984) should be regarded as no conclusive indication for surgical removal since these lesions, unlike those in sporadic adrenomedullary disease (Dralle et al. 1990), remain asymptomatic for many years, maybe for life. Prophylactic organ removal for asymptomatic , benign lesions does not seem to be acceptable today for the "well-disciplined patient living in a well-organized medical society" (Tibblin 1984), in so much as this procedure would lead to adrenocortical hormone substitution in the case of total bilateral adrenalectomy. Fatal complications of adrenomedullary

disease have been observed almost exclusively in symptomatic patients bearing big adrenal tumors but not in the screening population under medical observation with timely surgical removal of the tumor.
3. Malignant PCC is rare in MEN 2 (5.3%); it is no more frequent in families with one member bearing a malignant PCC and surgical radicality is not improved by bilateral adrenal gland resection.

Considering these biological prerequisites for adrenomedullary abnormalities in MEN 2, our present stategy in MEN 2 PCC may be summarized as follows (Fig. 3):

- Unilateral PCC nodule formation exceeding 15 mm in diameter, proven by CT scanning with 2-mm slice thickness, or MRI is treated by unilateral adrenalectomy. In young patients with unifocal PCC, which has to be established intraoperatively by complete exposure of the involved adrenal gland, organ resection may be limited to the neoplastic area preserving a well-vascularized, macroscopically normal tissue. The patient who was treated according to this approach is symptom free and has had normal catecholamine concentrations in urine and serum for 24 months. In multineoplastic unilateral adrenomedullary disease we would prefer total resection of the adrenal gland because of the increased risk of early local recurrence. However, experiences with partial adrenal gland resections in MEN 2 are limited (van Heerden et al. 1985; Hamberger et al. 1987); further results remain to be seen.
- Bilateral PCC, proven by the same criteria as unilateral PCC, has to be treated by bilateral adrenal gland resections. In two out of four patients with synchronous bilateral PCCs we were able to preserve adrenocortical function by unilateral total and contralateral subtotal adrenalectomy. Both patients have no adrenocortical supplementation and have shown no recurrence of the disease for 22 and 30 months respectively.
- Since routine exposure of the contralateral adrenal gland does not improve the detection of adrenomedullary abnormalities over the exactness of modern imaging techniques, an extraperitoneal approach is preferred for all patients with small (<5 cm) unilateral tumors.

Synchronous Multiorgan Involvement in MEN 2

Of our patients, 44% presented with synchronous bi- or triendocrinopathies in MEN 2 syndrome. Since a major proportion of patients in screened MEN 2 families are young people, one-stage procedures comprising neck and adrenal gland surgery can shorten the hospital stay without increasing surgical-related morbidity and may be performed with less individual discomfort than would be the case with a second surgical intervention. However, such procedures are appropriate only to selected persons after exact preoperative examination of physical status and analysis of the extent of the adrenomedullary disease and tumor stage of MTC. If neck surgery exceeds a three-compartment lymphadenectomy, or the patient's condition turns out to be impaired, two-stage procedures should be selected.

References

Bigner SH, Mendelsohn G, Wells SA, Cox EB, Baylin SB, Eggleston JC (1981) Medullary carcinoma of the thyroid in multiple endocrine neoplasia IIA syndrome. Am J Pathol 5:459–472

Block MA (1990) Surgical treatment of medullary carcinoma of the thyroid. Otolaryngol Clin North Am 23:453–473

Block MA, Jackson CE, Tashjian AH (1975) Management of parathyroid glands in surgery for medullary thyroid carcinoma. Arch Surg 110:617–624

Block MA, Jackson CE, Greenawald KA, Yott JB, Tashjian AH (1980) Clinical characteristics distinguishing hereditary from sporadic medullary thyroid carcinoma. Arch Surg 115:142–148

Brunt LM, Wells SA (1987) Advances in the diagnosis and treatment of medullary thyroid carcinoma. Surg Clin North Am 67:263–279

Carney JA, Sizemore GW, Sheps SG (1976a) Adrenal medullary disease in multiple endocrine neoplasia, type 2. Am J Clin Pathol 66:279–290

Carney JA, Sizemore GW, Lovestedt SA (1976b) Musosal ganglioneuromatosis, medullary thyroid carcinoma, and pheochromocytoma: multiple endocrine neoplasia, type 2b. Oral Surg 41:739–752

Carney JA, Sizemore GW, Hayles AB (1976c) Alimentary-tract ganglioneuromatosis. A major component of the syndrome of multiple endocrine neoplasia, type 2. N Engl J Med 295:1287–1291

Carney JA, Roth SI, Heath H III, Sizemore W, Hayles AB (1980) The parathyroid glands in multiple endocrine neoplasia type 2b. Am J Pathol 99:387–398

Cho KJ, Freier DT, McCormick TL, Nishiyama RH, Forrest ME, Kaufman A, Borlaza GS (1980) Adrenal medullary disease in multiple endocrine neoplasia type II. AJR 134:23–29

Chong GC, Beahrs OH, Sizemore GW, Woolner LH (1975) Medullary carcinoma of the thyroid gland. Cancer 35:695–704

Decker RA, Wells SA (1989) Multiple endocrine neoplasia. Jpn J Surg 19:645–657

Dralle H, Schürmeyer T, Kotzerke J, Kemnitz J, Grosse H, von zur Mühlen A (1989) Surgical aspects of familial pheochromocytoma. Horm Metab Res 21: 34–38

Dralle H, Schröder S, Gratz KF, Grote R, Padberg B, Hesch RD (1990) Sporadic unilateral adrenomedullary hyperplasia with hypertension cured by adrenalectomy. World J Surg 14:308–316

Dralle H, Damm I, Scheumann GFW, Kotzerke J, Kupsch E (1992a) Compartment-oriented microdissection of regional lymph nodes in medullary thyroid carcinoma. World J Surg

Dralle H, Damm I, Scheumann GFW, Kotzerke J, Kupsch E (1992b) Frequency and significance of mediastinal lymph node metastases in medullary thyroid carcinoma – results of a compartment-oriented microdissection method. Henry Ford Hosp Med J

Dralle H, Scheumann GFW, Hundeshagen H, Massmann J, Pidelmayr R (1992c) Die transsternale zervikomediastinale Primärtumorresektion und Lymphadenektomie beim Schilddrüsenkarzinom. Langenbecks Arch Chir 377:34–44

Duh QY, Sancho JJ, Greenspan FS, Hunt TK, Galante M, de Lorimier AA, Conte FA, Clark OH (1989) Medullary thyroid carcinoma. The need for early diagnosis and total thyroidectomy. Arch Surg 124:1206–1210

Farndon JR, Leight GS, Dilley WG, Baylin SB, Smallridge RC, Harrison TS, Wells SA (1986) Familial medullary thyroid carcinoma without associated endocrinopathies: a distinct clinical entity. Br J Surg 73:278–281

Gagel RF, Tashjian AH, Cummings T, Pathanasopoulos N, Kaplan MM, DeLellis RA, Wolfe HJ, Reichlin S (1988) The clinical outcome of prospective screening for multiple endocrine neoplasia type 2a. N Engl J Med 318:478–484

Gagel RF, Jackson CE, Ponder BAJ, Raue F, Simpson NE, Ziegler R (1989) Multiple endocrine neoplasia type 2 syndromes: nomenclature recommendation from the Workshop Organizing Committee. Henry Ford Hosp Med J 37:99

Grosse H, Schröder D, Schober O, Hansen B, Dralle H (1990) Die Bedeutung einer hochdosierten alpha-Rezeptorenblockade für Blutvolumen und Hämodynamik beim Phaeochromocytom. Anasthesist 39:313–318

Hamberger B, Telenius-Berg M, Cedermark B, Grondal S, Hansson BG, Werner S (1987) Subtotal adrenalectomy in multiple endocrine neoplasia type 2. Henry Ford Hosp Med J 35:127–128

Heath H III, Sizemore GW, Carney JA (1976) Preoperative diagnosis of occult parathyroid hyperplasia by calcitonin infusion in patients with multiple endocrine neoplasia, type 2a. J Clin Endocrinol Metab 43:428–435

Hermanek P, Sobin LH (eds) (1987) TNM classification of malignant tumors 4th edn. Springer, Berlin Heidelberg New York

Jackson CE, Talpos GB, Kambouris A, Yott JB, Tashjian AH, Block MA (1983) The clinical course after definitive operation for medullary thyroid carcinoma. Surgery 94:995–1001

Jackson CE, Talpos GB, Block MA, Norum RA, Lloyd RV, Tashjian AH (1984) Clinical value of tumor doubling estimations in multiple endocrine neoplasia type II. Surgery 96:981–987

Jansson S, Hansson G, Salander H, Stenström G, Tisell LE (1984) Prevalence of C-Cell hyperplasia and medullary thyroid carcinoma in a consecutive series of pheochromocytoma patients. World J Surg 8:493–500

Kakudo K, Carney JA, Sizemore GW (1985) Medullary carcinoma of thyroid. Biologic behavior of the sporadic and familial neoplasm. Cancer 55:2818–2821

Khairi MR, Dexter RN, Burzynski NT, Johnston CC (1975) Mucosal neuroma, pheochromocytoma and medullary thyroid carcinoma: multiple endocrine neoplasia type 3. Medicine (Baltimore) 54:89–112

Knudson AG (1971) Mutation and cancer: statistical study of retinoblastoma. Proc Natl Acad Sci USA 68:820–823

Lips KJM, van der Sluys Veer J, Struyvenberg A, Alleman M, Leo JR, Wittebol P, Minder WH, Kooiker CJ, Geerding RA, van Waes PFGM, Hackeng WHL (1981) Bilateral occurrence of pheochromocytoma on patients with the multiple endocrine neoplasia syndrome type 2A (Sipple's syndrome). Am J Med 70: 1051–1060

Marks AD, Channick BJ (1974) Extraadrenal pheochromocytoma and medullary thyroid carcinoma with pheochromocytoma. Arch Intern Med 134:1106–1109

Melicow MM (1977) One hundred cases of pheochromocytoma (107 tumors) at the Columbia-Presbyterian Medical Center, 1926–1976. A clinicopathological analysis. Cancer 40:1987–2004

Norton JA, Froome LC, Farrell RE, Wells SA (1979) Multiple endocrine neoplasia type IIb. The most aggressive form of medullary thyroid carcinoma. Surg Clin North Am 59:109–118

Raue F, Späth-Röger M, Winter J, Benker G, Buhr P, Dorn R, Dralle H, Frilling A, Herrmann J, Hörnig I, Meybier H, Klempa I, Kotzerke J, Pfannenstiel P, Reinwein D, Ritter M, Röher H-D, Schober O, Schröder S, Seif F, Trede M, Vogt H, Wahl R, Ziegler R (1990) Register für das medulläre Schilddrüsenkarzinom in der Bundesrepublik Deutschland. Med Klin 3:113–116

Russell CF, van Heerden JA, Sizemore W, Edis AJ, Taylor WF, ReMine WH, Carney JA (1983) The surgical management of medullary thyroid carcinoma. Ann Surg 197:42–48

Russell WO, Ibanez ML, Clark RL, White EC (1963) Thyroid carcinoma. Cancer 16:1425–1460

Saad MF, Ordonez NG, Rashid RK, Giudo JJ, Hill CST, Hickey RC, Samaan NA (1984) Medullary carcinoma of the thyroid. A study of the clinical features and prognostic factors in 161 patients. Medicine (Baltimore) 63:319–342

Samaan NA, Yang KPP, Schultz P, Hickey RC (1989) Diagnosis, management, and pathogenetic studies in medullary thyroid carcinoma syndrome. Henry Ford Hosp Med J 37:132–137

Schröder S, Böcker W, Baisch H, Bürk CG, Arps H, Meiners I, Kastendieck H, Heitz PU, Klöppel G (1988) Prognostic factors in medullary thyroid carcinomas. Survival in relation to age, sex, stage, histology, immunocytochemistry, and DNA content. Cancer 61:806–816

Sobol H, Narod SA, Schuffenecker I, Amos C, Ezekowitz RAB, Lenoir GM (1989) Hereditary medullary thyroid carcinoma: genetic analysis of three related syndromes. Henry Ford Hosp Med J 37:109–111

Steiner AL, Goodman AD, Powers SR (1968) Study of a kindred with pheochromocytoma, medullary thyroid carcinoma, hyperparathyroidism and cushing's disease: multiple endocrine neoplasia, type 2. Medicine (Baltimore) 47:371–409

Telander RL, Zimmermann D, Sizemore GW (1989) Medullary carcinoma in children. Results of early detection and surgery. Arch Surg 124:841–843

Telenius-Berg M, Ponder MA, Berg B, Ponder BAJ, Werner S (1989) Quality of life after bilateral adrenalectomy in MEN 2. Henry Ford Hosp Med J 37:160–163

Thompson NW (1984) Commentary to Jackson CE, Talpos GB, Block MA, Norum RA, Lloyd RV, Tashjian AH: Clinical value of tumor doubling estimations in multiple endocrine neoplasia type II. Surgery 96:981–987

Tibblin S (1984) Commentary to van Heerden JA, Sizemore GW, Carney JA, Grant CS, ReMine WH, Sheps SG: Surgical management of the adrenal glands in the multiple endocrine neoplasia type II syndrome. World J Surg 8:612–621

Tibblin S, Dymling JF, Ingemansson S, Telenius-Berg M (1983) Unilateral versus bilateral adrenalectomy in multiple endocrine neoplasia IIA. World J Surg 7:201–208

Tisell LE, Hansson G, Jansson S, Salander H (1986) Reoperation in the treatment of asymptomatic metastasizing medullary thyroid carcinoma. Surgery 99:60–66

Van Heerden JA, Sheps SG, Hamberger B, Sheedy PF II, Poston JG, ReMine WH (1982) Pheochromocytoma: current status and changing trends. Surgery 91:367–373

Van Heerden JA, Sizemore GW, Carney JA, Grant CS, ReMine WH, Sheps SG (1984) Surgical management of the adrenal glands in the multiple endocrine neoplasia type II syndrome. World J Sur 8:612–621

Van Heerden JA, Sizemore GW, Carney JA, Brennan MD, Sheps SG (1985) Bilateral subtotal adrenal resection for bilateral pheochromocytomas in multiple endocrine neoplasia, type 2a: a case report. Surgery 98:363–366

Van Heerden JA, Grant CS, Gharib H, Hay ID, Ilstrup DM (1990) Long-term course of patients with persistent hypercalcitonemia after apparent curative primary surgery for medullary thyroid carcinoma. Ann Surg 212:395–401

Wells SA, Dilley WG, Farndon JA, Leight GS, Baylin SB (1985) Early diagnosis and treatment of medullary thyroid carcinoma. Arch Intern Med 145:1248–1252

Westfried M, Mandel D, Alderete MN, Groopman J, Minkowitz ST (1978) Sipple's syndrome with a malignant pheochromocytoma presenting as a pericardial effusion. Cardiology 63:305–311

Woolner LB, Beahrs OH, Black BM, McConahey WM, Keating FR (1968) Thyroid carcinoma: general considerations and follow-up data on 1181 cases. In: Young S, Inman DR (eds) Thyroid neoplasia. Academic, New York, pp 51–79

*Postsurgical Follow-Up and Management**

F. Raue

Abteilung für Innere Medizin I – Endokrinologie und Stoffwechsel,
Universität Heidelberg, Luisenstraße 5, W-6900 Heidelberg 1, FRG

Postoperative Follow-Up

All patients with medullary thyroid carcinoma (MTC) should undergo calcitonin (CT) determination at regular intervals after total thyroidectomy. Within 6 weeks after operation serum CT measurement has to be performed to determine whether residual tumor or metastases are present (Fig. 1). Patients with normal basal and pentagastrin-stimulated CT levels suggest a tumor-free state where no further treatment is necessary. They can then be followed-up at half-year intervals with physical examinations, and once a year a pentagastrin stimulation test has to be done (Grauer et al. 1990).

The most difficult problem associated with the management of MTC is what to do with patients who have persistent elevation of serum CT concentration after apparently adequate surgical procedure. If the surgical procedure was inadequate, then reoperation with an appropriate surgical procedure is indicated (see H.J. Buhr et al., this volume). Prior to this type of procedure, a thorough evaluation should be done to define the extent of local and distant disease. Ultrasound examination has been particularly useful for the identification of nonpalpable metastases in the neck and can be used in conjunction with fine needle aspiration to positively identify metastatic disease before surgery (Schwerk et al. 1985; Frank et al. 1987; Gorman et al. 1987). Computerized tomography or magnetic resonance (MR) imaging techniques of neck, chest and abdomen, bone scan and other scanning techniques (see C. Reiners, this volume) help to make a decision regarding reoperation. Selective venous catheterization with blood sampling for serum CT determination also provides an anatomic region for the surgeon to either focus upon or exclude from surgery as a potential curative treatment modality in patients in whom metastatic disease (liver, lung) is

* This study was supported in part by a grant from the Baden-Württembergischer Krebsverband project *Prävention durch Screening*.

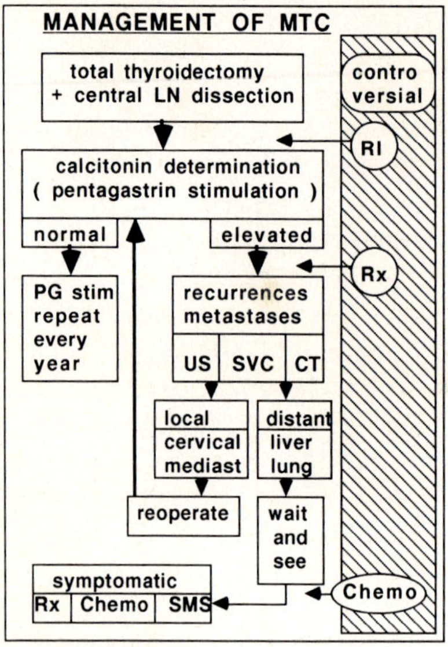

Fig. 1. Postoperative management of patients with MTC. *RI*, radioiodine treatment; *Rx*, external radiotherapy; *chemo*, chemotherapy; *PG*, pentagastrin; *US*, ultrasound; *SVC*, selective venous catheterization; *CT*, computerized tomography; *SMS*, somatostatin; *LN*, lymph node

found (Norton et al. 1980; Ben Mrad et al. 1989; Wells et al. 1982a; Gautvik et al. 1989; Frank-Raue et al. 1992). If there is no evidence of distant metastases and if local disease is found in the neck, reoperation is advocated using meticulous dissection and microsurgical techniques (Tisell et al. 1986; Buhr et al. 1990; see H.J. Buhr et al., this volume). With this procedure a cure rate of 25%–35% has been produced.

In patients remaining CT positive with evidence of nonoperable disease (distant metastases) or occult disease (no cervical recurrence is localized), close observation of the changes in CT and carcinoembryonic antigen (CEA) secretion is required. Many patients may exhibit a remarkably stable course and no further treatment is recommended; a "wait and see" approach is then advocated (van Heerden et al. 1990), as experience with nonsurgical therapy in the management of metastatic MTC has been disappointing. In those patients whose disease shows rapid or steady progress, intervention with chemotherapy, radiotherapy, or somatostatin (SRIF) can be considered as a palliative therapy modality (Fig. 1).

Radioiodine Treatment

The C-cells and MTC do not concentrate iodine (Ljungbert 1966) or generally respond to thyroid hormone and therefore the administration of ^{131}I has no role in the treatment of MTC. But there are some reports that after total thyroidectomy the ^{131}I treatment of patients with MTC further decreased the postoperatively still abnormally elevated CT levels (Hellmann et al. 1979; Deftos and Stein 1980). It could be speculated that follicular cells remaining in the thyroid bed after maximal thyroidectomy could trap sufficient isotope to permit accumulataion of ^{131}I in the tumor bed and thus destroy adjacent noniodine-trapping cancer cells. That depends on the assumption that adjacent tumor cells, if they are located within the short range of the β-radiation emitted by ^{131}I, could be radiated effectively in this manner. There are some experimental data confirming these assumptions: neonatal rat thyroid C-cells are very sensitive to ^{131}I; pathology of the irradiated gland showed a dramatic reduction in the number of C-cells (Thurston and Williams 1982). A decrease in circulating CT levels, and a reduced number of spontaneously developing MTC was demonstrated in rats that had undergone low-dose radiation with ^{131}I (Shah et al. 1983; Ott et al. 1987). Mice receiving ^{131}I in amounts sufficient to completely destroy the thyroid tissue also destroyed C-cells without any signs of their recovery (Feinstein et al. 1986).

Also radioiodine treatment for hyperthyroidism in patients with Graves' disease or toxic goiter showed a decrease in basal and calcium stimulated CT levels (Body et al. 1988; Bayraktar et al. 1990). Therefore radioiodine treatment might be useful in hereditary MTC, where all C-cells appear to have increased malignant potential and it is important that all possible thyroid tissue be removed. For this reason any remaining thyroid tissue can be treated with ^{131}I to achieve total ablation and destruction of C-cells adjacent to iodine-trapping follicular cells. But there is no convincing evidence of the effectiveness of such prophylactic postoperative radiotherapy. ^{131}I ablation does not improve survival in patients with MTC nor reduce recurrences (Nieuwenhuijzen-Krusemann et al. 1984; Saad et al. 1983).

The failure of ^{131}I to alter the serum CT levels and thus residual MTC is most probably due to the presence of lymph node metastases too distant from the thyroid remnant to become affected by the β emission of ^{131}I accumulated in the thyroid follicular cells. In patients with abnormal preoperative basal CT levels, cervical lymph nodes metastases are usually present and they are often not completely removed even after a modified neck dissection (Wells et al. 1982a,b).

In rare cases ^{131}I uptake in MTC metastases of bone (Rasmusson and Hansen 1979) or lung (Nusynowitz et al. 1982) was demonstrated, which disappeared after the administration of a therapeutic dose of ^{131}I. However, these authors did not exclude the possibility that their patient could have a mixture of follicular carcinoma and MTC, in which the follicular part concentrated iodine (Hales et al. 1982). The mixed medullary and follicular pattern of the primary tumor could be confirmed in a patient with MTC and pulmonary metastases with radioiodine uptake (Ruhlmann et al. 1987). The majority of MTC cases have, however, been found not to concentrate iodine. Therefore ^{131}I administration is not recommended postoperatively nor in the treatment of metastatic MTC (Saad et al. 1983).

External Radiotherapy

The role of regional external radiotherapy in the treatment of MTC continues to be controversial because the growth rate of MTC is very slow; the tumor stages of patients receiving radiotherapy are often not comparable (prophylactic postoperatively, after incomplete surgery, or for inoperable disease); and only small numbers of patients are studied. Some earlier reports have shown a favorable response of MTC to radiotherapy in a small series of patients (Halnan 1975; Simpson 1975; Steinfeld 1977). In a retrospective study 29 patients who received postoperative cervical radiotherapy had a survival rate similar to those who received surgery alone, despite having more advanced local disease (Rougier et al. 1983). In contrast, Samaan et al. (1988) found that patients with a similar extent of disease who received external radiotherapy had a worse prognosis than those who did not. They speculated that the high death rate in patients who received radiotherapy may be related to the extensive recurrence of the disease in these patients beyond the field of radiation, and the difficulties of second surgery for recurrence within the field of radiation. New techniques in localization of the disease and more meticulous dissection and microsurgical techniques have produced a higher cure rate in patients with inadequate primary surgical procedure. Surgical reintervention is often more difficult after external radiation because of scarring and fibrosis of adjacent structures. This has to be kept in mind before recommendation of postoperative radiotherapy. If appropriate surgical procedure has been performed, then sometimes no further treatment is warranted.

In patients with inoperable tumor, radiotherapy can give prolonged palliation and can achieve local tumor control (Sarrazin et al. 1984). Radiotherapy may be helpful for any expanding final stage lesion or for painful osseous metastases, but the response is poor. Therapy for each patient must be individualized.

Chemotherapy

MTC represents a neoplasm of low aggressiveness and good prognosis. Long-term survival even in advanced disease is not unusual. Due to the rarity of this disease with good results from initial surgical treatment few data regarding chemotherapy for advanced MTC are available. Most of these studies have been done with a small number of patients, summarizing the results of advanced thyroid cancer including a variety of histological types of tumor. The definition of a favorable response is often not given exactly. Sometimes several drugs have been used in the same trial; sometimes a combination of drugs in the same patient and somewhat arbitrary doses (Bukowski et al. 1983). Some potentially active agents, namely doxorubicin (adriamycin), bleomycin and cisplatin have been identified (Poster et al. 1981; Shimoaka 1980).

Table 1. Response of MTC to adriamycin plus cisplatin

Total no. of patients	No. of patients			Reference
	CR	PR	MR	
6	0	2		Schimoaka 1985
6	0	0		Williams et al. 1986
6	0	0		Athanassiades et al. 1988
3	0	0	2	Droz et al. 1985
10	0	1		Scherübl et al. 1990
31	0	3	2	Summary of all studies

CR, complete response; PR, partial response; MR, minor response.

Gottlieb and Hill (1974) indicated that adriamycin produced incomplete tumor remission in 30% of all histological types among three of six patients with MTC. Similar results with an overall response of 34% have been published by Benker and Reinwein (1983) (four out of ten patients with MTC had partial remission). Other single agent chemotherapy has not cured patients and generally has not produced greater than a 33% partial response. Combinations of agents have also been employed in small numbers of patients with varying success (Table 1). An anecdotal report described the complete response of MTC under the treatment of dacarbazine and 5-fluorouracil lasting 10 months (Petursson 1988). Hoskin and Harmer (1987) reported only one complete response in their series of 29 patients with differentiated advanced thyroid carcinoma. The results from the French group (Droz et al. 1990) over the last 10 years with five successive chemotherapeutic protocols in 49 patients were very disappointing with only two objective responses (3%). In contrast to the study of Shimoaka (1985), who showed that the quality of response achieved by the combination of doxorubicin and cisplatin is far superior to that achieved by doxorubicin alone, others could not confirm the better role of combination chemotherapy (Williams et al. 1986; Bukowski et al. 1983; Scherubl et al. 1990a). Concerning the response rate of MTC, it has been similar in all studies – between 10% (1 of 10 patients) (Scherübl et al. 1990a) and 30% (3 of 10 patients) (Shimoaka et al. 1985). Due to its lower toxicity, particulary cardiotoxicity, 4′-epiadriamycin or aclarubicin can be used instead of adriamycin (Samonigg et al. 1988; Ahuja and Ernst 1987). During chemotherapy serial determination of the tumor makers CT and CEA proved to be a valuable parameter of the course of the disease. In patients with partial remission, tumor markers decreased (Raue et al. 1985; Scherübl et al. 1990b). Life quality, toxic side effects and survival have to be taken into account when chemotherapy is recommended. The mean survival time of patients responding to treatment may be longer (about 18 months) than in nonresponders (about 6 months); toxicity is considerable. As MTC is relatively insensitive to chemotherapy it cannot be recommended for patients with asymptomatic disease which resides after surgery as tumor mass, and serum CT and CEA levels may remain stable for years. It might only be indicated when tumor mass seems to have escaped local control and entered a more aggressive growth phase. As improvement has not been obtained consistently with any traditional chemotherapy agent treatment of each patient with advanced MTC should be individualized based on clinical grounds; palliative surgery, radiotherapy or chemotherapy are all considered.

Somatostatin

SRIF, a tetradecapeptide originally found in the hypothalamus as an inhibitor of pituitary growth hormone secretion is also synthesized and secreted from the C-cells (Laurberg 1984; Gagel et al. 1986). SRIF seems to play an important physiological role in auto- and paracrine regulation of CT secretion. By immunohistochemical methods the presence of positive SRIF staining has been reported in 40%–60% of primary MTC; in at least 30% of cases, elevated SRIF concentration in the peripheral circulation has been measured (Pacini et al. 1989). Thus SRIF must be added to the long list of tumor markers secreted by MTC, although it may act as a regulatory peptide in normal as well as tumoral conditions (Modigliani et al. 1990).

Exogenous infusion of SRIF or the stable analogue SMS 201-995 is able to reduce the secretion of several hormones in normal subjects and to suppress the secretion of a variety of hyperfunctioning endocrine tumors (Lamberts et al. 1990b). Parallel to the inhibitory property on peptide hormone secretion a marked clinical improvement in symptoms related to the excess of hormone could be documented. In addition to the effect on hormone secretion, SMS also has an inhibitory effect on tumor growth; tumor regression of pancreatic tumors, carcinoids, and pituitary adenomas has been observed (Kvols et al. 1988; Kraenzlin et al. 1985). As a nontoxic drug without important side effects SMS could provide superior palliative treatment in advanced metastatic MTC.

Contradictory results of the acute effect on basal and stimulated CT secretion are reported: A 40%–70% reduction of basal and pentagastrin-stimulated CT levels in most patients with MTC treated with 0.4–1.5 mg SMS has been observed (Gordin et al. 1987; Bertagna et al. 1980; Clements et al. 1986; Pacini et al. 1989; Guliana et al. 1989; Mahler et al. 1990); no effect was observed with 0.05–0.1 mg SMS (Schrezemeir et al. 1986; Ahlman et al. 1987; Modigliani et al. 1988; Raue et al. 1976). One reason why some MTC patients respond and other do not might be the doses of SMS.

Also a long-term effect on CT secretion can be obtained in at least some patients (Mahler et al. 1990; Libroia et al. 1989); this correlated with a symptomatic improvement, and diarrhea and flushing ameliorated. Long-term alleviation of diarrhea in patients with advanced MTC despite unchanged levels of CT and CEA may occur (Geelhoed et al. 1986; Keeling and Basso 1988). Increasing the dose of SMS might be required to control the syndromes. The mechanism responsible for this tachyphylaxis is unknown.

Whether treatment with octreotide will be associated with the arrest of tumor growth or longer survival of patients with MTC remains questionable. Regression of measurable tumor has occasionally been reported in carcinoid tumors (Kvols et al. 1988) and vipomas (Kraenzlin et al. 1985). The way in which SRIF or SMS acts on C-cells has to be clarified. SRIF receptors coupled to Gi protein are known to inhibit the cAMP- and Ca-dependent pathway on C-cells (Raue et al., this volume), thereby inhibiting Ca- and pentagastrin-stimulated CT secretion. Whether or not inhibition of tumor growth is directly influenced by SRIF is controversial. In a recently done observation it could be shown that patients with SRIF expression in the primary tumor had better survival rates than patients with SRIF-negative tumors. Its presence in the tumor could exert an inhibitory effect on the growth of adjacent neoplastic C-cells through a para- or autocrine mechanism, or could act by inhibiting some, as yet unknown, growth factors implicated in the proliferation of MTC cells (Pacini et al. 1991). The antiproliferative effect might be mediated via inhibition of insulin-like growth factor I (IGF-I) or tumor growth factor through the SRIF receptor. The presence of the SRIF receptor might therefore be of considerable importance in predicting which tumor respond favorably to chronic treatment with SMS; SMS receptor-positive tumor could be imaged by ^{123}radioiodine-labelled SMS. This might be also important for localizing metastases of MTC (Reichlin 1990; Lamberts et al. 1990). Long-term treatment of metastatic MTC with high doses of SMS improved symptomatic diarrhea and reduced CT levels in some but not all patients; effects on tumor mass could not yet be confirmed. Based on these observations further studies are necessary to clarify the role of SMS in MTC.

Prognostic Factors

The natural history of sporadic MTC is variable. The spectrum of aggressiveness ranges from years of dormant residual disease after surgery to rapidly progressing disseminated disease and death related to either metastatic thyroid tumor or pheochromocytoma. There is general agreement that surgical management has a favorable influence on the clinical course of the disease. Early detection and treatment of MTC is likely to be curative; more than 95% of patients detected at early stage of disease remain disease free (normal or undetectable CT values). Early total thyroidectomy will alter the natural course of the disease to the extent that death from metastatic carcinoma will be unlikely.

Table 2. Reported survival rates in MTC

Reference	No. of patients	Survival rate (%)	
		5 years	10 years
Hazard et al. 1959	21	63	25
Woolner et al. 1961	77	76	62
Fletcher 1970	249	48	12
Gordon et al. 1973	40	71	58
Chong et al. 1975	139	80	67
Normann et al. 1976	57	65	61
Rougier et al. 1983	75	72	54
Saad et al. 1984	161	78	61
Schröder et al. 1988	60	67	47
Bergholm et al. 1990	249	80	68
Kohlwagen et al. 1991	480	81	61

Table 3. Prognostic factors influencing survival

Criterion	Survival rate (%)	
	5 years	10 years
All patients	80.2	61.5
Male	75.0	47.5
Female	86.8	72.8
<40 years	88.2	75.0
>40 years	75.0	53.3
Sporadic	77.5	57.7
Familial	91.5	72.4
– Only MTC	96.0	
– MEN 2A	87.0	75.6
– MEN 2B	75.0	50.0
Stage I	100.0	
Stage II	84.2	
Stage III	74.7	
Stage IV	75.0	

Data calculated from the registry German MTC Study Group, $n = 480$ patients, December 1990.
MEN, multiple endocrine neoplasia; MTC, medullary thyroid carcinoma.

The overall survival rate based on retrospective studies is approximately 75% after 5 years and 55% after 10 years of observation (Table 2). The overall prognosis is intermediate between either differentiated papillary and follicular carcinoma and the more aggressive anaplastic thyroid cancer. Thus it is important to analyze the principle prognostic factors in MTC to adapt the aggressiveness of treatment to that of the disease. The main factors that influence survival are the stage of the disease at the time of diagnosis (size of tumor and lymph node involvement), the type of MTC (sporadic, familial), and the age and sex of the patient (Table 3). Other factors having a negative effect on survival are high CT concentration during initial evaluation and diarrhea on presentation.

The stage of the disease at presentation is a major prognostic factor (Chong et al. 1975; Rougier et al. 1983; Saad et al. 1984; Schröder et al. 1988; Wells et al. 1982a,b). Stage I disease (tumor localized to the thyroid gland) has a much better survival rate than stage IV (distant metastases); this confirms the prognostic importance of distant metastases. The prognostic impact of cervical lymph node involvement is controversial. Rougier et al. (1983) and Saad et al. (1984) found that the presence of cervical lymph node metastases does not affect survival adversely; these data differ from findings of Chong et al. (1975), Normann et al. (1976), Bergholm et al. (1989) and Schröder et al. (1988). The difference in survival between patients with a small tumor (<1 cm) and those with a large one (>3 cm) observed in univariate analysis disappeared in the multivariate analysis when adjustment was made for confounding factors (Bergholm et al. 1990). It is less likely that lymph node metastases will be found at surgery when the primary tumor is small while a large tumor is significantly more often associated with palpable cervical lymph nodes and distant metastases (Bergholm et al. 1989).

Patients with MEN 2A had a much better survival rate than those with sporadic disease (Kakuda et al. 1985). In fact the difference in survival may be more related to the stage at which the disease is detected rather to the inherited differences in biological behavior of tumor. After adjustment for age alone there is only a difference between patients with sporadic MTC and those with familial disease detected by screening. The patient in the latter group were younger than those with the sporadic type of MTC. They were diagnosed at an earlier stage of the disease, when the tumors were smaller and there were fewer signs of involvement of the cervical lymph nodes, than the patients diagnosed from symptoms, both in the sporadic and familial group (Bergholm et al. 1989). The favorable stage distribution and prognosis might not be due entirely to the earlier diagnosis.

The prognostic value of gender in MTC is not yet settled. Several authors have reported a better prognosis among females then among males of corresponding ages. It seems that women have longer survival duration and lower incidence of recurrence (Rougier et al. 1983; Saad et al. 1984; Schröder et al. 1988; Bergholm et al. 1990); other authors have found no sex differences (Chong et al. 1975). However when all other factors were taken into account in the multivariate analysis, this difference disappeared (Bergholm et al. 1990). More women presented with stage I disease, indicating that stage of disease at diagnosis was a more important prognostic factor than sex (Saad et al. 1984). Patients younger than 40 years old at the time of diagnosis of MTC had a significantly better survival rate than those who were older. Older patients more often had a less favorable tumor stage than younger patients. The youngest patient detected by screening had the smallest tumor size, rare cervical lymph node involvement, and no distant metastases (Bergholm et al. 1989). The type of treatment was not a significant prognostic factor, and the type of surgery did not influence survival (Saad et al. 1984; Chong et al. 1975; Rougier et al. 1983). However, patients who had total thyroidectomy and modified neck dissection had a lower incidence of recurrence. Patients who had surgery alone had a better survival rate than those who had surgery and radiotherapy. Adjunct postoperative radioactive iodine therapy did not improve the prognosis (Saad et al. 1984). Prognosis of MTC was found not to be related to histological features or immunocytochemical pattern (Schröder et al. 1988). This is in contrast to findings that CT-rich tumor appears to have a better prognosis that CT-poor neoplasms and those with intermediate reactivity (Lippman et al. 1982). Diarrhea is a bad prognostic sign but did not appear as a significant prognostic factor. It occurs more commonly in patients with advanced disease and its presence may reflect the presence of a larger tumor mass (Saad et al. 1984).

Conclusion

The definitive treatment of MTC is surgical removal of the entire thyroid gland and its primary lymphatic drainage. Following surgical treatment a CT stimulation test with pentagastrin should be performed. Patients with normal or undetectable CT levels on two follow-up evaluations are likely to be free of disease. Adjunctive forms of therapy in patients with persistent elevation of serum CT levels after adequate surgical procedure is controversial. Many patients may exhibit a remarkably stable course without further treatment. Overall survival rate is approximately 75% after 5 years and 55% after 10 years of observation. This has to be kept in mind when nonsurgical therapy such as radioiodine treatment, external radiotherapy, chemotherapy, and SRIF is recommended. None of these different treatments is curative and they do not influence survival. The main prognostic factor is the stage of disease at the time of diagnosis. Therefore, early detection and adequate surgical treatment is likely to be curative in MTC.

Acknowledgements. The author wishes to express his gratitude to the members of the German Medullary Thyroid Carcinoma Study Group who collected the information about patients with MTC for calculating the prognostic factors influencing the survival rate (see Table 3): V. Bay, Hamburg; W. Becker, Erlangen; H. Buhr, Heidelberg; R. Dorn, Munich; H. Dralle, Hanover; A. Frilling, Düsseldorf; H.G. Heinze, Karlsruhe; E. Heissen, Mülheim; J. Herrmann, Bielefeld; R. Höfer, Vienna; I. Hörnig, Münster; F. Kallinowski, Heidelberg; F.S. Keck, Ulm; I. Klempa, Bremen;

J. Kotzerke, Hanover; H.-J. Langer, Homburg; H. Neumann, Freiburg; A. Passath, Graz; P. Pfannenstiel, Wiesbaden/Mainz Kastel; D. Reinwein, Essen; M. Ritter, Munich; H. Röher, Düsseldorf; O. Schober, Münster; S. Schröder, Hamburg; F. Seif, Tübingen; M. Späth-Röger, Mannheim; H. Stracke, Gießen; M. Trede, Mannheim; H. Vogt, Augsburg; R. Wahl, Frankfurt; K.F. Weinges, Homburg; J. Winter, Mannheim; S. Zabransky, Homburg; R. Ziegler, Heidelberg.

References

Ahlman H, Tisell LE (1987) The use of a long acting somatostatin analogue in the treatment of advanced endocrine malignancies with gastrointestinal symptoms. Scand J Gastroenterol 22:938–942

Ahuja S, Ernst H (1987) Chemotherapy of thyroid carcinoma. J Endocrinol Invest 10:303–310

Athanassiades P, Piperingos G, Pandos P, Koutras D, Moulopoulos S (1988) Serial serum calcitonin concentrations to evaluate responses to therapy of patients with medullary thyroid carcinoma. Chemotherapy 7:195–197

Bayraktar M, Gedik O, Akalin S, Usman A, Adalara N, Telatar F (1990) The effect of radioactive iodine treatment on thyroid C-cells. Clin Endocrinol (Oxf) 33: 625–630

Benker G, Reinwein D (1983) Ergebnisse der Chemotherapie des Schilddrüsen-carcinoms. Dtsch Med Wochenschr 108:403–406

BenMrad MD, Gardet P, Roche A, Rougier P, Calmettes C, Motte P, Parmentier C (1989) Value of venous catheterization and calcitonin studies in the treatment and management of clinical inapparent medullary thyroid carcinoma. Cancer 63: 133–138

Bergholm U, Adami HO, Bergström R, Johannsson H, Lundell G, Telenius-Berg M, Ackerström G (1989) Clinical characteristics in sporadic and familial medullary thyroid carcinoma, a nationwide study of 249 patients in Sweden from 1959 through 1981. Cancer 63:1196–1204

Bergholm U, Adami HO, Bergström R, Bäckdahl M, Ackerström G (1990) Long-term survival in sporadic and familial medullary thyroid carcinoma with special reference to clinical characteristics as prognostic factors. Acta Chir Scand 156:37–46

Bertagna XY, Bloomgarden ZT, Rabin D, Roberts LJ, Orth DN (1980) Molecular weight forms of immunoreactive calcitonin in a patient with medullary carcinoma of the thyroid: dynamic studies with calcium, pentagastrin, and somatostatin. Clin Endocrinol (Oxf) 13:115–123

Body JJ, Mirkine NLD, Corvilain J (1988) Calcitonin deficiency after radioactive iodine treatment. Ann Intern Med 109:590–591

Buhr HJ, Lehnert T, Raue F (1990) New operative strategy in the treatment of metastasizing medullary carcinoma of the thyroid. Eur J Surg Oncol 16:366–369

Bukowski RM, Brown L, Weik JK, Groppe CW, Purvis J (1983) Combination chemotherapy of metastatic thyroid cancer, phase II study. Am J Clin Oncol 6:579–581

Chong GC, Beahrs OH, Sizemore GW, Woolner LH (1975) Medullary carcinoma of the thyroid gland. Cancer 35:695–704

Clements D, Webb J, Heath D, McMaster P, Elias E (1986) SMS 201-995 and endocrine tumours. Scand J Gastroenterol 21 Suppl 119:251–255

Deftos LJ, Stein MF (1980) Radioiodine as an adjunct to the surgical treatment of medullary thyroid carcinoma. J Clin Endocrinol Metab 50:967–968

Droz JP, Schlumberger M, Rougier P, Caillon B, Godefroy W, Gardet P, Parmentier C (1985) Phase II trials of chemotherapy with adriamycin, cisplatin and their combination in thyroid cancer – a review of 44 cases. In: Jaffiol C, Milhaud G (eds) Thyroid cancer. Elsevier, Amsterdam, pp 203–208

Droz JP, Schlumberger M, Rougier P, Ghosu M, Gardet P, Parmentier C (1990) Chemotherapy in metastatic non anaplastic thyroid cancer: experience at the Institut Gustave-Roussy. Tumori 76:480–483

Feinstein RE, Gimeno EJ, el-Salhy M, Wilander E, Walinder G (1986) Evidence of C-cell destruction in the thyroid gland of mice exposed to high 131-I doses. Acta Radiol [Oncol] 25:199–202

Fletcher JR (1970) Medullary (solid) carcinoma of the thyroid gland, a review of 249 cases. Arch Surg 100:257–262

Frank K, Raue F, Lorenz D, Herfarth C, Ziegler R (1987) Importance of ultrasound examination for the follow-up of medullary thyroid carcinoma: comparison with other localization methods. Henry Ford Hosp Med J 35:122–123

Frank-Raue K, Raue F, Buhr HJ, Baldauf G, Lorenz D, Ziegler R (1992) Localization of occult medullary thyroid carcinoma before microsurgical reoperation: high sensitivity of selective venous catheterization. Thyroid 2:113–117

Gagel RF, Palmer WN, Leonhart K, Chan L, Leong SS (1986) Somatostatin production by a human medullary thyroid carcinoma cell line. Endocrinology 118:1643–1651

Gautvik KM, Talle K, Hager B, Jørgensen OG, Aas M (1989) Early liver metastases in patients with medullary carcinoma of the thyroid gland. Cancer 63:175–180

Geelhoed GW, Bass BL, Mertz SL, Becker KL (1986) Somatostatin analog: effect on hypergastrinemia and hypercalcitoninemia. Surgery 100:962–970

Gordin A, Lamberg BA, Pelkonen R, Almquists (1987) Somatostatin inhibits the pentagastrin induced release of serum calcitonin in medullary carcinoma of the thyroid. Clin Endocrinol (Oxf) 8:289–293

Gordon PR, Huvos AG, Strong EW (1973) Medullary carcinoma of the thyroid gland, a clinicopathologic study of 40 cases. Cancer 31:915–924

Gorman B, Charbonean JW, James EM (1987) Medullary thyroid carcinoma: Role of high-resolution ultrasound. Radiology 162:147–150

Gottlieb JA, Hill CS (1974) Chemotherapy of thyroid cancer with adriamycin: experience with 30 patients. N Engl J Med 290:193–197

Grauer A, Raue F, Gagel RF (1990) Changing concepts in the management of hereditary and sporadic medullary thyroid carcinoma. Endocrinol Metab Clin North Am 19:613–635

Guliana JM, Guillausseau PJ, Caron J, Siame-Mourot, Calmettes C, Modigliani E (1989) Effects of short-term subcutaneous administration of SMS 201-995 on calcitonin plasma levels in patients suffering from medullary thyroid carcinoma. Horm Metab Res 21:584–586

Hales M, Rosenau W, Okerlund MD, Galante M (1982) Carcinoma of the thyroid with a mixed medullary and follicular pattern. Morphologic, immunhistochemical, and clinical laboratory studies. Cancer 50:1352–1359

Halnan KE (1975) The nonsurgical treatment of thyroid cancer. Surgery 62:769–771

Hazard JB, Hawk WA, Crile G (1959) Medullary (solid) carcinoma of the thyroid – a clinicopathologic entity. J Clin Endocrinol Metab 19:152–161

Hellmann DE, Kartchner M, van Antwerp JD, Salmon SE, Patton D, O'Mara R (1979) Radioiodine in the treatment of medullary carcinoma of the thyroid. J Clin Endocrinol Metab 48:4–11

Hoskin PJ, Harmer C (1987) Chemotherapy for thyroid cancer. Radiother Oncol 10:187–194

Kakuda K, Carney A, Sizemore GW (1985) Medullary thyroid carcinoma of the thyroid, biological behavior of the sporadic and familial neoplasm. Cancer 55:2818–2821

Keeling CA, Basso LV (1988) Iodine-131 MIBG uptake in metastatic medullary carcinoma of the thyroid. A patient treated with somatostatin. Clin Nucl Med 13:260–263

Kohlwagen R, Raue F, Winter J (1991) Register of medullary thyroid carcinoma in Germany. Acta Endocrinol (Copenh) 124, Suppl 1:Abstr 7

Kraenzlin ME, Ch'ng JLC, Wood SM, Carr DH, Bloom SRC (1985) Long-term treatment of a VIPoma with somatostatin analogue resulting in remission of symptoms and possible shrinkage of metastases. Gastroenterology 88:185–187

Kvols LK (1988) The carcinoid syndrome: a treatable malignant disease. Oncology 2:22–41

Lamberts SWJ, Hofland LJ, van Koetsveld PM, Reubi JC, Bruining HA, Bakker WH, Krenning EP (1990a) Parallel in vivo and in vitro detection of functional somatostatin receptors in human endocrine pancreatic tumors, consequences with regard to diagnosis, localisation and therapy. J Clin Endocrinol Metab 71: 566–574

Lamberts SWJ, Krenning EP, Klijn JGM, Reubi JC (1990b) Clinical applications of somatostatin analogs. Trends Endocrinol Metab 1:139–145

Laurberg P (1984) Somatostatin and calcitonin release from perfused dog thyroid lobes; studies with calcium and pentagastrin. Endocrinology 114:2234–2241

Libroia A, Verga U, di Sacco G, Piolini M, Muratori F (1989) Use of somatostatin analog SMS 201-995 in medullary thyroid carcinoma. Henry Ford Hosp Med J 37:151–153

Lippman SM, Mendelsohn G, Trump DL, Wells SA, Baylin SB (1982) The prognostic and biological significance of cellular heterogeneity in medullary thyroid carcinoma: a study of calcitonin, L-dopa decarboxylase and histaminase. J Clin Endocrinol Metab 54:233–240

Ljungberg O (1966) Medullary carcinoma of the human thyroid gland: autoradiographic localization of radioiodine. Acta Pathol Microbiol Scand 68:476–484

Mahler C, Verhelst J, de Longueville M, Harris A (1990) Long-term treatment of metastatic medullary thyroid carcinoma with the somatostatin analogue octreotide. Clin Endocrinol (Oxf) 33:261–269

Modigliani E, Chayvialle JA, Cohen R, Perret G, Guliana JM, Vassy R, Roger P, Siame-Mourot C, Bennet M, Bentata-Pessayre M, Baulieu JL, Charpentier G, Rusniewsky P, Deidier A, Calmettes C (1988) Effect of a somatostatin analog (SMS 210-995) in perfusion on basal and pentagastrin stimulated calcitonin levels in medullary thyroid carcinoma. Horm Metab Res 20:773–775

Modigliani E, Alamowith C, Cohen R, Calmettes C, Guliana JM, Franc B, Bernard C, Chayvialle JA (1990) The intratumoral immunoassayable somatostatin concentration is frequently elevated in medullary thyroid carcinoma, results in 34 cases. Cancer 65:224–228

Nieuwenhuijzen-Kruseman AC, Bussemarker JK, Frölich M (1984) Radioiodine in the treatment of hereditary medullary carcinoma of the thyroid. J Clin Endocrinol Metab 59:491–494

Normann T, Gautvik KM, Johannessen JV, Brennhood IO (1976) Medullary carcinoma of the thyroid in Norway. Acta Endocrinol (Copenh) 83:71–85

Norton JA, Doppmann JL, Brennan MF (1980) Localization and resection of clinical inapparent medullary carcinoma of the thyroid. Surgery 87:616–622

Nusynowitz ML, Pollard E, Benedetto AR, Lecklitner ML, Ware RW (1982) Treatment of medullary carcinoma of the thyroid with I-131. J Nucl Med 23:142–146

Ott RA, Hofmann C, Oslaps R, Naggar R, Palogan E (1987) Radioiodine sensitivity of parafollicular C-cells in aged long-evens rats. Surgery 102:1043–1048

Pacini F, Elisei R, Anelli S, Basolo F, Cola A, Pincera A (1989) Somatostatin in medullary thyroid cancer, in vitro and in vivo studies. Cancer 63:1186–1195

Pacini F, Basolo F, Elisei R, Fugazzola L, Cola A, Pincera A (1991) Medullary thyroid cancer, an immunohistochemical and humoral study using sex separate antigens. Am J Clin Pathol 95:300–308

Petursson SR (1988) Metastatic medullary thyroid carcinoma, complete response to combination chemotherapy with dacarbazine and 5-fluorouracil. Cancer 62: 1899–1903

Poster DS, Bruno S, Penta J, Pina K, Catane R (1981) Current status of chemotherapy in the treatment of advanced carcinoma of the thyroid gland. Cancer Clin Trial 4:301–307

Rasmusson B, Hansen HS (1979) Treatment of medullary carcinoma of the thyroid: Value of calcitonin as tumor marker. Acta Radiol [Oncol] 18:521–534

Raue F, Minne H, Bayer JM (1976) Studies in endogenous hypercalcitoninaemia in man. 5th International Congress on Endocrinology, Hamburg, Abstr 386

Raue F, Minne H, Ziegler R (1985) Cisplatin, adriamycin und vindesin, eine Kombinationschemotherapie beim differenzierten Schilddrüsencarcinom. Tumor Diagn Ther 6:134–138

Reichlin S (1990) Clinical application of somatostatin receptor imaging (Editorial). J Clin Endocrinol Metab 71:564–565

Rougier P, Parmentier C, Laplanche A, Lefevre M, Travagli JP, Caillou B, Schlumberger M, Lacour J, Tubiana M (1983) Medullary thyroid carcinoma: prognostic factors and treatment. Int J Radiat Oncol Biol Phys 9:161–169

Ruhlmann J, Vogel J, Bockisch A, Biersack HJ (1987) Metastasen eines medullären Schilddrüsencarcinoms (folliculäre Variante) Diagnostik und Therapie mit Radiojod. Dtsch Med Wochenschr 112:1170–1172

Saad MF, Guido JJ, Samaan NA (1983) Radioactive iodine in the treatment of medullary carcinoma of the thyroid. J Clin Endocrinol Metab 57:124–128

Saad MF, Ordonez NG, Rashid RK, Guido JJ, Hill CS, Hickey RC, Samaan NA (1984) Medullary carcinoma of the thyroid, a study of the clinical feature and prognostic factors in 161 patients. Medicine (Baltimore) 63:319–342

Samaan NA, Schultz PN, Hickey R (1988) Medullary thyroid carcinoma: prognosis of familial versus sporadic disease and the role of radiotherapy. J Clin Endocrinol 67:801–805

Samonigg H, Hossfeld DK, Spehn J, Fill H, Leb G (1988) Aclarubicin in advanced thyroid cancer: a phase II study. Eur J Cancer Clin Oncol 24:1271–1275

Sarrazin D, Fontaine F, Rougier P, Gardet P, Schlumberger M, Travagli JP, Bounik H, Parmentier C, Tubiana M (1984) The role of external radiotherapy in the treatment of medullary thyroid carcinoma. Bull Cancer 71:200–208

Scherübl H, Raue F, Ziegler R (1990a) Combination chemotherapy of advanced medullary and differentiated thyroid cancer, phase II study. J Cancer Res Clin Oncol 116:21–23

Scherübl H, Raue F, Ziegler R (1990b) Kombinationstherapie von Adriamycin, Cisplatin und Vindesin beim C-Zell-Karzinom der Schilddrüse. Onkologie 13:198–202

Schrezemeir J, Plewe G, Sturmer W, Kahaly G, Opperman D, Krause U, del Pozo E, Kaspar H, Beyer J (1986) Treatment of APUDomas with the longacting somatostatin analogue SMS 201-995. Scand J Gastroenterol 21 Suppl 119:223–227

Schröder S, Böcker W, Baisch H, Bürk CG, Arps H, Meiners I, Kustendieck H, Heitz PU, Klöppel G (1988) Prognostic factors in medullary thyroid carcinomas, survival in relation to age, sex, stage, history, immunocytochemistry, and DNA content. Cancer 61:806–816

Schwerk WB, Grün R, Wahl R (1985) Ultrasound diagnosis of C-cell carcinoma of the thyroid. Cancer 55:624–630
Shah KH, Oslapas R, Calandra DB, Prinz RA, Ernst K, Hofmann C, Smith M, Chejfec, Lawrence AM, Polagan E (1983) Effects of radiation on parafollicular C-cells of the thyroid gland. Surgery 94:989–994
Shimoaka K (1980) Adjunctive management of thyroid cancer: chemotherapy. J Surg Oncol 15:283–286
Shimoaka K, Schoenfeld DA, de Wys WD, Creech RH, de Conti R (1985) A randomized trial of doxorubicin versus doxorubicin plus cisplatin in patients with advanced thyroid carcinoma. Cancer 56:2155–2160
Simpson WJK (1975) Radiotherapy in thyroid cancer. Can Med Assoc J 113: 115–118
Steinfeld AD (1977) The role of radiation therapy in medullary thyroid carcinoma of the thyroid. Radiology 123:745–746
Thurston V, Williams ED (1982) The effect of radiation on thyroid C-cells. Acta Endocrinol (Copenh) 92:72–78
Tisell L, Hansson G, Jansson S, Salander H (1986) Reoperation in the treatment of asymptomatic metastasizing medullary thyroid carcinoma. Surgery 99:60–66
Van Heerden JA, Grant CS, Gharib H, Hay ID, Ilstrup DM (1990) Long-term course of patients with persistant hypercalcitoninemia after apparent curative primary surgery for medullary thyroid carcinoma. Ann Surg 212:395–401
Wells SA, Baylin SB, Johnsrude JS, Harrington DP, Mendelsohn G, Ontjes DJ, Cooper CW (1982a) Thyroid venous catheterization in the early diagnosis of familial medullary thyroid carcinoma. Ann Surg 196:505–511
Wells SA, Baylin SB, Leight GS, Dale JK, Dilley WG, Farndon JR (1982b) The importance of early diagnosis in patients with hereditary medullary thyroid carcinoma. Ann Surg 195:595–602
Williams SD, Birch R, Einhorn LH (1986) Phase II evaluation of doxorubicin plus cisplatin in advanced thyroid cancer: a southeastern cancer study group trial. Cancer Treat Rep 70:405–407
Woolner LB, Beahrs OH, Blach BM, McConahey WM, Keating FR (1961) Classification and prognosis of thyroid carcinoma, a study of 885 cases observed in a thirty year period. Am J Surg 102:354–387

Subject Index